MANAGING DIABETES AND HYPERGLYCEMIA IN THE HOSPITAL SETTING

A Clinician's Guide

Boris Draznin, MD, PhD

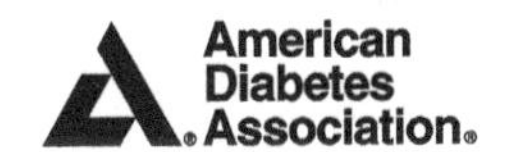

Director, Book Publishing, Abe Ogden; *Managing Editor*, Rebekah Renshaw; *Acquisitions Editor*, Victor Van Beuren; *Production Manager*, Melissa Sprott; *Production Services*, Cenveo Publisher Services; *Cover Design*, Lawrence Marie, Inc.; *Printer*, Data Reproduction Corp.

Printed in the United States of America
1 3 5 7 9 10 8 6 4 2

The suggestions and information contained in this publication are generally consistent with the *Standards of Medical Care in Diabetes* and other policies of the American Diabetes Association, but they do not represent the policy or position of the Association or any of its boards or committees. Reasonable steps have been taken to ensure the accuracy of the information presented. However, the American Diabetes Association cannot ensure the safety or efficacy of any product or service described in this publication. Individuals are advised to consult a physician or other appropriate health care professional before undertaking any diet or exercise program or taking any medication referred to in this publication. Professionals must use and apply their own professional judgment, experience, and training and should not rely solely on the information contained in this publication before prescribing any diet, exercise, or medication. The American Diabetes Association—its officers, directors, employees, volunteers, and members—assumes no responsibility or liability for personal or other injury, loss, or damage that may result from the suggestions or information in this publication.

∞ The paper in this publication meets the requirements of the ANSI Standard Z39.48-1992 (permanence of paper).

Jane Chiang, MD, conducted the internal review of this book to ensure that it meets American Diabetes Association guidelines.

ADA titles may be purchased for business or promotional use or for special sales. To purchase more than 50 copies of this book at a discount, or for custom editions of this book with your logo, contact the American Diabetes Association at the address below or at booksales@diabetes.org.

American Diabetes Association
1701 North Beauregard Street
Alexandria, Virginia 22311

DOI: 10.2337/9781580406086

Library of Congress Cataloging-in-Publication Data
Names: Draznin, Boris, editor. | American Diabetes Association, issuing body.
Title: Managing diabetes and hyperglycemia in the hospital setting / Boris Draznin, editor.
Description: Alexandria : The American Diabetes Association, [2016] | Includes bibliographical references and index.
Identifiers: LCCN 2015045525 | ISBN 9781580406086 (alk. paper)
Subjects: | MESH: Hyperglycemia—therapy. | Diabetes Mellitus—therapy. | Hospitalization. | Hyperglycemia—prevention & control.
Classification: LCC RC660.7 | NLM WK 880 | DDC 616.4/62—dc23 LC record available at http://lccn.loc.gov/2015045525

Contents

Contributors

Sara Alexanian, MD
Jill Apel, MD
David Baldwin, Jr., MD
Susan S. Braithwaite, MD
Elizabeth O. Buschur, MD
Enrico Cagliero, MD
Jorge Calles-Escandón, MD
Amy Diesburg-Stanwood, DNP, FNP-BC
Boris Draznin, MD, PhD
Andjela Drincic, MD
Elizabeth Dubois, PA-C
Kathleen Dungan, MD, MPH
Emma M. Eggleston, MD
Kathryn Evans Kreider, DNP, APRN, FNP-BC
Mercedes Falciglia, MD, FACP
Eileen Faulds, CNP, CDE
M. Kathleen Figaro, MD
Linda M. Gaudiani, MD, FACP, FACE
Roma Gianchandani, MD
Janice L. Gilden, MS, MD, FCP, FACE
J. Sonya Haw, MD
R. Matthew Hawkins, PA-C, MMSc
Sara J. Healy, MD
Richard Hellman, MD, FACP, FACE
Irl B. Hirsch, MD, MACP
Silvio E. Inzucchi, MD
Jane Jeffrie Seley, DNP, MSN, MPH, GNP, BC-ADM, CDE, CDTC
Abhishek Kansara, MD
Sarah Kim, MD
Kenneth L. Koch, MD
Mary Korytkowski, MD
Kristen Kulasa, MD
Lillian F. Lien, MD
Ildiko Lingvay, MD, MPH, MSCS
Cecilia C. Low Wang, MD
Michelle Magee, MD, MBBCh, BAO, LRCPSI
Umesh Masharani, MD
Nestoras Mathioudakis, MD
Greg Maynard, MD, MSc, SFHM
Marie E. McDonnell, MD
Carlos E. Mendez, MD, FACP
Luigi F. Meneghini, MD, MBA
Etie Moghissi, MD, FACE
Carine M. Nassar, MS, RD, CDE
Patricia Peter, MD
Neda Rasouli, MD
Jodie Reider, MD
John J. Reyes-Castano, MD
Kellie Rodriguez, MSN, MBA, CDE
Daniel J. Rubin, MD, MSc, FACE
Robert J. Rushakoff, MD
Archana Sadhu, MD, FACE
Stacey Seggelke, RN, MS, CDE
Guillermo E. Umpierrez, MD
Amisha Wallia, MD
Alicia Lynn Warnock, MD, FACP
Heidemarie Windham MacMaster, PharmD, CDE, FCSHP

Preface

As the number of patients with diabetes, both diagnosed and as yet undiagnosed, increases annually, it is not surprising that the number of patients with diabetes who are admitted to the hospital also increases. The prevalence of overt diabetes is estimated to exceed 30% among individuals who are 60 years of age and older. Because individuals in this age-group account for a large number of hospital admissions for a variety of medical and surgical conditions, even conservative estimates suggest that ~25 to 30% of all hospitalized patients on any given day in any given hospital in the U.S. have diabetes. The percentage of hospitalized patients outside the U.S. who have diabetes is likely to show the same trend.

Even though patients with diabetes may be admitted to the hospital with acute or chronic complications of diabetes, most frequently they are hospitalized for other medical and surgical problems and their diabetes becomes a significant comorbidity that may affect the outcome of their hospitalization. Moreover, patients with prediabetes or undiagnosed diabetes are frequently hyperglycemic either on admission to the hospital or in the course of their hospital stay, adding to the complexity of their medical or surgical problems. The treatment of diabetes and hyperglycemia in these situations requires the utmost attention and specialized knowledge.

Once in the hospital, patients with diabetes or hyperglycemia may be admitted to the intensive care unit, require urgent or elective surgery, enteral or parenteral nutrition, intravenous insulin infusion, and therapies that have a significant impact on glycemic control (e.g., steroids). Because many clinical outcomes are profoundly influenced by the degree of glycemic control, knowledge of the best practice in inpatient diabetes management assumes paramount importance.

In the twenty-first century, in most U.S. community hospitals, hospitalist physicians provide medical care to these patients. In some hospitals, particularly academic and other tertiary care hospitals, hospitalists share this task with endocrinologists. A small number of hospitals have established specialized glycemic (diabetes) management teams led by either a physician or a mid-level provider, such as a nurse practitioner or a physician assistant, to help control blood glucose levels in hospitalized patients. These teams prove to be of great importance not only for successful management of patients with diabetes, but also for diabetes education of patients, nursing staff, and house staff.

The field of inpatient management of diabetes and hyperglycemia has grown substantially in the last several years, accumulating and disseminating important clinical knowledge. This body of knowledge is summarized in this book, so it can reach the audience of hospitalists and endocrinologists, both in practice and in training—the very physicians who take care of hospitalized patients with diabetes and hyperglycemia.

Boris Draznin, MD, PhD, Editor,
The Celeste and Jack Grynberg Professor of Medicine
University of Colorado School of Medicine

The Management of Diabetes and Hyperglycemia in the Hospital Setting: A Practical Guide

INTRODUCTION

As the number of patients with diabetes, both diagnosed and as yet undiagnosed, increases annually, it is not surprising that the number of patients with diabetes who are admitted to the hospital also increases. The prevalence of overt diabetes is estimated to exceed 30% among individuals who are 60 years of age and older. Because individuals in this age-group account for a large number of hospital admissions for a variety of medical and surgical conditions, even conservative estimates suggest that ~25 to 30% of all hospitalized patients on any given day in any given hospital in the U.S. have diabetes. The percentage of hospitalized patients outside the U.S. who have diabetes is likely to show the same trend.

Even though patients with diabetes may be admitted to the hospital with acute or chronic complications of diabetes, most frequently they are hospitalized for other medical and surgical problems and their diabetes becomes a significant comorbidity that may affect the outcome of their hospitalization. Moreover, patients with prediabetes or undiagnosed diabetes are frequently hyperglycemic either on admission to the hospital or in the course of their hospital stay, adding to the complexity of their medical or surgical problems. The treatment of diabetes and hyperglycemia in these situations requires the utmost attention and specialized knowledge.

Once in the hospital, patients with diabetes or hyperglycemia may be admitted to the intensive care unit, require urgent or elective surgery, enteral or parenteral nutrition, intravenous insulin infusion, and therapies that have a significant impact on glycemic control (e.g., steroids). Because many clinical outcomes are profoundly influenced by the degree of glycemic control, knowledge of the best practice in inpatient diabetes management assumes paramount importance.

In the twenty-first century, in most U.S. community hospitals, hospitalist physicians provide medical care to these patients. In some hospitals, particularly academic and other tertiary care hospitals, hospitalists share this task with endocrinologists. A small number of hospitals have established specialized glycemic (diabetes) management teams led by either a physician or a mid-level provider, such as a nurse practitioner or a physician assistant, to help control blood glucose levels in hospitalized patients. These teams prove to be of great importance not only for successful management of patients with diabetes, but also for diabetes education of patients, nursing staff, and house staff.

The field of inpatient management of diabetes and hyperglycemia has grown substantially in the last several years, accumulating and disseminating important clinical knowledge. This body of knowledge is summarized in this book, so it can reach the audience of hospitalists and endocrinologists, both in practice and in training—the very physicians who take care of hospitalized patients with diabetes and hyperglycemia.

Chapter 1

The Evolution of Glycemic Control in the Hospital Setting

Etie Moghissi, MD, FACE,[1] and Silvio Inzucchi, MD[2]

INTRODUCTION

Patients with diabetes are hospitalized three times more frequently than those without diabetes, and hyperglycemia in the hospital setting is associated with increased mortality, morbidity, longer hospital stays, and cost. Yet at the turn of the twenty-first century, few appreciated the risk of acute hyperglycemia among hospitalized patients. There were no clinical practice guidelines or recommended glycemic targets for inpatients, and every hospital relied on sliding-scale insulin therapy to manage hyperglycemia.

Early observational studies and the seminal 2001 randomized clinical trial of intensive insulin therapy in critically ill patients[1] paved the way for diabetes organizations to issue calls for tight glycemic control in the critically ill patients.[2–4] Investigations published after these initial recommendations, however, called into question the benefit of maintaining near-normal glycemic control in the critically ill and raised concerns regarding the prevalence of incremental hypoglycemia associated with such an approach.[5–8] Notably, the Normoglycemia in Intensive Care Evaluation Using Glucose Algorithm Regulation (NICE-SUGAR) study actually showed that a 14% increased risk of death accompanied dramatically increased rates of severe hypoglycemia in patients whose glucose was controlled to the euglycemic range,[9] the latter confirmed by meta-analysis of multiple studies involving the critically ill.[8] These findings prompted the American Association of Clinical Endocrinologists (AACE)/American Diabetes Association (ADA) consensus group to evaluate all related published studies and update their recommendations for glycemic targets in hospitalized patients,[10] with the goal of recommending reasonable, achievable, and safe glycemic targets. The consensus group chose a target of 140–180 mg/dL for critically ill patients based on the best available evidence. The group's primary concern was maintaining patient safety, especially the avoidance of hypoglycemia. The panel recommended insulin as the treatment of choice for the majority of hospitalized patients. Continuous intravenous (IV) insulin infusion was recommended for those patients in the intensive care unit (ICU), and scheduled insulin in the form of basal, nutritional, and supplemental injections was preferred for the noncritically ill (Table 1.1). Echoing these

[1]Associate Clinical Professor, Department of Medicine, University of California Los Angeles, Los Angeles, CA. [2]Professor of Medicine Section of Endocrinology, Yale School of Medicine, New Haven, CT.

DOI: 10.2337/9781580406086.01

Table 1.1—Summary of ADA/AACE Recommendations for Management of Hyperglycemia among Hospitalized Patients

	Critically ill	Noncritically ill
Blood glucose target	■ 140 to 180 mg/dL (7.8 to 10.0 mmol/L)	■ Premeal: <140 mg/dL (<7.8 mmol/L)* ■ Random: <180 mg/dL (<10.0 mmol/L)*
Preferred treatment regimen	■ Intravenous insulin infusion of regular insulin ■ Use validated insulin infusion protocol ■ Frequently monitor blood glucose to minimize hypoglycemia	■ Scheduled subcutaneous administration of insulin, with basal, nutritional, and correction components ■ Prolonged therapy with sliding-scale insulin as the sole regimen is discouraged ■ Noninsulin antihyperglycemic agents are not appropriate for most hospitalized patients who require therapy for hyperglycemia

*Provided these targets can be safely achieved. More stringent targets may be appropriate in stable patients with previous tight glycemic control; less stringent targets may be appropriate in terminally ill patients or those with severe comorbidities.

recommendations, in 2012 The Endocrine Society issued an updated guidance focused on noncritically ill patients,[11] with similar recommendations as the AACE/ADA consensus group. Both groups emphasize that clinical judgment, individualized regimens tailored to each patient, and ongoing assessment of clinical status must be incorporated into day-to-day decisions regarding the management of hyperglycemia.[10,11]

STRESS HYPERGLYCEMIA

Approximately one-third of hospital inpatients experience hyperglycemia, with up to a third of these individuals having no previous history of diabetes.[12–14] Although a substantial portion of these patients likely have prediabetes or undiagnosed diabetes, acute injury and illness clearly can lead to glucose elevations in those with previously normal glucose tolerance. This stress hyperglycemia results from a complex interplay between inflammatory cytokines, catecholamines, the oxidative stress resulting from gluco- and lipotoxicity, and activation of the hypothalamic-pituitary-adrenal axis, all resulting in insulin resistance and insufficient pancreatic insulin secretion. Treatments commonly used among inpatients, such as glucocorticoids, enteral and parenteral nutrition, and vasopressors also may lead to or exacerbate glucose elevations.[15] Regardless of the cause, however, hyperglycemia, particularly when severe, must be treated to reduce adverse outcomes, including dehydration, electrolyte disturbance, infectious complications, and poor wound healing.

HYPERGLYCEMIA AND ADVERSE HOSPITAL OUTCOMES

Epidemiologic studies began to establish a clear link between increasing blood glucose levels and hospital mortality in the late 1990s and early 2000s. In a 1999 publication from the Diabetes and Insulin-Glucose Infusion in Acute Myocardial Infarction (DIGAMI) study, the risk of death among 620 patients with diabetes admitted for acute myocardial infarction (MI) rose by 8% with each 18 mg/dL increase in admission blood glucose (relative risk [RR] 1.08, 95% confidence interval [CI] 1.05–1.11; $P < 0.001$).[16] A 2003 retrospective review of data from ICU patients revealed that the mortality rate approximately doubled among patients with a mean glucose value during hospitalization between 160 and 199 mg/dL and roughly tripled among patients with mean glucose between 200 and 299 mg/dL. Above 300 mg/dL, the rate of death was approximately fourfold higher.[17] In a large retrospective study of more than 250,000 admissions to 173 hospitals published in 2009, the risk of death nearly doubled for patients with blood glucose 146–199 mg/dL during hospitalization (odds ratio [OR] 1.31; 95% CI 1.26–1.36), independent of severity of illness. The odds of death, adjusted for illness severity, more than doubled at 200–299 mg/dL (OR 1.82; 95% CI 1.74–1.90), and almost tripled for glucose values >300 mg/dL (OR 2.85; 95% CI 2.58–3.14).[18] Other observational and controlled studies have unequivocally supported the association between hyperglycemia and inpatient mortality risk.[14,19–21] In addition, patients with hyperglycemia are more likely to have prolonged hospital stays, infections, and greater degrees of disability after hospital discharge.[14,21–23] Data from outside the ICU further establish the association of hyperglycemia with adverse outcomes. For example, in a study of 2,471 patients with community acquired pneumonia, blood glucose levels >200 mg/dL during hospitalization were associated with higher rates of mortality and in-hospital complications than blood glucose levels <200 mg/dL.[24]

Patients at greatest risk for adverse hospital outcomes may be those *without* a previous history of diabetes, which emphasizes the importance of treating inpatient hyperglycemia regardless of the cause. A retrospective review of medical records of more than 2,000 critically ill patients showed significant increases in mortality among patients with new hyperglycemia, that is, those without previously diagnosed diabetes. The mortality rate was about eight times higher among patients with hyperglycemia as those with normal glucose levels ($P < 0.01$) and about five times higher than patients with diagnosed diabetes ($P < 0.01$).[14] In the aforementioned retrospective study of 250,000 admissions, the odds of mortality were significantly higher for patients with no previous history of diabetes than for those with diagnosed diabetes ($P < 0.01$). Compared with normoglycemic patients, those without diagnosed diabetes had a 35% increased risk of death if their glucose was 111–145 mg/dL (OR 1.35; 95% CI 1.30–1.41). Successively increasing glucose ranges were associated with a doubled, tripled, and quadrupled mortality risk (146–199 mg/dL: OR 2.14, 95% CI 2.04–2.24; 200–299 mg/dL: OR 2.91, 95% CI 2.71–3.11; >300 mg/dL: OR 4.04, 95% CI 3.44–4.75).[18] Observational studies such as these can only be considered hypothesis generating. Indeed, because the degree of illness will be associated with the level of stress hyperglycemia, studies such as these are particularly prone to influence by unmeasured confounders. It is only through randomized clinical trials that one may know whether glucose control actually improves the risk of adverse outcomes in hospitalized patients with hyperglycemia.

EFFECTS OF GLYCEMIC CONTROL ON INPATIENT OUTCOMES

Both retrospective and prospective controlled studies have brought us to our current understanding of optimal glucose control for both critically ill and noncritically ill patients. In the DIGAMI study, 1-year mortality significantly decreased by 29% ($P = 0.027$) in patients with diabetes randomly assigned to insulin-glucose infusion for the first 24 h after acute MI compared with patients given standard therapy of the time, in which insulin was given during the first 24 h only if it was deemed clinically necessary.[25] Other early controlled trials comparing tight glucose control to standard treatment approaches also demonstrated significant reductions in mortality and morbidity among both ICU and noncritical inpatient populations. In an often-cited 2001 prospective, randomized clinical trial involving 1,548 surgical ICU patients in Belgium, intensive insulin therapy to maintain glycemia between 80 and 110 mg/dL significantly reduced mortality risk by 32% ($P < 0.04$) compared with standard treatment of the time, in which insulin was given only when patients' blood glucose exceeded 215 mg/dL, with the goal of maintaining blood glucose values of 180-200 mg/dL. In addition, intensive insulin therapy also significantly reduced the duration of ICU stays and ventilatory support, need for dialysis, and episodes of septicemia.[1] These results were supported by a retrospective analysis of ICU patients who had undergone coronary artery bypass grafting (CABG). The investigators compared hospital records from two time periods during which different glucose control approaches had been used. During the earlier period, subcutaneous (SQ) insulin had resulted in a mean glucose value of 213 mg/dL among CABG patients, whereas a later protocol using insulin infusion resulted in a mean glucose value of 177 mg/dL. Insulin infusion reduced the risk of death by 57% (OR 0.43; $P = 0.001$).[19]

Further investigations, however, were not able to confirm the benefit of near normalization of glucose and raised concerns regarding the risk of hypoglycemia with this approach. In 2003, the same Belgian investigators published results from a second clinical trial, showing that tight glucose control did *not* significantly reduce mortality in the medical (as opposed to surgical) ICU, except among patients whose ICU stays exceeded 5 days.[26] Subsequently, the NICE-SUGAR study highlighted the dangers of hypoglycemia that accompany tight glucose control. This international investigation compared 90-day mortality in a cohort of 6,104 patients who were admitted to medical and surgical ICUs at 42 different hospitals where they were assigned randomly to glycemic targets of 81–108 mg/dL and 144–180 mg/dL. Rates of severe hypoglycemia were ~15 times greater among intensively treated patients (OR 14.7, 95% CI 9.0–25.9; $P < 0.001$), and mortality was 14% higher in the same group compared with patients whose glucose was less intensively controlled ($P = 0.02$).[9] A meta-analysis of 26 randomized controlled trials involving 13,567 ICU patients (including the NICE-SUGAR cohort) supported the NICE-SUGAR finding that the risk of hypoglycemia is too great to justify near-normal glucose values, especially in medical ICU patients. In the pooled analysis of studies reporting hypoglycemia, the relative risk of hypoglycemia was 6.0 (95% CI 4.5–8.0) for intensive insulin therapy compared with conventional glucose control. Meanwhile, the overall relative risk of death was 0.93 (95% CI 0.83–1.04).[8] As a result of these findings, recommendations for target glucose levels were relaxed from the euglycemic range to the values shown in Table 1.1.

PROTOCOLS FOR GLUCOSE MANAGEMENT

A major goal of treating hyperglycemia in the hospital is patient safety, because overtreatment and undertreatment of hyperglycemia represents major quality concerns. Well-defined, validated protocols for the management of hyperglycemia will include provisions for glucose monitoring and the treatment of hypoglycemia as well as guidance on matching insulin administration to blood glucose levels and nutrition (either meals or enteral or parenteral nutrition) in a dynamic fashion.

Changing patient circumstances also drive modifications to insulin regimens in the hospital. These include transitions from ICU to noncritical care settings, which call for changes from IV infusion to SQ injections of insulin; nutrition therapy transitions between enteral or parenteral therapy and solid foods; or perioperative glycemic control. Patients admitted for diabetic hyperglycemic crises (diabetes ketoacidosis or hyperglycemic hyperosmolar state) also will require insulin therapy along with close monitoring of blood glucose values to reduce the risk of hypoglycemia. Of course, these patients also require extensive management decisions related to fluids and electrolytes, beyond mere glycemic control.

Monitoring the patient's glycemic status falls to point-of-care (POC) capillary blood glucose meters, which provide nearly instantaneous results and have become the standard measurement technique at the hospital bedside. Caution is required in interpreting the results from POC meters in patients who have anemia, polycythemia, or hypoperfusion or who use certain medications. Newer technologies, including continuous glucose monitoring, are under study.

Ongoing education of hospital personnel in these protocols is essential not only to ensure proper implementation but also to gain support of those involved in the care of inpatients with hyperglycemia, including the hospital administration. Evidence supporting the cost-effectiveness of a rational systems approach to inpatient glycemic management will help persuade administrators to provide necessary financial and operational support.[27,28]

STATUS OF GLYCEMIC CONTROL IN THE HOSPITAL SETTING

The health-care community at large now generally accepts that both hyperglycemia and hypoglycemia are markers of poor clinical outcomes, and many institutions have made important strides to improve glycemia at their facilities. Multiple barriers persist, however, and the frequency of poor glycemic control remains high. In an analysis of a database containing information on 70,000 admissions of patients with diabetes, an HbA_{1c} was recorded for only 18% of cases.[29] The authors of this study found that, when A1C was measured, a value >8% prompted a change in antihyperglycemic regimen for only two-thirds of patients (64%). Additionally, several studies have documented failures to reliably follow hypoglycemia management protocols, with long delays in glucose retesting after hypoglycemic events, poor documentation of the hypoglycemic and subsequent treatment, and long intervals before hypoglycemia resolution.[30–32] The root of the problem may be in poor *communication and coordination* between health-care teams,[30,33] but knowledge gaps also appear to contribute. In a recent survey of health-care professionals working in an urban, community teaching hospital, only about half of questions regarding best practices for managing inpatient hyperglycemia were answered correctly by physicians, nurses, and dietitians (mean scores of 53%, 52%, and 48%, respectively). Pharmacists performed somewhat better (mean score 64%), whereas patient care assistants correctly answered only about a third of the questions (38%). In general, this group of health-care workers acknowledged the importance of controlling hyperglycemia, but they still preferred the perceived convenience of sliding-scale insulin, and this preference influenced clinical decision making.[34]

Many institutions rely on a systematic analysis of their glucose measurements to address these problems. Sometimes referred to as "glucometrics," this approach incorporates the tracking of glycemic exposure, the efficacy of glycemic control, and the rates of adverse events and allows hospitals to measure the success of inpatient glucose management efforts. Individual health-care professionals can use glucometrics to identify and address the causes of hyper- and hypoglycemia. Institutions can use these metrics to identify opportunities for improvement in glycemic management across the health system. A goal of 85% of blood glucose levels within the target range has been proposed as a gold standard, and some groups recommend use of the patient-day unit of measure, because it may more accurately reflect the frequency of hypoglycemia and severe hyperglycemic events. Glucometric approaches have not been standardized, however, and various methods continue to be implemented. Of course, merely tracking glycemic values does not appear to improve outcomes.[35] The data obtained must be used to guide the actions of health-care professionals across disciplines[10,11,36] and to advise institutions to make strategic decisions regarding support staff, protocol development, and practitioner education.

EMERGING EVIDENCE TO CONTROL GLUCOSE IN THE INPATIENT SETTING

Recent interest has focused on the potential of incretin-based therapies as a supplement or alternative to insulin therapy in the hospital setting. These agents carry a low risk of hypoglycemia and may offer cardioprotective benefits.[37] One pilot study involving 90 patients randomly assigned general medical and surgery patients with type 2 diabetes to glucose management with the dipeptidyl peptidase 4 (DPP-4) inhibitor sitagliptin alone, sitagliptin plus insulin glargine, or a basal-bolus insulin regimen. Overall, the three treatment groups experienced similar glycemic control, although basal-bolus insulin provided better control in patients whose admission glucose was >180 mg/dL.[38] In addition, patients in the sitagliptin-only group required correction doses with rapid-acting insulin as often as patients in the other groups to maintain target glucose levels. Rates of hypoglycemia were also similar among the three groups.

Glucagon-like peptide 1 (GLP-1) receptor agonists for inpatient management have shown some potential to control glucocorticoid-induced and stress hyperglycemia in several small studies, but so far no randomized, controlled trials have been conducted.[37] In one pilot study involving 40 patients in a cardiac ICU, exenatide infusion successfully maintained a steady-state glucose value of 132 mg/dL without incidence of hypoglycemia; however, a large proportion of patients experienced nausea.[39]

Areas for future research include investigations of the following:

1. Glycemic quality measures needed to improve patient outcomes
2. Safe and effective methods of point-of-care testing for the management of glycemia in critically ill patients
3. The role of continuous glucose monitoring in the inpatient setting
4. Appropriate glycemic targets for different patient populations in the hospital setting
5. Efficacy and safety of incretin-based therapies in the management of hyperglycemia in the hospital setting

CONCLUSION

Management of glycemic control in the hospital setting continues to evolve. We have witnessed several shifts in treatment paradigms over the past two decades, from essentially ignoring blood glucose levels except for extremes, to overly stringent approaches stemming from initial clinical trials that reported benefits from achieving euglycemia, to a more rational approach over the past several years. Professional organizations and leading experts now advise controlling glucose, especially in the ICU, within the high-normal to mildly elevated range, while avoiding hypoglycemia. The overriding primary goal of treating hyperglycemia among hospital inpatients is now patient *safety*, because overtreatment and undertreatment of hyperglycemia are associated with adverse outcomes. Any validated protocols for the management of hyperglycemia should include provisions for glucose monitoring and the treatment of hypoglycemia as well as guidance on dynamically matching insulin doses to glucose levels. Smooth transitioning between IV and SQ insulin regimens is also important. Discharge planning, which should begin at hospital admission, is equally vital. A clear plan for outpatient glucose management, including transition to previous antihyperglycemic therapy before discharge, patient education about diabetes self-management, and clear communication with outpatient providers, will ensure a safe and successful transition to the outpatient arena. Developing reliable diabetes management systems in our hospitals, developed and tracked by a multidisciplinary group of key stakeholders, will ensure best practice in each of these domains.

REFERENCES

1. Van den Berghe G, Wouters P, Weekers F, Verwaest C, Bruyninckx F, Schetz M, et al. Intensive insulin therapy in critically ill patients. *N Engl J Med* 2001;345:1359–1367
2. American College of Endocrinology, American Diabetes Association. American College of Endocrinology and American Diabetes Association consensus statement on inpatient diabetes and glycemic control. *Endocr Pract* 2006;12:458–468
3. Garber AJ, Moghissi ES, Bransome ED, Jr., Clark NG, Clement S, Cobin RH, et al. American College of Endocrinology position statement on inpatient diabetes and metabolic control. *Endocr Pract* 2004;10:77–82
4. Clement S, Braithwaite SS, Magee MF, Ahmann A, Smith EP, Schafer RG, et al. Management of diabetes and hyperglycemia in hospitals. *Diabetes Care* 2004;27:553–591
5. Wiener RS, Wiener DC, Larson RJ. Benefits and risks of tight glucose control in critically ill adults: a meta-analysis. *JAMA* 2008;300:933–944
6. Brunkhorst FM, Engel C, Bloos F, Meier-Hellmann A, Ragaller M, Weiler N, et al. Intensive insulin therapy and pentastarch resuscitation in severe sepsis. *N Engl J Med* 2008;358:125–139
7. Krinsley JS, Grover A. Severe hypoglycemia in critically ill patients: risk factors and outcomes. *Crit Care Med* 2007;35:2262–2267
8. Griesdale DE, de Souza RJ, van Dam RM, Heyland DK, Cook DJ, Malhotra A, et al. Intensive insulin therapy and mortality among critically ill patients: a meta-analysis including NICE-SUGAR study data. *CMAJ* 2009;180:821–827
9. NICE-SUGAR Study Investigators, Finfer S, Chittock DR, Su SY, Blair D, Foster D, et al. Intensive versus conventional glucose control in critically ill patients. *N Engl J Med* 2009;360:1283–1297
10. Moghissi ES, Korytkowski MT, DiNardo M, Einhorn D, Hellman R, Hirsch IB, et al. American Association of Clinical Endocrinologists and American Diabetes Association consensus statement on inpatient glycemic control. *Endocr Pract* 2009;15:353–369
11. Umpierrez GE, Hellman R, Korytkowski MT, Kosiborod M, Maynard GA, Montori VM, et al. Management of hyperglycemia in hospitalized patients in non-critical care setting: an Endocrine Society clinical practice guideline. *J Clin Endocrinol Metab* 2012;97:16–38
12. Kosiborod M, Rathore SS, Inzucchi SE, Masoudi FA, Wang Y, Havranek EP, et al. Admission glucose and mortality in elderly patients hospitalized with acute myocardial infarction: implications for patients with and without recognized diabetes. *Circulation* 2005;111:3078–3086
13. Swanson CM, Potter DJ, Kongable GL, Cook CB. Update on inpatient glycemic control in hospitals in the United States. *Endocr Pract* 2011;17:853–861

14. Umpierrez GE, Isaacs SD, Bazargan N, You X, Thaler LM, Kitabchi AE. Hyperglycemia: an independent marker of in-hospital mortality in patients with undiagnosed diabetes. *J Clin Endocrinol Metab* 2002;87:978–982
15. Dungan KM, Braithwaite SS, Preiser JC. Stress hyperglycaemia. *Lancet* 2009;373:1798–1807
16. Malmberg K, Norhammar A, Wedel H, Ryden L. Glycometabolic state at admission: important risk marker of mortality in conventionally treated patients with diabetes mellitus and acute myocardial infarction: long-term results from the Diabetes and Insulin-Glucose Infusion in Acute Myocardial Infarction (DIGAMI) study. *Circulation* 1999;99:2626–2632
17. Krinsley JS. Association between hyperglycemia and increased hospital mortality in a heterogeneous population of critically ill patients. *Mayo Clin Proc* 2003;78:1471–1478
18. Falciglia M, Freyberg RW, Almenoff PL, D'Alessio DA, Render ML. Hyperglycemia-related mortality in critically ill patients varies with admission diagnosis. *Crit Care Med* 2009;37:3001–3009
19. Furnary AP, Gao G, Grunkemeier GL, Wu Y, Zerr KJ, Bookin SO, et al. Continuous insulin infusion reduces mortality in patients with diabetes undergoing coronary artery bypass grafting. *J Thorac Cardiovasc Surg* 2003;125:1007–1021
20. Frisch A, Chandra P, Smiley D, Peng L, Rizzo M, Gatcliffe C, et al. Prevalence and clinical outcome of hyperglycemia in the perioperative period in noncardiac surgery. *Diabetes Care* 2010;33:1783–1788
21. Kwon S, Thompson R, Dellinger P, Yanez D, Farrohki E, Flum D. Importance of perioperative glycemic control in general surgery: a report from the Surgical Care and Outcomes Assessment Program. *Ann Surg* 2013;257:8–14
22. Golden SH, Peart-Vigilance C, Kao WH, Brancati FL. Perioperative glycemic control and the risk of infectious complications in a cohort of adults with diabetes. *Diabetes Care* 1999;22:1408–1414
23. Latham R, Lancaster AD, Covington JF, Pirolo JS, Thomas CS, Jr. The association of diabetes and glucose control with surgical-site infections among cardiothoracic surgery patients. *Infect Control Hosp Epidemiol* 2001;22:607–612
24. McAlister FA, Majumdar SR, Blitz S, Rowe BH, Romney J, Marrie TJ. The relation between hyperglycemia and outcomes in 2,471 patients admitted to the hospital with community-acquired pneumonia. *Diabetes Care* 2005;28:810–815
25. Malmberg K, Ryden L, Efendic S, Herlitz J, Nicol P, Waldenstrom A, et al. Randomized trial of insulin-glucose infusion followed by subcutaneous insulin treatment in diabetic patients with acute myocardial infarction (DIGAMI study): effects on mortality at 1 year. *J Am Coll Cardiol* 1995;26:57–65
26. Van den Berghe G, Wilmer A, Hermans G, Meersseman W, Wouters PJ, Milants I, et al. Intensive insulin therapy in the medical ICU. *N Engl J Med* 2006;354:449–461

27. Magee MF. Hospital protocols for targeted glycemic control: Development, implementation, and models for cost justification. *AJHP* 2007;64:S15–S20; quiz S1–S3

28. Braithwaite SS, Magee MF, Sharretts JM, Schnipper JL, Amin A, Maynard G. *The Case for Supporting Inpatient Glycemic Control Programs Now: The Evidence and Beyond.* Philadelphia, Society of Hospital Medicine, 2008. Available from http://www.hospitalmedicine.org/ResourceRoomRedesign/html/02First_Steps/03_The_Case_for_Support.cfm. Accessed 25 February 2016

29. Strack B, DeShazo JP, Gennings C, Olmo JL, Ventura S, Cios KJ, et al. Impact of HbA_{1c} measurement on hospital readmission rates: analysis of 70,000 clinical database patient records. *Biomed Res Int* 2014;2014:781670

30. Maynard G, Kulasa K, Ramos P, Childers D, Clay B, Sebasky M, et al. Impact of a hypoglycemia reduction bundle and a systems approach to inpatient glycemic management. *Endocr Pract* 2014:1–34

31. Garg R, Bhutani H, Jarry A, Pendergrass M. Provider response to insulin-induced hypoglycemia in hospitalized patients. *J Hosp Med* 2007;2:258–260

32. Varghese P, Gleason V, Sorokin R, Senholzi C, Jabbour S, Gottlieb JE. Hypoglycemia in hospitalized patients treated with antihyperglycemic agents. *J Hosp Med* 2007;2:234–240

33. Rousseau MP, Beauchesne MF, Naud AS, Leblond J, Cossette B, Lanthier L, et al. An interprofessional qualitative study of barriers and potential solutions for the safe use of insulin in the hospital setting. *Can J Diabetes* 2014;38:85–89

34. Beliard R, Muzykovsky K, Vincent W, 3rd, Shah B, Davanos E. Perceptions, barriers, and knowledge of inpatient glycemic control: a survey of health care workers. *J Pharm Pract* 2015; doi: 10.1177/0897190014566309

35. Efird LE, Golden SH, Visram K, Shermock K. Impact of a pharmacy-based glucose management program on glycemic control in an inpatient general medicine population. *Hosp Pract (1995)* 2014;42:101–108

36. Cobaugh DJ, Maynard G, Cooper L, Kienle PC, Vigersky R, Childers D, et al. Enhancing insulin-use safety in hospitals: Practical recommendations from an ASHP Foundation expert consensus panel. *AJHP* 2013;70:1404–1413

37. Umpierrez GE, Schwartz S. Use of incretin-based therapy in hospitalized patients with hyperglycemia. *Endocr Pract* 2014;20:933–944

38. Umpierrez GE, Gianchandani R, Smiley D, Jacobs S, Wesorick DH, Newton C, et al. Safety and efficacy of sitagliptin therapy for the inpatient management of general medicine and surgery patients with type 2 diabetes: a pilot, randomized, controlled study. *Diabetes Care* 2013;36:3430–3435

39. Abuannadi M, Kosiborod M, Riggs L, House JA, Hamburg MS, Kennedy KF, et al. Management of hyperglycemia with the administration of intravenous exenatide to patients in the cardiac intensive care unit. *Endocr Pract* 2013;19:81–90

Chapter 2

The Diagnosis and Classification of Diabetes in Nonpregnant Adults

Irl B. Hirsch, MD, MACP,[1] and Linda M. Gaudiani, MD, FACP, FACE[2]

Much has been learned about the diverse pathogenesis of diabetes over the previous two decades resulting in alterations in the traditional classification of this disease. Although former classifications focused largely on age at onset of initial clinical presentations, such as acute diabetic ketoacidosis (DKA) versus chronic hyperglycemia, the newer position statements on classification by the American Diabetes Association (ADA) have focused on etiologies rather than phenotype. New genetic testing capabilities, expanded immunologic characterizations, and case reports of novel presentations in special disease states have further expanded diagnostic and classification schemes. This has resulted in nomenclature that is more complex than type 1 diabetes (T1D) and type 2 diabetes (T2D), recognizing the heterogeneous characteristics of the major classes of diabetes as well as the phenotypic and mechanistic overlap both initially and over the course of the disease state. Although assigning a type of diabetes to any given patient may be confounded by the circumstances at the time of diagnosis or by acute illness in the hospitalized patient, misdiagnosis of the type of diabetes, failure to attempt to classify the patient accurately, or failure to recognize that the hospitalized patient has diabetes all are critical errors that may affect treatment decisions in the hospital and following discharge and also may contribute to readmissions. An incorrect diabetes classification during the hospital admission and discharge could have especially significant consequences in our current protocol-driven system of diabetes management and certainly on safe transitions of aftercare.

Unfortunately, misclassification of diabetes is not uncommon. Reasons include the fact that age and obesity are traditional discriminating factors for T1D and T2D. Although the exact number is not known, it is estimated that as many as 50% of patients with T1D are diagnosed after the age of 18 years. The impact of this change in the demographics of T1D is not yet clear; however, misdiagnosis of T1D is responsible for admissions for DKA and the development of DKA in the hospital setting.

Several other issues are contributing to a more complex classification of diabetes type. The recent increase in the use of insulin to treat T2D has blurred the prior differentiating schemes based on therapy, as has the expanded uses of noninsulin injectable and oral agents to augment insulin therapy in select

[1]Professor of Medicine, University of Washington School of Medicine, Seattle, WA. [2]Medical Director, Braden Diabetes Center, Marin Endocrine Care and Research, Greenbrae, CA; Associate Clinical Professor of Medicine, University California San Francisco, CA.

DOI: 10.2337/9781580406086.02

individuals with T1D. Additionally, the expanded descriptions and differentiations of the various forms of monogenic diabetes, pancreatic diabetes, and lipodystrophic and syndromic diabetes now often require the assistance of sophisticated laboratory testing for diagnosis[1-3] and often provoke controversy even among endocrinologists. Even with appropriate genetic or antibody analysis, classification is not always clear, available, or timely, resulting in movement between diagnostic categories over time.[4]

It is critical that significant hyperglycemia in the hospitalized patient be promptly recognized and addressed with therapies and education to ensure safe glycemic targets that support best clinical outcomes for the admission. An adequate history must be obtained and testing tailored to guide inpatient management and discharge planning. These goals can be best met by thoughtful consideration of accurate diabetes classification and reconsideration of patients' prior classification as they present clinically.

This chapter reviews the current diagnostic criteria and classification scheme of diabetes for nonpregnant adults with a focus on areas of special interest in the hospital setting. We also hope to acknowledge the areas of controversy and confusion in the current nomenclature and to clarify and further define the various nomenclatures in a schema that is useful, intuitive, and flexible. It is our expectation that as understanding about the pathogenesis and genetic influences of the various forms of diabetes expands, future classifications will continue to evolve.[5]

DIAGNOSIS

Because more than 8 million people (nearly a third) in the U.S. with diabetes are not diagnosed,[6] many patients admitted with hyperglycemia will have undiagnosed diabetes. Those with previously undiagnosed diabetes are more likely to require admission to the hospital compared with those without diabetes.[7] Furthermore, at each level of hyperglycemia, those without a previous diagnosis of diabetes have been shown to be less likely to receive insulin and have greater adverse events compared with those with known diabetes before admission.[8] Unfortunately, diabetes can remain undiagnosed or unattended during hospitalization[9] and the nondiagnosis of diabetes or the undertreatment of stress-induced hyperglycemia in the hospital represents a "missed opportunity" and confers increased mortality risk.[10]

The current diagnostic criteria for diabetes mellitus pose special challenges for the admitting health-care provider. All of the three recently proposed diagnostic glucometric tests for diabetes, except for the HbA_{1c}, are specific for nonill, nonstressed individuals, rendering a new diagnosis of diabetes during hospitalization problematic. The traditional glucose tolerance tests are impractical in the hospital setting and random plasma and fasting plasma glucose values can be distorted by dextrose-containing intravenous (IV) fluids, steroids, stress, illness, and fluctuations in nutrition. The HbA_{1c} test has the advantages of speed, convenience (fasting is not required), and fewer perturbations from recent stress and illness. Table 2.1 notes the current ADA criteria for diabetes.[5]

Of the three diagnostic glucose tests for diabetes, all of which have limitations in hospitalized patients, the most recently added is HbA_{1c}.[5] Despite its advantages,

Table 2.1—Criteria for the Diagnosis of Diabetes

HbA_{1c} ≥6.5% (The test should be performed in a laboratory using a method that is National Glycohemoglobin Standardization Program certified* and standardized to the Diabetes Control and Complications Trial assay.**)
OR
Fasting plasma glucose ≥126 mg/dL (fasting is defined as no caloric intake for at least 8 h)
OR
2-h postprandial plasma glucose ≥200 mg/dL during a 75-g oral glucose tolerance test
OR
In a patient with classic symptoms of hyperglycemia or hyperglycemic crisis, a random plasma glucose ≥200 mg/dL

*See NGSP.org; **in the absence of unequivocal hyperglycemia, the results should be confirmed by repeat testing.

Table 2.2—Etiologies of Falsely High or Low HbA_{1c} Levels

Falsely high
Iron deficiency (with or without anemia)
Anemia
Hemoglobinopathies
Race: African American, Hispanic, Asian
Falsely low
Hemolysis
Reticulocytosis
Hemoglobinopathies
Posthemorrhage or post-transfusion
Drugs: iron, erythropoietin, dapsone
Uremia
Splenomegaly

a number of cautions still pertain to the reliability and accuracy of this test in the acutely ill population, especially when critical illness is superimposed on chronic comorbidities.[11] There are numerous clinical scenarios in which the HbA_{1c} may be falsely high or more commonly low and therefore not actually reflect the glycemic history that usually relates to changes in red blood cell survival times (Table 2.2). This obviously makes the HbA_{1c} difficult to utilize as a diagnostic tool in the hospital setting without careful consideration. In one study, just treating an iron-deficiency anemia can lower the HbA_{1c} from 10.1% to 8.2% in a population with diabetes and from 7.6% to 6.2% in a population without diabetes.[12]

Cardiac valvulopathies and valve replacements with both aortic or mitral valves can cause a microhemolysis resulting in a falsely low HbA_{1c}.[11] Thus, despite the fact many hospitals now require admission HbA_{1c} measurements on patients with and without known diabetes entering the hospital, the test has inherent problems, resulting in the potential for misdiagnosis and mismanagement. Nonetheless, a significantly high HbA_{1c} level (e.g., >8.0%) in the context of hyperglycemia (>180–200 mg/dL) makes the diagnosis of diabetes highly probable.

Plasma glucose is another test that can be used for the diagnosis of diabetes. In the outpatient setting, a fasting glucose of 126 mg/dL or higher or a 75-g oral glucose tolerance test with a 2-h glucose ≥200 mg/dL confirms the diagnosis of diabetes.[5] It is recommended that two such tests are performed in the absence of unequivocal hyperglycemia. The third diagnostic test using glucose is a random plasma glucose >200 mg/dL with classic symptoms of hyperglycemia (polyuria, polydipsia).[5] In addition to a significantly high HbA_{1c}, only this last diagnostic test can be used definitively to confirm the diagnosis of diabetes for the hospitalized patient.

Consider the patient with an HbA_{1c} of 6.8%, anemia, and renal insufficiency who is admitted with pneumonia and fasting and postprandial glucose levels in the 130–140 mg/dL and 200–220 mg/dL range, respectively. This patient may or may not meet the criteria for diabetes once discharged from the hospital. Nonetheless, the inpatient strategy for the treatment of this patient's hyperglycemia should be to meet the goals for optimal inpatient glycemic control and should not be influenced by diagnostic ambiguity. It is critical that "stress hyperglycemia versus diabetes" be included on the discharge problem list so both the patient and the outpatient care team appreciates the specific diagnosis clarifications to be investigated once the acute illness has resolved.

In addition to the diagnostic categories of diabetes and stress-induced hyperglycemia, the Expert Committee on Diagnosis and Classification of Diabetes now recognizes a significant group of patients who are at increased risk of developing future diabetes. The term "prediabetes" is used to describe these individuals with impaired fasting glucose or impaired glucose tolerance (Table 2.3).[5] Although these patients do not meet the diagnostic criteria for diabetes, their glucose values are too high to be considered normal, and numerous prospective studies have shown a strong association between HbA_{1c} and progression to diabetes. In the hospital setting, these patients can develop significant hyperglycemia and are at

Table 2.3—Categories of Increased Risk for Diabetes (Prediabetes)*

Fasting plasma glucose 100–125 mg/dL (impaired glucose tolerance)
OR
2-h plasma glucose in the 75-g oral glucose tolerance test 140–199 mg/dL
OR
HbA_{1c} 5.7–6.4%

*For all three tests, risk is continuous, extending below the lower limit of the range and becoming disproportionately greater at higher ends of the range.

increased risk for complications while hospitalized and subsequently for cardiovascular disease.

CLASSIFICATION

The goal of classifying a patient with a particular type of diabetes in the hospital setting should be to provide useful information about the pathogenesis, natural history, genetics, and phenotype of their disease to optimize safe and appropriate treatments, monitoring, education, patient expectations, and quality of life. Additionally, proper classification of hospitalized patients with hyperglycemia assists in appropriate transitions of aftercare.

Recent classifications have broadly distinguished the types of diabetes into two groups—autoimmune (T1D) and nonautoimmune (T2D)—with all other types being classified in an "other" category. The other category includes monogenic, gestational, pancreatic, steroid-induced, HIV-associated, hepatitis C–associated, polycystic ovarian syndrome–related, and endocrinopathy-associated (acromegaly and Cushing's syndrome) diabetes. This general schema is useful despite considerable overlap in classic phenotypic presentation in each major class and will guide the knowledgeable health-care provider to make prudent decisions on whom to consider for more specific assignment. In addition to sophisticated testing, it is highly useful to obtain accurate and detailed histories of presentation and family history to advise further evaluation.

TYPE 1 DIABETES

T1D accounts for ~5–10% of diabetes and is the result of cellular-mediated autoimmune destruction of the pancreatic β-cells,[13] resulting in moderate to severe insulin deficiency. It classically but not invariably manifests with acute and severe symptoms of hyperglycemia, dehydration, and ketoacidosis. Although the presence of autoantibodies assists in identifying autoimmune versus nonautoimmune diabetes, these antibodies usually but not always disappear over a variable amount of time. The most common antibody in the adult population is glutamic acid decarboxylase 65 (GAD65).[14] Other antibodies that are quickly becoming commercially available include antibodies to tyrosine phosphatase IA-2 and zinc transporter 8 (ZnT8). Traditional islet cell antibodies (ICA) generally are not used because of the assay's subjectivity. Insulin autoantibodies rarely are seen in adults (although they cross-react with antibodies from exogenous insulin). T1D has strong human leukocyte antigen (HLA) associations, which may be either predisposing or protective in most cases.

Although severe insulin deficiency and the tendency to ketosis and acute onset of symptoms are the hallmarks of T1D, the time of progression to absolute insulin deficiency is variable. Particularly in adults with newly diagnosed T1D, residual endogenous insulin secretion may still be present decades after the diagnosis[15] and appears to be protective to the complications of the disease.[16] This is significant to the health-care provider in the hospital setting because the measurement of c-peptide, while helpful in some circumstances, does not necessarily differentiate T1D from T2D as previously thought and may be misleading. Because a number of factors significantly influence the accurate measurement of c-peptide (antecedent hyperglycemia leading to glucotoxicity, nonstandardization of c-peptide measurement and assay), it generally is not recommended as a helpful test to classify the inpatient with hyperglycemia and may be misleading.

Age and BMI do not invariably discriminate T1D and T2D. Although most commonly presenting in childhood and adolescence, T1D can manifest at any decade of life and with extended life spans in the T1D population combined with the increased frequency of T2D in the young adult obese population, age is no longer a reliable discriminatory factor in the classification between T1D and T2D. Similarly, recent data show that the BMI breakdown for the T1D population is now identical to that of the general population, a shift thought to be related to more intensive insulin regimens and secondary weight gain in the T1D population.[17]

Patients with T1D may have personal or family histories of one or more autoimmune disorders. These include Graves' disease, Hashimoto's thyroiditis, Addison's disease, celiac disease, myasthenia gravis, vitiligo, and pernicious anemia. Other historical features may be helpful, such as family history of associated endocrinopathies, or features at initial disease presentation, but these facts may not be available to the treating health-care provider in the hospital setting.

Classic T1D is now appreciated to include factors of β-cell dysfunction as well as β-cell loss and the understanding of the mechanisms that trigger these processes is still incomplete but rapidly expanding.

One of the most confusing controversies in the nomenclature of T1D classification is latent autoimmune diabetes of adults (LADA). Originally described in patients over the age of 30 years, who were GAD65 antibody positive,[18] but who did not require insulin treatment in the first 6 months after diagnosis, these patients eventually required insulin for survival similarly to what was seen in individuals with complete insulin deficiency. LADA also has been called "slowly progressive insulin dependent diabetes," "latent T1D," "antibody-positive, noninsulin-dependent diabetes," and "type 1.5 diabetes." Not all adults who develop autoimmune diabetes have LADA, however, progression to complete β-cell deficiency and even ketosis can be rapid in some adults or may be provoked suddenly by acute illness, infection, hyperthyroidism, or other stress.

It is estimated that between 2 and 12% of all diabetes in adults is LADA. In the United Kingdom Prospective Diabetes Study (UKPDS), ~10% of adults presumed to have T2D at diagnosis had evidence of positive GAD or ICA[19] and most of these progressed to require insulin within 6 years. These patients should be sought for accurate diagnosis because they require vigilance as to the timing of beginning insulin and optimal therapies to preserve β-cell function. Some authors consider all adult-diagnosed patients with diabetes who are antibody positive to have LADA or type 1.5 diabetes. We suggest it may be useful to differentiate the classical nonobese (noninsulin-resistant) adult with positive diabetes autoantibodies and not requiring insulin 6 months after diagnosis as LADA,[18] and those adults who are antibody positive but exhibit classic insulin resistance with phenotypic features of metabolic syndrome as type 1.5 diabetes. This differentiation may inform more effective and specific treatment strategies based on pathogenesis. Despite widespread use of these diabetes classifications in the literature, neither LADA nor type 1.5 diabetes is included in the current ADA classification scheme.[5]

For the typical LADA patient, basal-bolus insulin therapy has been shown to retard the progression to more profound β-cell failure.[20] The obese, antibody-positive patients classified as having type 1.5 diabetes may respond to all of the T2D agents, although these individuals will likely progress to profound insulin deficiency more rapidly than if they were antibody negative.[21] Patients with LADA and type 1.5 diabetes generally will require insulin in the hospital setting.

Another group of adult autoantibody-positive patients is seen more frequently in the early 21st century with a phenotype rarely seen 30 years ago and variously called "double diabetes" or "hybrid diabetes," but to keep the nomenclature consistent, we call this "type 3 diabetes." This class refers to adults who developed classic T1D autoimmune diabetes as children but because of all of the genetic and environmental issues that have resulted in the current obesity epidemic, as they reach adolescence and adulthood, these individuals also become obese and develop features of the metabolic syndrome.[22] Although they may appear to be the same, the factor differentiating these patients from those with type 1.5 diabetes is the history of being diagnosed initially with classic childhood diabetes and having relatively rapid β-cell failure as opposed to the more recently diagnosed adults with autoimmune diabetes who tend to have less profound β-cell destruction and slower development of insulin deficiency.

Admittedly, there is no consensus on these various T1D subcategories as yet, but classifying patients as LADA (diagnosed as an adult, normal body weight, normal insulin resistance, gradually deficient in endogenous insulin, and antibody positive), type 1.5 (diagnosed as an adult, obese, insulin resistant, and antibody positive), or type 3 (diagnosed as a child, obese, insulin deficient, and resistant) may be useful if this classification results in a more clear appreciation of the pathogenesis and institution of optimal treatments

A minority of T1D occurs without evidence of autoimmunity as in the cause of the insulin deficiency, which nonetheless can be profound and develop rapidly. This is referred to as idiopathic diabetes, previously called "type 1b diabetes." Included in the category of idiopathic diabetes is "fulminant type 1 diabetes,"[23] most commonly described in Asian patients[24] and usually presenting after a viral infection or during pregnancy. Onset is acute, usually with DKA despite HbA_{1c} levels that are near normal because of the rapid onset of the hyperglycemia. Of special relevance to treating health-care providers in the emergency room and hospital, death from DKA may occur within 24 h if insulin therapy is not initiated immediately upon presentation.[23]

TYPE 2 DIABETES

T2D accounts for the majority of diabetes in the world, accounting for ~90% of all cases. Uncontrolled hyperglycemia in T2D often goes undiagnosed for many years because of the absence of symptoms or presence of vague symptoms. In the hospitalized setting, DKA can occur, but it is almost always associated with stress of another illness, such as infection or ischemia. Undiagnosed diabetes is particularly common in patients admitted for myocardial infarction.[25] An inpatient admission can be an important opportunity for diagnosis and initiation of treatment in such high-risk individuals. Even patients with previously well-controlled T2D usually will require discontinuation of prior diabetes oral agents and noninsulin injectable therapies during hospitalizations and treatment with IV or subcutaneous insulin therapies to optimally and safely control hyperglycemia.

Individuals with T2D are resistant to insulin and have relative, as opposed to absolute, insulin deficiency. Over time, they can become profoundly insulin deficient. Depending on the individual and the situation, insulin and c-peptide levels may be high, normal, or low. Autoimmune destruction of the β-cells does not occur, and patients are antibody negative. The risk of developing T2D increases with age, obesity, sedentary lifestyle, and positive family history. It occurs more frequently in women with previous gestational diabetes and polycystic ovarian syndrome; post-menopause, it is seen in individuals with dyslipidemia and hypertension; and it is seen in many ethnic groups (African American, Native American, Hispanic, Pacific Islander, and Asian American). Approximately 85% of individuals with T2D are obese or overweight, and those who are not obese often have an increased percentage of body fat distributed in the abdominal region. The obesity definition is ethnicity-related. For example, although Caucasians are considered obese with a BMI ≥30 kg/m², the World Health Organization defines obesity <30 kg/m² for most Asians and the recent ADA standards changed the BMI cut point for screening overweight Asian Americans for T2D to 23 kg/m², from the previous 25 kg/m².[5]

Multiple genetic mutations have been associated with T2D but in clinical practice it is not possible to identify a specific genetic abnormality. One specific example of a poorly understood genetic entity of T2D is atypical diabetes, also called Flatbush diabetes. This is a ketosis-prone diabetes, initially described in African Americans who presented with DKA, but the subsequent disease course more closely resembles classic T2D.[26] The underlying pathogenesis is unclear, but studies have shown a transient secretory defect of β-cells at the time of presentation with remarkable recovery of insulin-secretory capacity.[27] Ketosis-prone diabetes also has been described in other ethnicities.

MONOGENIC DIABETES SYNDROMES

These patients represent a small fraction of diabetes (<5%), which is the result of a single genetic defect and generally presents before the age of 25 years. They usually are negative for the antibodies commonly found in T1D. The two main subtypes of monogenic diabetes are neonatal diabetes and maturity onset diabetes of youth (MODY). When diagnosed within the first 6 months of life, diabetes is called neonatal diabetes, which is not a form of T1D. The diabetes in these neonates may be transient or permanent, with the latter most commonly having a mutation on the gene encoding the Kir6.2 subunit of the β-cell K_{ATP} channel. Despite the early onset, these individuals can be well managed with sulfonylureas instead of insulin as children and, if eventually diagnosed later, even as adults. For this reason, all patients diagnosed with diabetes before the age of 6 months should have genetic screening for neonatal diabetes, even if the history of age of onset is discovered decades later.

MODY is a heterogeneous group of antibody-negative, autosomal-dominant inherited, youth-onset disorders of the β-cell. MODY is characterized by impaired insulin secretion but no (or minimal) defects in insulin action. To date, six different gene mutations are identified on different chromosomes, each one resulting in a different clinical entity.[28] One of these genes encodes the enzyme glucokinase (associated with MODY 2), whereas the other five loci encode transcription factors. The most common is hepatic nuclear factor 1-α (associated with MODY 3). Differentiating MODY from T1D is important given the autosomal-dominant inheritance of the former and the observation that many of these patients can be controlled with sulfonylureas. Furthermore, those with glucokinase MODY generally need no therapy (except during pregnancy). Specialty commercial lab testing is now available to identify the gene mutations for clinical (nonresearch) diagnosis to accurately diagnose youth who have MODY and to facilitate prompt identification of other potentially affected family members.

PANCREATIC DIABETES

Many diseases of the pancreas affect endocrine function. Formally termed "pancreatic diabetes," the etiologies, degree of insulin sensitivity, and the subsequent risk for hypoglycemia vary.

For example, cystic fibrosis (CF) patients have a high frequency of diabetes called cystic fibrosis–related diabetes (CFRD). This occurs in 40–50% of adult patients with CF.[29] Insulin sensitivity is generally normal or only slightly decreased except in the setting of acute illness when insulin resistance can be severe.[30] The frequent intervention of lung transplantation requiring use of corticosteroids and calcineurin inhibitors further increases the prevalence of diabetes in this population. Conversely, the diabetes secondary to chronic pancreatitis mainly occurs from the destruction of islet cells by pancreatic inflammation. There is also an idiopathic variety of chronic, calcific pancreatitis associated with malnutrition that has been termed "tropical chronic pancreatitis." Both of these latter forms of chronic pancreatitis also are associated with glucagon deficiency and thus more marked sensitivity to insulin with increased risks of hypoglycemia associated with insulin therapy.

Hereditary hemochromatosis is another etiology of pancreatic diabetes, with up to 23% of hemochromatosis patients in one study diagnosed with diabetes.[31]

Surgical pancreatectomy is particularly common in hospitals with busy oncology centers. Immediately after surgery, insulin deficiency in these patients can be reasonably easy to control with basal-bolus insulin therapy. These patients, however, are extremely prone to the risk of devastating hypoglycemia because of glucagon deficiency, and reducing insulin dosing by 20–25% at discharge from the hospital is suggested.

Ideally, patients scheduled for pancreatectomy should meet with a diabetes team or endocrinologist before the surgery and focused diabetes education is needed after this procedure. Because the pancreatectomy is due to a malignancy (or in some cases pancreatic dysplasia[32]), the diabetes often is not the main focus of the patient or the family. Especially for those patients who have a good prognosis, the importance of good glycemic control and avoidance of hypoglycemia, even more so than the newly diagnosed patient with T1D, should be stressed. The glucagon deficiency, besides leading to abnormal glucose counterregulation, also results in overall increased insulin sensitivity, meaning extra precaution is required for exercise. Although exact data are not available, there are anecdotal reports of death resulting from hypoglycemia in this population possibly related to physical activity, lack of blood glucose testing, alcohol, or a combination. Continuous glucose monitoring should be strongly considered for these patients.

DRUG-INDUCED DIABETES

Many drugs are known to cause diabetes. Some drugs, such as streptozotocin and IV pentamidine can permanently destroy pancreatic β-cells. More commonly, the ubiquitously useful glucocorticoid therapies (including IV, oral, intra-articular, inhaled, and even topical) can result in hyperglycemia or frank diabetes. Glucocorticoids cause hyperglycemia by increasing insulin resistance by several mechanisms, including inducing an increase in visceral fat and direct actions on muscle and liver resulting in decreased insulin activity. Atypical antipsychotics also can result in diabetes in part because of the effects of increasing appetite and food intake resulting in obesity, although the exact mechanisms are complex.[33] DKA has been described as resulting from these agents and should be considered by the health-care providers when someone taking one of these medications presents with this metabolic emergency.[34] Table 2.4 lists medications often used in the hospital that can cause hyperglycemia or diabetes.

Table 2.4—Drugs Often Used in the Hospital That Can Cause Hyperglycemia or Diabetes

- Antibiotics
  - Quinolones
    - Gantifloxicin (can also cause hypoglycemia)
    - Levofloxicin
- Atypical antipsychotics
  - Most risky
    - Clozapine
    - Olanzapine
  - Intermediate
    - Paliperidone
    - Risperidone
- β-Blockers (carvedilol not associated with hyperglycemia)
  - Atenolol
  - Metoprolol
  - Propranolol
- Calcineurin inhibitors
  - Cyclosporin
  - Sirolimus
  - Tacrolimus
- Corticosteroids
- Diazoxide
- Nicotinic Acid
- Protease inhibitors
- Thiazide and thiazide-like diuretics

LIPODYSTROPHIC DIABETES

Lipodystrophies are heterogeneous-heterogeneously acquired or inherited disorders characterized by selective loss of adipose tissue. These patients have severe insulin resistance, dyslipidemia, and hepatic steatosis.[35] Interestingly, insulin resistance but not hyperglycemia is the norm in those patients with lipodystrophy related to protease inhibitors. Conversely, congenital generalized lipodystrophy usually is associated with severe hypertriglyceridemia prone to pancreatitis.

OTHER FORMS OF DIABETES OFTEN SEEN IN THE HOSPITAL

The etiology of the diabetes is multifactorial. As noted, other conditions are associated with diabetes, and one that often is seen in the hospital is diabetes associated with hepatitis C infection.[36] These patients are at high risk for stress hyperglycemia or already may have undiagnosed T2D when admitted.

CONCLUSION

The classification of diabetes remains a work in progress. Attempts to classify our patients will lead to better understanding of the pathophysiology of the common diabetes types, the genetic mutations causing diabetes in rare forms of diabetes, and greater recognition of the vast heterogeneity in this disease. It is clear that for some patients, accurately classifying diabetes in the hospital may not be possible, whereas for others, more sophisticated lab testing may be required to confirm

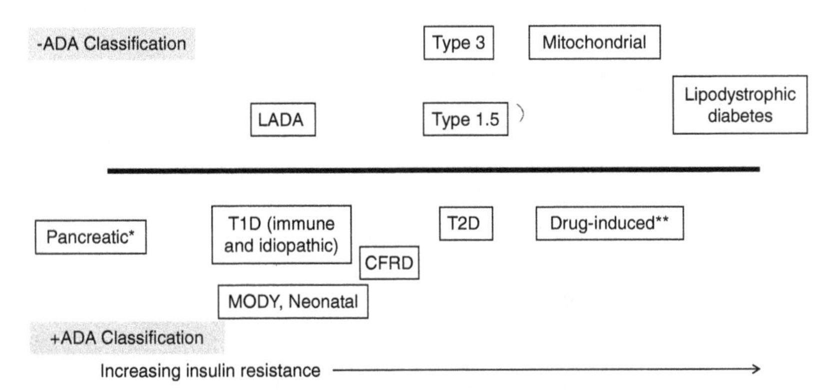

Figure 2.1—A conceptual classification for diabetes mellitus. Above the dark line are those classes not included in the 2015 ADA classification; below the line are those that are included. Moving left to right moves to greater degrees of insulin resistance.

*Depending on etiology, may have different degrees of insulin resistance and does not include CFRD; **wide degrees of insulin resistance depending on etiology.

both diagnosis as well as classification. Occasional patients will be difficult to classify. Nevertheless, while in the hospital, the primary goal will remain to thoughtfully consider classification of diabetes and to treat the hyperglycemia to accepted targets, and this usually will require insulin therapy.

We acknowledge that the various subtypes of autoimmune diabetes have an evolving consensus in their classification. Figure 2.1 illustrates our conceptualization for how a health-care provider in the hospital can think about the classification of diabetes, taking into account what is now accepted by the ADA and what often is used clinically.

REFERENCES

1. Pihoker C, Gilliam LK, Ellard S, et al. Prevalence, characteristics, and clinical diagnosis of maturity onset diabetes of the young due to mutations in HNF1A, HNF4A, and glucokinase: results for the SEARCH for diabetes in youth. *J Clin Metabol Endocrinol* 2013;4055–4062
2. Thewitchcharoen Y, Wanothavaro E, Himathongkam T, et al. Permanent neonatal diabetes misdiagnosed as type 1 diabetes in a 28-year-old female: a life-changing event. *Diabetes Res Clin Pract* 2014;106:e22–e24
3. Hardt PD, Brendel MD, Kloer HU, et al. Is pancreatic diabetes (type 3c diabetes) underdiagnosed and misdiagnosed? *Diabetes Care* 2008;31(Suppl. 2): S165–S169
4. Reinehr T, Schober E, Wiegand S, et al. β-cell autoantibodies in children with type 2 diabetes mellitus: subgroup or misclassification? *Arch Dis Child* 2006;91:473–477
5. American Diabetes Association. Classification and diagnosis of diabetes. *Diabetes Care* 2015;38(Suppl. 1):S8–S16
6. Centers for Disease Control and Prevention. 2014 National diabetes statistics report. http://www.cdc.gov/diabetes/data/statistics/2014StatisticsReport.html. Accessed 20 January 2015
7. Young K, Mustard CA. Undiagnosed diabetes: does it matter? *CMAJ* 2001;164:24–28
8. Kotagal M, Symons R, Hirsch IB, et al. Perioperative hyperglycemia and risk for adverse events among patients with and without diabetes. *Ann Surg* 2015;261:97–103
9. Levetan CS, Passaro M, Jablonski K, et al. Unrecognized diabetes among hospitalized patients. *Diabetes Care* 1998;21:246–249
10. Umpierrez GE, Isaacs SD, Bazargan N, et al. Hyperglycemia: an independent marker of in-hospital mortality in patients with undiagnosed diabetes. *J Clin Endocrinol Metab* 2002;87:978–982
11. Rubinow KB, Hirsch IB. Reexamining metrics for glucose control. *JAMA* 2011;305:1132–1133

12. Tarim O, Kucukerdgan A, Gunay U, et al. Effects of iron deficiency anemia on hemoglobin A_{1c} I type 1 diabetes mellitus. *Pediatr Inter* 1999;41:357–362
13. Atkinson MA, Eisenbarth GS, Michels AW. Type 1 diabetes. *Lancet* 2014; 383:69–82
14. Knip M, Siljander H. Autoimmune mechanisms in type 1 diabetes. *Autoimmun Rev* 2008;7:550–557
15. Davis AK, Dubose SN, Haller MJ, et al. Prevalence of detectable c-peptide according to age of diagnosis and duration of type 1 diabetes. *Diabetes Care* 2015;38:476–481
16. Sun JK, Keenan HA, Cavallerano JD. Protection from retinopathy and other complications in patients with type 1 diabetes of extreme duration: the Joslin 50-year medalist study. *Diabetes Care* 2011;34:968–974
17. Miller KM, Foster NC, Beck RW, et al. Current state of type 1 diabetes treatment in the US: updated data from the T1D Exchange Clinic Registry. *Diabetes Care* 2015;38:971–978
18. Zimmet P, Tuomi T, Mackay IR, et al. Latent autoimmune diabetes of adults (LADA): the role of antibodies to glutamic acid decarboxylase in diagnosis and prediction of insulin dependency. *Diab Med* 1994;11:294–303
19. UK Prospective Diabetes Study Group. UK prospective diabetes study 16: overview of 6 years' therapy of type II diabetes: a progressive disease. *Diabetes* 1995;44:1249–1258
20. DCCT Research Group. Effect of intensive therapy on residual beta-cell function in patients with type 1 diabetes in the diabetes control and complications trial. A randomized, controlled trial. *Ann Intern Med* 1998;128:517–523
21. Turner R, Stratton I, Horton V, et al. UKPDS 25: autoantibodies to islet-cell cytoplasm and glutamic acid decarboxylase for prediction of insulin requirement in type 2 diabetes. *Lancet* 1997;350:1288–1293
22. Pozzilli P, Guglielmi C, Caprio S, Buzzetti R. Obesity, autoimmunity, and double diabetes in youth. *Diabetes Care* 2011;34(Suppl. 2):S166–S170
23. Hanafusa T, Imagawa A. Fulminant type 1 diabetes: a novel entity requiring special attention by all medical practitioners. *Nature Clin Pract Encrinol* 2007;3:36–45
24. WHO Expert Consultation. Appropriate body mass index for Asian populations and its implications for policy and intervention strategies. *Lancet* 2004;363:157–163
25. Norhammar A, Tenerz A, Nilsson G, et al. Glucose metabolism in patients with acute myocardial infarction and no previous diagnosis of diabetes mellitus: a prospective study. *Lancet* 2002;359:2140–2144
26. Winter WE, Maclaren NK, Riley WJ. Maturity-onset diabetes of youth in black Americans. *N Engl J Med* 1987;316:285–291

27. Mauvas-Jarvis F, Sobngwi E, Porcher R, et al. Ketosis-prone type 2 diabetes in patients of Sub-Saharan African origin clinical pathophysiology and natural history of b-cell dysfunction an insulin resistance. *Diabetes* 2004;53:645–653

28. Fajans SS, Bell GI, Polonsky KS. Molecular mechanisms and clinical pathophysiology of maturity-onset diabetes of the young. *N Engl J Med* 2001;345:971–980

29. Moran A, Dunitz J, Nathan B, et al. Cystic fibrosis-related diabetes: current trends in prevalence, incidence, and mortality. *Diabetes Care* 2009;32:1626–1631

30. Ode LK, Moran A. New insights into cystic fibrosis-related diabetes in children. *Lancet Diabetes Endocrinol* 2013;1:52–58

31. McClain DA, Abraham D, Rogers J, et al. High prevalence of abnormal glucose homeostasis secondary to decreased insulin secretion in individuals with hereditary hemochromatosis. *Diabetologia* 2006;49:1661–1669

32. Templeton AW, Brentnall TA. Screening and surgical outcomes of familial pancreatic cancer. *Surg Clin North Am* 2013;93:629–645

33. Goncalves P, Araujo JR, Martel F. Antipsychotics-induced metabolic alterations: focus on adipose tissue and molecular mechanisms. *Eur Neuropsychlpharmacol* 2015;25:1–16

34. Jin H, Meyer JM, Jeste DV. Phenomenology of and risk factors for new-onset diabetes mellitus and diabetic ketoacidosis associated with atypical antipsychotics: an analysis of 45 published cases. *Ann Clin Psychiatry* 2002;14:59–64

35. Garg A. Acquired and inherited lipodystrophies. *N Engl J Med* 2004;350: 1220–1234

36. Lacube A, Hernadez C, Genesca, Simo R. Glucose abnormalities in patients with hepatitis C virus infection. *Diabetes Care* 2006;29:1140–1149

Chapter 3

Perils of Glycemic Variability and Rapid Correction of Chronic Hyperglycemia

Susan S. Braithwaite, MD,[1] and Irl B. Hirsch, MD[2]

INTRODUCTION

The objective of this chapter is to discuss evidence among hospitalized patients supporting or discrediting each of two propositions, in contexts other than hyperglycemic emergencies:

- Glycemic variability, independent of hyperglycemia and hypoglycemia, may causally contribute to risk of harm among hospitalized patients.
- Aggressive correction of chronic hyperglycemia may cause short-term harm for hospitalized patients experiencing uncontrolled diabetes.

Under each of several definitions, glycemic variability, independently from hypoglycemia and hyperglycemia, in the hospital has been recognized to be a risk factor associated with adverse outcomes.[1–12] Although supporting evidence has been collected mostly in the intensive care setting, limited data collected in the general hospital setting suggest a similar relationship.[10] Glycemic variability is not restricted to patients having preexisting diabetes, whereas rapid correction of chronic hyperglycemia occurs only among patients having preexisting uncontrolled diabetes.[1] With respect to predictive value or physiology, it is not clear to what extent glycemic variability actually resembles rapid correction of chronic hyperglycemia. Therefore, we do not classify a one-time hospital-based correction of chronic hyperglycemia as an example of glycemic variability. Present-day therapeutic tools may permit the provider to control the rate of correction of chronic hyperglycemia. Importantly, we have only early evidence suggestive of therapeutic approaches that could reduce glycemic variability in the hospital.

GLYCEMIC VARIABILITY

GLYCEMIC VARIABILITY AND OUTCOMES IN THE INPATIENT SETTING

The goal of this section is to discuss evidence that harms occurring in the hospital are associated with glycemic variability, independent of hyperglycemia and

[1]Presence Saint Joseph Hospital, Chicago, IL; Presence Saint Francis Hospital, Evanston, IL; West Suburban Medical Center, Oak Park, IL; Westlake Hospital, Melrose Park, IL; Clinical Professor of Medicine, University of Illinois at Chicago, Chicago, IL. [2]Professor of Medicine University of Washington Medical Center–Roosevelt, Seattle, WA.

DOI: 10.2337/9781580406086.03

hypoglycemia (Table 3.1). The definition of variability and choice of metrics may determine whether or not a pattern of glycemia within a population is identified as showing increased patient-level glycemic variability.[2–12] Intuitively, for this discussion, glycemic variability is understood as a propensity of a single patient to develop repeated episodes of excursions of hyperglycemia or troughs of hypoglycemia over a relatively short period of time that exceed the amplitude expected in normal physiology.[13]

To characterize or compare groups of patients, it is desirable to choose metrics that will quantify the variability experienced by typical group members. The choice of metrics used to identify variability has been controversial. When standard deviation (SD) or coefficient of variability (CV) is used as a variability metric, all of the data points are used, thus optimizing the power of the metric to make comparisons. For inferential or predictive purposes, SD should be applied to data sets exhibiting Gaussian distribution. Recognizing the predictive value of CV with respect to risk for hypoglycemia, and depending on whether the absolute magnitude of excursions is important or the magnitude of excursions relative to the mean, some authorities favor CV over SD.[14,15] The SD is highly correlated with the mean BG.[16] In a study of 18,563 patients having myocardial infarction, an association of variability with mortality risk, noted by five metrics in unadjusted analyses, was not upheld after reexamination with adjustment for patient factors, including mean BG.[7] Recognizing that a single major change of glycemia during an observation interval can yield a high SD, we favor caution on the use of the SD or CV during intervals of rapidly changing average of blood glucose. Alternative metrics should be considered, such that glycemic variability can be differentiated by the chosen metrics from rapid correction of chronic hyperglycemia.[5,13] Nevertheless, some of the earliest and strongest evidence linking variability to outcomes in the critical care setting is based on the use of SD.[2,3]

During an era in which the inpatient use of continuous glucose monitoring (CGM) has not yet become a standard of care, the study of inpatient glycemic variability has suffered from irregularity of timing and infrequency of monitoring of blood glucose. When applied to CGM, the problem of autocorrelations introduces a caveat for the use of SD with traditional statistics. Kovatchev and Clarke[17] report that the autocorrelation coefficients become insignificant at a time lag of approximately 1 h, such that CGM readings more than 1 h apart could be considered linearly independent.

Outcome studies about variability in the hospital generally confirm an association of variability, identified by at least some measures, with adverse outcomes. Although variability is associated with hyperglycemia and hypoglycemia, in multivariate analyses, variability has remained an independent predictor of adverse hospital outcomes.[6,8] The outcomes have included nosocomial infection rate, hospital length of stay, and mortality.[13] The relationship between glycemic variability and outcomes in the hospital may be stronger among patients not having known diabetes than among those with diagnosed diabetes and, depending on the study, may be attenuated or not discernable in the presence of diabetes.[4,9–11] As a caution on interpretation, it is noted that a one-time correction of BG with insulin during the time frame of data collection may inflate the SD or CV, thus complicating comparisons of these metrics among patients who did or did not experience such one-time corrections of overall glycemia. Additionally, in the analysis of large

Table 3.1—Outcomes Associated with Glycemic Variability

Reference	Number of patients	Variability metric	Overall findings	Findings in the absence of confirmed diabetes	Findings among patients having diabetes
Krinsley 2009[4]	Mortality outcomes were studied at a single site among 4,084 adult intensive care unit (ICU) patients.*	SD and CV of central lab glucose readings	Patients with diabetes had higher mean glucose, SD and CV than did those without diabetes ($P < 0.0001$ for all comparisons).	CV had a strong, independent association with mortality among 3,142 critically ill patients without diabetes. A CV of 50+ was associated with adjusted odds ratio for mortality of 2.39 (95% CI, 1.48–3.86).	There was no association between CV and mortality among 942 patients having diabetes using the same multivariable model.
Lipska et al.[7]	Five different variability metrics were studied among 18,563 patients having acute myocardial infarction.* Data were captured from an electronic medical record used by 61 participating hospitals.	Range, standard deviation, mean amplitude of glycemic excursions, mean absolute glucose change, average daily risk range	When mean BG was included among variables used to control for multiple patients factors, none of the examined variability metrics predicted in-hospital mortality.		
Meynaar et al.[8]	Variability metrics were evaluated as predictors of mortality among 20,375 patients admitted to 37 Dutch ICUs.*	SD and three other metrics were evaluated as predictors of mortality after adjustment for severity of illness, hypoglycemia, mean glucose, and other variables	The median (IQR) for SD in mmol/L was 1.66 (1.2–2.4) among 15,962 survivors and 1.97 (1.4–2.8) among 4,413 nonsurvivors. The SD was independently associated with hospital mortality in surgical and medical patients.		

continued

Table 3.1—Outcomes Associated with Glycemic Variability *(continued)*

Reference	Number of patients	Variability metric	Overall findings	Findings in the absence of confirmed diabetes	Findings among patients having diabetes
Krinsley et al.[9]	Mortality data were analyzed in relation to hypoglycemia, hyperglycemia, glycemic variability, and presence or absence of diabetes for 44,964 patients admitted to 23 ICUs from nine countries.	CV of BG according to bands (<20%, 20–40%, >40%), with hypoglycemia and diabetes status included as variables in the multivariable model	For the entire cohort, hypoglycemia was independently associated with increased risk of mortality.	Within the cohort of 32,084 patients not having diabetes, glycemic variability <20% was independently associated with decreased risk of mortality compared with increased risk at 20–40% or >40%.	Within the cohort of 12,880 patients having diabetes, increased CV in multivariable analysis was not independently associated with risk of mortality.
Mendez et al.[10]	935 nonacute admissions to a single VA hospital were evaluated for relationship of variability with length of stay and 90-day mortality.	SD and CV	For every 10 mg/dL increase in SD and 10% increase in CV, length of stay increased by 4.4 and 9.7%, respectively. After multivariate adjustment, mortality at 90 days increased by 8% for every 10-mg/dL increase in SD.		
Farrokhi et al.[11]	At a single site, 276 medical and surgical patients receiving TPN were studied for the relationship between glycemic variability and mortality.	SD and mean BG daily delta change (daily max – daily minimum)	Overall hospital mortality was 27.3%. SD was 48±25 among deceased patients vs. 34±18 mg/dL among survivors, $P < 0.01$; mean delta change was 75±39 vs. 51±29, $P < 0.01$. Glycemic variability was higher among those with known diabetes ($P < 0.01$ for both variability metrics).	Among 223 patients without diabetes, mortality rate was 26%, not significantly different from those having diabetes. Daily delta change was 53±29, and SD was 34±19 mg/dL. The association between glycemic variability and mortality was significant for patients without a history of diabetes ($P = 0.02$).	Among 53 patients with diabetes, mortality rate was 30%. Daily delta change was 79±41, and SD was 51±23 mg/dL. The association between GV and mortality was not significant for patients with a history of diabetes ($P = 0.32$).

*At least 3 BG measurements were required.
See also Braithwaite.[13]

groups, it is likely that patient factors should be considered that may acutely change overall glycemia and degree of insulin resistance, including underlying diagnosis, use of glucocorticoids, nutritional treatment plan, and choice of antihyperglycemic therapy.

Technology and newer treatments may be at hand that have the potential to reduce glycemic variability, thus permitting both design of randomized trials and ultimately therapeutic intervention to reduce variability.[18–21] The expected opportunities for improvement include refinement of insulin-based treatment algorithms, hypoglycemia protocols, use of glucose monitoring technology to improve the effectiveness of insulin delivery systems,[22] new insulins, and use of incretin-based therapy.[23]

GLYCEMIC TARGETS AND RATE OF CORRECTION

As is well appreciated, the strongest evidence showing causal relationship between hyperglycemia and complications of diabetes arose from randomized trials of the 20th century, including the Diabetes Control and Complications Trial Research Group (DCCT) and UK Prospective Diabetes Study (UKPDS), enrolling patients having type 1 diabetes (T1D) and type 2 diabetes (T2D), respectively.[24,25] These trials demonstrated, in comparison to control groups receiving less intensive treatment, that there was reduction in the risk of microvascular complications for patients receiving more intensive glycemic management. Each intensively treated group experienced a greater event rate for hypoglycemia. Reductions in the microvascular complications in these studies are thought to result from exposure to hyperglycemia experienced over the long term, in time frames measured in years (also termed "glycemic exposure"). A separate question is whether immediate beneficial consequences of glycemic exposure, in the absence of a hyperglycemic emergency, also would be realized by hospitalized patients vulnerable to a different set of specific risks that potentially would be realized in the short term. Theoretically, the improvement of hyperglycemia and glycemic variability could reduce reactive oxygen species accumulation and inflammatory activation, resulting in both short-term and long-term benefits.

Glycemic Targets and Rate of Correction in the Ambulatory Setting

In the ambulatory setting, during initial correction of chronic hyperglycemia, a patient may experience painful neuropathic symptoms.[26–30] Similarly, during intensification of therapy, early worsening of retinopathy may be observed. Risk factors for early worsening include the duration of diabetes, severity of the diabetic retinopathy at baseline, higher HbA_{1c}, and magnitude of HbA_{1c} reduction, such that specific cautions on monitoring have been recommended.[31,32] The temporary problems of acute painful sensory neuropathy or early worsening of retinopathy are seen as a tolerable price to pay for the long-term benefits expected from improved glycemic control. In the ACCORD trial, however, in an older population with more cardiovascular disease than among subjects studied in the UKPDS, intensification of therapy of T2D was accompanied by increased mortality.[33–35] With acknowledgment that mechanisms of harm would be different in each situation, and that comorbidities and concomitant therapies must be considered, these experiences are mentioned as analogies when discussing whether treatment guidelines for hyperglycemia in the inpatient setting might differ according to the presence or absence of diabetes. Furthermore, among patients with diabetes, one needs to consider whether the target and rate of correction of hyperglycemia might differ according to severity of chronic hyperglycemia before admission, as reflected by the HbA_{1c} or other indicators of preadmission control, including other biomarkers, such as fructosamine, glycated albumin, home blood glucose monitoring, or CGM. As we enter the era of personalized medicine, it is quite possible that glycemic targets may differ based on the preexisting metabolic status of the patient.

Glycemic Targets and Rate of Correction among Subgroups of Hospitalized Patients

Many observational studies of hyperglycemia in the hospital setting include both patients with diabetes and patients not known to have diabetes. Overall, the findings show that hospital hyperglycemia is associated with adverse outcomes, including mortality (see Chapter 1).[36] If diabetes can be discounted, then hospital hyperglycemia may be designated as stress hyperglycemia.[37] In the critical care setting, randomized trials of strict glycemic control have not produced consistent evidence for benefit among mixed intensive care unit (ICU) populations, but overall these trials have demonstrated increased risk for hypoglycemia. In some but not all reviews or meta-analyses of interventional trials among critically ill patients, a signal suggesting benefit persisted according to subpopulation, with beneficial outcomes most readily observable among surgical patients.

Relationship of Outcomes to Hyperglycemia in the Presence of Diabetes

In some but not all observational studies of patients confirmed to have diabetes, the severity of hyperglycemia at the time of admission or during the course of hospitalization has been found to correlate with adverse outcomes. Among surgical patients, an increased risk of surgical site infection, myocardial infarction, stroke, and death, associated with the presence of diabetes, has been thoroughly reviewed.[38] There have been exceptions to a general observation that severity of chronic hyperglycemia may be associated with adverse surgical outcomes. Among surgical patients with diabetes, however, most studies reporting glucose levels before elective surgery, or preoperative HbA_{1c}, do find a relationship between severity of chronic hyperglycemia and adverse outcomes. Despite the lack of randomized controlled trials that might define any impact of preoperative correction of hyperglycemia, guidelines have been issued suggesting an upper limit of acceptable HbA_{1c} between 8 and 9% before elective procedures.[39] However, there is no true consensus on this point.

Over the years during which health-care-provider protocols for the reduction of perioperative hyperglycemia were increasingly utilized in patients with diabetes having cardiothoracic surgery, a downward trend was noted for adverse outcomes in the population having diabetes (see Chapter 1).[36] During the same time frame, however, other aspects of care also changed. Although studied prospectively, much of the data in the cardiac surgery population with diabetes has been observational, such that a clear causal relationship between attainment of specific glycemic targets and improvement of outcomes cannot be inferred with confidence.

Outside of the ICU, an effective glycemic treatment protocol among surgical patients with diabetes also signaled a benefit. Some of the benefits included reduction of infection, reoperation, and mortality. A randomized trial among general surgical patients with T2D showed improvement of a composite end point of postoperative complications, including wound infection, pneumonia, bacteremia, and respiratory and acute renal failure.[40]

Among noncritically ill admissions with T2D having a cardiac or infection-related diagnosis, a recent retrospective analysis of the impact of glycemic control on hospital outcomes of 378 patients was divided into two groups according to mean point-of-care glucose for evaluation of adverse events, including death during hospitalization, ICU transfer, initiation of enteral or parenteral nutrition, line infection, new in-hospital infection, or infection lasting >20 days of hospitalization, deep venous thrombosis or pulmonary embolism, qualifying rise of creatinine, or readmission. In the group having mean BG <180 mg/dL, there were lower SD of BG and lower admission HbA_{1c}, with overall 1.00 events per patient, compared with 1.46 ($P < 0.0004$) for the group with mean BG ≥180 mg/dL.[41]

Comparison of Stress Hyperglycemia and Diabetes

In studies that classify hyperglycemia according to presence or absence of chart history of diabetes or preadmission antihyperglycemic medication use, some hyperglycemic patients will have diagnosed or undiagnosed diabetes and others will have stress hyperglycemia. A study of burn patients showed greater length of stay for burn victims admitted with diabetes compared with those who had acute hyperglycemia.[42] A meta-analysis of observational and interventional studies between May 2005 and May 2010 involving 12,489,574 critically ill patients, of whom 2,327,178 had diabetes, suggested increased mortality among patients with diabetes and admitted to the surgical ICU, with odds ratio (OR) for ICU mortality (95% confidence interval [CI]) being 1.48 (1.04 to 2.11), in-hospital mortality 1.59 (1.28 to 1.97), and 30-day mortality 1.62 (1.13 to 2.34). Otherwise, in this meta-analysis, the presence of diabetes showed no overall association with mortality.[43] In the general critical care setting, a number of studies have found that diabetes itself is not a predictor of increased mortality.[9,42,44–47] In many studies, hyperglycemia without a history of diabetes has been associated with outcomes worse than those outcomes observed among patients known to have diabetes.[9,38,48–56] In a seminal report, although mean BG on admission of 223 patients with new hyperglycemia did not differ significantly compared with that of 495 patients with known diabetes, higher hospital mortality was observed in the new hyperglycemia group.[48] Details of studies contrasting the impact of diabetes versus stress hyperglycemia upon outcomes are shown in Table 3.2.

Some studies refine the comparison between stress hyperglycemia and diabetes by focusing on given levels of hyperglycemia, which may be associated with harms experienced among patients not having diabetes, and which may be associated with less risk among those known to have diabetes. Among 8,727 cardiac surgery patients, when the adjusted ORs for specific complications were considered at each of three bands of glycemia (good, moderate, or poor control) according to the presence or absence of diabetes, the difference in complication rates between those having or not having diabetes was greatest for those with poor BG control (peak glucose >250 mg/dL in the first 60 h postoperatively), such that the

Table 3.2—Outcomes Associated with Diagnosis of Diabetes, Compared to Stress Hyperglycemia, in Relation to Hyperglycemia

Reference	Study design	Principal hyperglycemia measures	Outcomes of complete cohort, including patients having and not having diabetes	Relation to glycemia, patients not having known diabetes	Relation to glycemia, patients having diabetes
Umpierrez et al.[48]	A single site study was conducted on the relation between hyperglycemia and the presence or absence of known diabetes with in-hospital mortality, length of stay, and disposition at discharge.	Any FBG >125 mg/dL or random BG ≥200 mg/dL on two or more determinations	Among 2030 consecutive admissions, normoglycemia was present in 1,168 patients (62%); new hyperglycemia was present in 223 (12%); and known diabetes was present in 495 (26%). The group with new hyperglycemia had higher hospital mortality at 16%, compared with those with history of diabetes (3%), or those with normoglycemia (1.7%), $P < 0.01$.	BG on admission for 223 patients with new hyperglycemia was 10.5 ± 1 mmol/L, not significantly different from those with known diabetes. Among the 36 deceased patients, admission BG was 10.1 ±1, mean FBG was 9.7 ±0.4, and mean random BG was 10.6 ±0.6. Values are in mmol/L ± SEM.	BG on admission for 495 patients with known diabetes was 12.8 ±1 mmol/L. Among the 15 deceased patients, admission BG was 13 ±2 ($P < 0.01$ vs. new hyperglycemia), FBG was 9.7 ±1.4, and random BG was 14.3 ±1.8 ($P < 0.01$ vs. new hyperglycemia). Values are in mmol/L ± SEM.
Ascione et al.[52]	Single site in-hospital mortality and morbidities were observed among cardiac surgery patients, in relation to diagnosis of diabetes and hyperglycemia.	Peak BG over first 60 postoperative hours; BG control was classified as good (<200 mg/dL), moderate (200–250 mg/dL), or poor (>250 mg/dL)	Control was good in 85.4%, moderate in 10.6%, and poor in 4.2% of 8,727 patients. Hospital mortality rates according to BG control were 131/7,457 (1.8%) for good control ; 38/905 (4.2%) for moderate control; 35/365 (9.6%) for poor control; adjusted odds ratio for poor versus good BG control, 3.90 (95% confidence interval [CI], 2.47–6.15); moderate vs. good BG control, 1.68 (95% CI, 1.25–2.25). In-hospital mortality was not associated with diabetes, with OR (95% CI) being 0.93 (0.53-1.61), P=0.79.	Inadequate BG control was associated with postoperative myocardial infarction, with odds ratio, poor versus good BG control, 2.73 (95% CI, 1.74–4.26) and with pulmonary and renal complications, with odds ratio, poor versus good BG control, 2.27 (95% CI, 1.65–3.12) and 2.82 (95% CI, 1.54–5.14), respectively.	For patients having diabetes, across the three BG control groups the risk of pulmonary and renal complications was similar ($P > 0.07$). No significant interaction between BG control and diabetes was found for myocardial infarction.

Falciglia et al.[54]	Association between hyperglycemia and risk–adjusted mortality was studied retrospectively among critically ill patients with evaluation of subgroups.	Mean glucose for ICU stay, excluding admission glucose, by ranges 70–110, 111–145, 146–199, 200–300, and >300 mg/dL	259,040 admissions had unadjusted hospital mortality rate of 11.2%. Hyperglycemia was independently associated with increased mortality after adjustment for severity of illness ($P < 0.0001$), and the risk of death increased in proportion to blood glucose levels.	The mortality risk from hyperglycemia was greater in those without diabetes ($P < 0.01$). For 180,084 patients not having diabetes, compared with those having mean BG 70–110 mg/dL, the adjusted OR (95% CI) for mortality increased progressively to reach 4.04 (3.44–4.75) for those having mean BG >300 mg/dL.	For 77,850 patients having diabetes, compared with those having mean BG 70–110 mg/dL, the adjusted OR (95% CI) for mortality increased progressively to reach 2.76 (2.38–3.20) for those having mean BG >300 mg/dL.
Frisch et al.[55]	A single site observational study was conducted on the relationship of perioperative hyperglycemia to hospital complications and 30-day mortality after noncardiac surgery.	BG before surgery, BG on day of surgery, average BG after surgery	Among 3,112 patients, there were 72 deaths (2.26%), without significant difference among those having or not having diabetes. Among the 643 patients with diabetes compared with the 2,469 without diabetes, there were higher rates of pneumonia, wound infection, sepsis/bacteremia, urinary tract infection, acute myocardial infarction, and acute renal failure, and length of stay.	There was a positive association between hyperglycemia and mortality for both preoperative and postoperative BG ($P < 0.001$ for both), for patients without a history of diabetes.	There was not a significant association between hyperglycemia and mortality, either for preoperative BG ($P = 0.78$) or for postoperative glucose ($P = 0.51$), for patients with known diabetes.
Krinsley et al.[9]	Retrospectively evaluated mortality data that was prospectively collected for 44,964 patients admitted to 23 ICUs from nine countries.	Mean BG according to bands (80–110, 110–140, 140–180, >180 mg/dL), with hypoglycemia and diabetes status included as variables in the multivariable model	For the combined cohorts, diabetes was independently associated with decreased risk of mortality.	Within the cohort of 32,084 patients not having diabetes, mean BG of 80–140 mg/dL was independently associated with lowest risk of mortality.	Within the cohort of 12,880 patients having diabetes, mean BG 80–110 mg/dL was independently associated with increased mortality and mean BG 110–180 mg/dL with decreased mortality.

continued

Table 3.2—Outcomes Associated with Diagnosis of Diabetes, Compared to Stress Hyperglycemia, in Relation to Hyperglycemia *(continued)*

Reference	Study design	Principal hyperglycemia measures	Outcomes of complete cohort, including patients having and not having diabetes	Relation to glycemia, patients not having known diabetes	Relation to glycemia, patients having diabetes
Kotagal et al.[38]	A statewide cohort having abdominal, vascular, and spine surgery, 2010–2012 (complete cohort), was examined for diagnosis of diabetes, peak perioperative glucose, and adverse events.	Diabetes by history; availability of peak glucose within 48 h after surgery (study cohort); hyperglycemia BG ≥180 mg/dL defining hyperglycemia; composite adverse event metric composed of cardiac and noncardiac events and death	40,836 patients, 47% with perioperative BG available (34.2% with and 65.8% without diabetes), of whom 18% had peak value ≥180 mg/dL; patients having diabetes had higher rate of adverse events than nondiabetes patients (12.0% vs. 8.9%, $P < 0.001$).	80.8% of complete cohort (N = 33,003), of whom 38% had BG performed (N = 12,663), and of whom 6% (N = 756) had peak value >180 mg/dL; compared with having BG ≤125 mg/dL, OR (95% CI) for adverse event in multivariate analysis according to peak BG was 1.26 (10.8–1.47) for BG 125<BG<180, and 1.63 (1.27–2.10) for BG ≥180 mg/dL.	19.2% of complete cohort (N = 7,833), of whom 84% (N = 6,595) had BG performed, and of whom 40% (N = 2,627) had peak value >180 mg/dL; compared with having BG ≤125 mg/dL, OR (95% CI) for adverse event in multivariate analysis according to peak BG was 0.66 (0.49–0.91) for BG 125<BG<180, and 0.78 (0.58–1.04) for BG ≥180 mg/dL.

diabetes group had the lower rate for each type of several complications (see Figure 3.1).[52]

In a case-control single-center ICU study, after implementation of an insulin-based glycemic management protocol for BG >150 mg/dL, the rate of death in the hospital was 10% (95% CI, 9–12%) for patients without diabetes who required glycemic control, higher than the rate of 6% (95% CI, 4–7%) for patients with diabetes, or 5% (95% CI, 4–6%) for controls ($P < 0.001$). Mortality increased for patients without diabetes at mean blood glucose of 144 mg/dL and for patients with diabetes at 200 mg/dL ($P < 0.001$).[49] In another mixed ICU study, when glucose readings were examined by several metrics among 4,946 admissions, the degree of hyperglycemia was found to be associated with mortality among the patients without diabetes but, at similar levels, not among the 728 patients with diabetes. Hyperglycemia showed no significant association with outcome in the patients with diabetes.[53] Under some methods of analysis, hyperglycemia in the presence of diabetes even may seem to confer a "protective" effect when compared with similar degrees of hyperglycemia in the control population.[38,52,55] In a large multicenter international observational study of 44,964 patients admitted to 23 ICUs with 12,880 patients identified as having diabetes, diabetes was associated

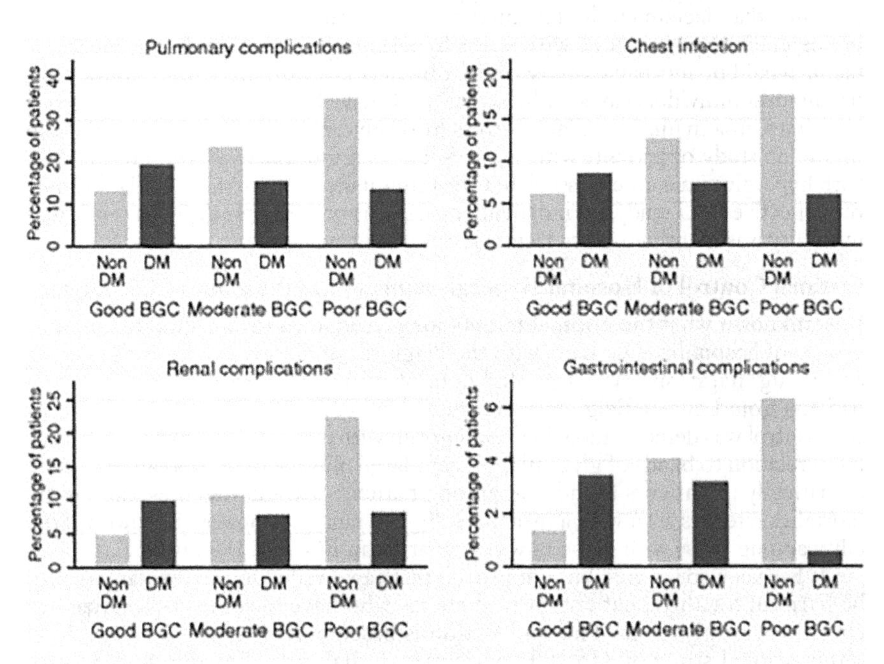

Figure 3.1—Prevalence of complications by blood glucose concentrations and diabetes status.

Source: With permission from Ascione et al.[52]

independently with a slightly lower mortality rate, with OR (95% CI) of 0.93 (0.87–0.97); among patients with mean BG 80–110 mg/dL, diabetes was independently associated with increased risk of mortality, but among patients with mean BG of 110–140 mg/dL, diabetes was independently associated with decreased risk of mortality, leading the authors to speculate that those with antecedent diabetes may have developed a tolerance for hyperglycemia that was lacking among those experiencing stress hyperglycemia.[9]

Of course, such an interpretation that diabetes confers a "protective effect" implies that hyperglycemia as a stress response does itself contribute to adverse outcomes. Another speculation, more relevant on general wards, would be that the beneficial actions of insulin are more likely to be experienced by patients with diabetes, because of greater readiness to introduce insulin therapy.[38,57] Difficulty of interpretation results from the observational design of most studies. There is uncertainty on diagnosis of diabetes in some reports; uncertainty whether stress hyperglycemia in general is simply a marker of severity of illness or other downstream consequence of the illness or its treatment, possibly even beneficial[58]; and, conversely, uncertainty whether stress hyperglycemia at some given level of severity becomes maladaptive, itself contributing to adverse outcomes.

It has been suggested that stress hyperglycemia may be no worse a prognostic indicator than lactate levels. The incremental overall increase of lactate observed in hospitalized populations with stress hyperglycemia is so small that measurements would be incapable of discriminating between normal or stressed physiology in most individual cases. Still, lactate levels have been shown to correlate with outcomes, in a manner similar to stress hyperglycemia.[59–61] An emergency room follow-up study of patients with sepsis found that mortality risk did not increase with hyperglycemia unless associated with simultaneous hyperlactatemia.[60] In one retrospective ICU study, no independent association between hyperglycemia and mortality was identified, once lactate levels were considered.[62]

Optimal Control of Hospital Hyperglycemia in the Presence of Diabetes

It is unknown what the optimal targets for glycemic control should be for subgroups of hospitalized patients with the diagnosis of diabetes along with another admitting diagnosis. When pooled data of critically ill medical and surgical patients from Leuven, Belgium, were studied, no mortality reduction from intensive control was demonstrable in the subgroup with diabetes.[63] Examining mortality in relation to bands of glycemia, a recent large multicenter observational study of critically ill patients found that among patients without diabetes, the lowest mortality rate was seen with a mean BG 80–140 mg/dL, whereas the lowest mortality among those with diabetes was seen at mean BG 110–180 mg/dL.[9]

It has been speculated but not proven that rapid reduction to low targets may be harmful for those patients with diabetes who have become acclimatized to chronic hyperglycemia. The speculation is based partly on a two-center ICU observational study of 415 ICU patient with diabetes, showing that if time-weighted hospital glycemia was in a higher rather than lower range, then patients with diabetes with higher HbA_{1c} (>7%) had a lower mortality rate than those with diabetes with lower HbA_{1c} (≤7%) (see Figure 3.2).[64] For those with HbA_{1c} >7%, among the nonsurvivors, there was a lower time-weighted average BG than among the survivors. At lower HbA_{1c}, the mortality difference according to

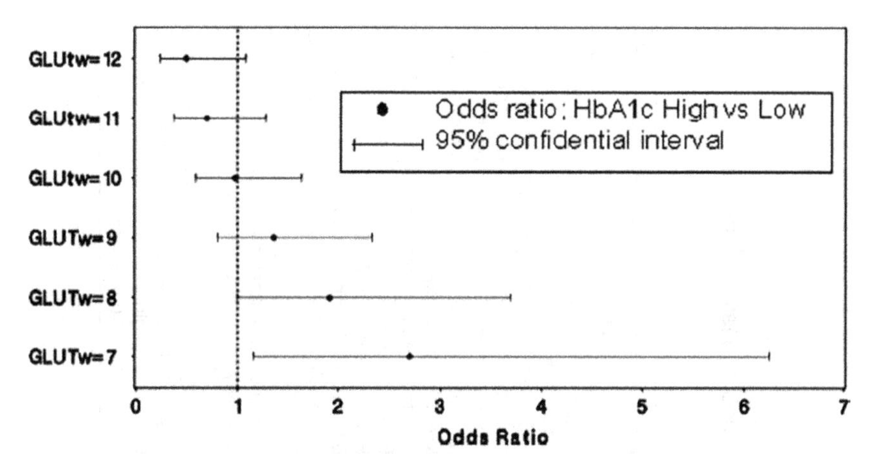

Figure 3.2—Among patients having diabetes and admitted to intensive care units, odds ratios for hospital mortality are shown comparing those with higher (>7%) versus lower (≤7%) HbA_{1c}, according to time-weighted average of blood glucose control in mMol/L.

Source: From Egi et al.[64]

time-weighted average BG was not apparent. The authors speculated that rapid reduction of hyperglycemia, among patients habituated to chronic hyperglycemia, might be acutely harmful. By not capturing the glucose on first admission to compare against the HbA_{1c}, however, the effects of medical stress could have been underestimated.[64]

Among patients with diabetes, it may be necessary to differentiate between those admitted with chronic hyperglycemia and those experiencing acute worsening of hyperglycemia upon admission, whose physiology might more closely resemble that of a person having stress hyperglycemia. The abnormalities of physiology that might cause stress hyperglycemia also may exist in a patient with diabetes. Among patients with diabetes, little published information examines outcomes separately for those with or without exacerbation of preadmission glycemic control, which might be taken as the equivalent of stress hyperglycemia among patients with diabetes.

It must be acknowledged that exacerbation of hyperglycemia in diabetes is not readily definable in a quantitative manner that would permit comparison to stress-induced hyperglycemia among people without diabetes. When HbA_{1c} results are considered, hyperglycemia detected during admission may have the greater adverse prognostic significance among those patients with diabetes who formerly had the more satisfactory control.[64–67] Although the numbers of patients examined so far has been small, a great step forward is taken by those studies that refer to HbA_{1c} to identify acute changes of glycemia, including rapid reduction or stress-induced exacerbation of hyperglycemia among patients with diabetes, and their relationship to outcomes (Table 3.3). In a study of mortality among patients

Table 3.3—Glycemic Gap: Hospital Complications among Patients Confirmed to Have Diabetes, in Relation to Acute Hospital Hyperglycemia

Reference	Design	Outcomes, complete cohort	Relation to change of glycemia, patients having diabetes
Egi et al.[64]	Retrospective observational study was conducted at two sites, 415 diabetes patients with HbA_{1c} admitted to ICU, time-weighted average glucose concentration (TWBG).	Among those having diabetes with evaluable HbA_{1c}, there were 318 survivors and 97 nonsurvivors.	Those with HbA_{1c} ≤7% had TWBG (SD) = 8.8 (1.9) mmol/L, and those with HbA_{1c} >7% had TWBG (SD) = 10.3 (3.0) mmol/L, $P < 0.0001$. The ICU and hospital mortality did not differ by HbA_{1c}. However, the odds ratio for mortality, according to higher vs. lower HbA_{1c} category, showed trend of a progressive decrease according to TWBG from 1.99 (0.93–4.25), $P = 0.07$ at BG = 7 mmol/L to 0.52 (0.27–1.00), $P = 0.05$ at BG 11 mmol/L and to a significant value 0.37 (0.16–0.86), $P = 0.02$ at BG 12 mmol/L.
Hirata et al.[65]	Observational study was conducted of 185 patients having diabetes and pneumonia treated at a community hospital between 2005-2011.	Overall there were 171 survivors and 14 deaths. Among those having diabetes with both evaluable HbA_{1c} and mean glucose data ($N = 151$), there were 140 survivors and 11 deaths.	In multivariable analysis, OR for 30 day mortality by admission glucose (per 1 mg/dL) was 1.00 (0.996–1.01), $P = 0.35$, and OR for 30-day mortality by HbA_{1c} (per 1%) was 1.05 (0.77–1.43), $P = 0.75$. However, OR by mean glucose (per 1 mg/dL) was 1.02 (1.01–1.04), $P = 0.004$.

Liao et al.[66]	Retrospectively, among 329 patients having pyogenic liver abscess, the presence or absence of diabetes and, among those having diabetes, the glycemic gap*, were examined as possible predictors of an adverse outcome.	Among 164 without and 165 with known history of diabetes, there were adverse outcomes among 70 (42.7%) of patients without diabetes and 67 (40.6%) of patient with diabetes, $P = 0.70$.	Among those having diabetes, percentages having adverse outcomes did not differ by HbA_{1c}, being 11/33 (33.3%) with HbA_{1c} ≤7%, 16/39 (41.0%) with 7%<HbA_{1c} ≤9%, and 23/63 (35.9%) with HbA_{1c} ≥9%, $P = 0.78$. Among those having diabetes with both evaluable HbA_{1c} and admission BG ($N = 131$ patients), for glycemic gap <72 mg/dL ($N = 78$) there were 15 (19.2%) having an adverse outcome, and for glycemic gap ≥72 mg/dL ($N = 53$) there were 22 (41.5%) having adverse outcomes, $P = 0.005$.
Plummer et al.[67]	Among 1,000 consecutively admitted critically ill patients, hospital mortality was examined as a function of peak BG in the first 48 h. Unrecognized diabetes was identified by HbA_{1c} ≥6.5%.	220 patients had recognized diabetes and 55 had unrecognized diabetes. When those having diabetes with HbA_{1c} <6% were evaluated together with those not known to have diabetes, the total group of 672 patients showed increased risk of death by 20% (95% CI 1.12, 1.28) for each increase in peak BG of 1 mmol/L ($P < 0.001$). After adjustment for confounders, the association between peak glucose and mortality was no longer significant, and the only variable that indicated an independent association with mortality was APACHE II (OR 1.16, CI 1.13–1.20, $P < 0.001$).	The 129 patients having HbA_{1c} ≥7% showed no relationship between mortality and peak BG ($P = 0.95$). The 199 patients having 6 ≤HbA_{1c} <7% showed an intermediate relationship.

*Glycemic gap = difference between HbA_{1c}-derived estimated average glucose (eAG) and observed plasma glucose measured at initial presentation. See also a discussion of "background hyperglycemia" in relation to acute hospital hyperglycemia.[68]

having known diabetes admitted with pneumonia, the 30-day mortality was not predicted by admission glucose, hypoglycemia during hospitalization, or HbA_{1c}, but rather was predicted by mean glucose during the admission.[65] In an observational study of 329 pyogenic liver abscess patients with diabetes, the HbA_{1c} alone did not predict adverse outcomes. Among 131 patients having available both an HbA_{1c} within 1 week of admission and also an evaluable admission BG, the "glycemic gap" (admission BG minus estimated average BG) was shown to be associated with adverse outcomes. In a receiver operating characteristic (ROC) analysis, a glycemic gap cutoff value of 72 mg/dL was optimal for predicting adverse outcomes.[66] One center has shown that among patients with diabetes, peak glucose predicts adverse ICU outcomes for those having lower HbA_{1c}, but not for those having higher HbA_{1c} (see Figure 3.3).[67] The study of 1,000 critically ill patients showed significantly higher mortality for those having diabetes with HbA_{1c} >7%, but no relationship to peak hyperglycemia. Among the patients with HbA_{1c} <7% and those having stress hyperglycemia, the mortality risk increased according to severity of peak hyperglycemia in the first 48 h. In a multivariable analysis, however, these relationships no longer were seen, and only the Acute Physiology and Chronic Health Evaluation II (Apache II) score was independently associated with mortality.[67] In a search for metrics that might be used to assess the importance of exacerbation of both acute and chronic hyperglycemia, the stress hyperglycemia ratio (SHR) has been defined by one group as the ratio of admission glucose divided by estimated average glucose derived from HbA_{1c}.[68] From a study

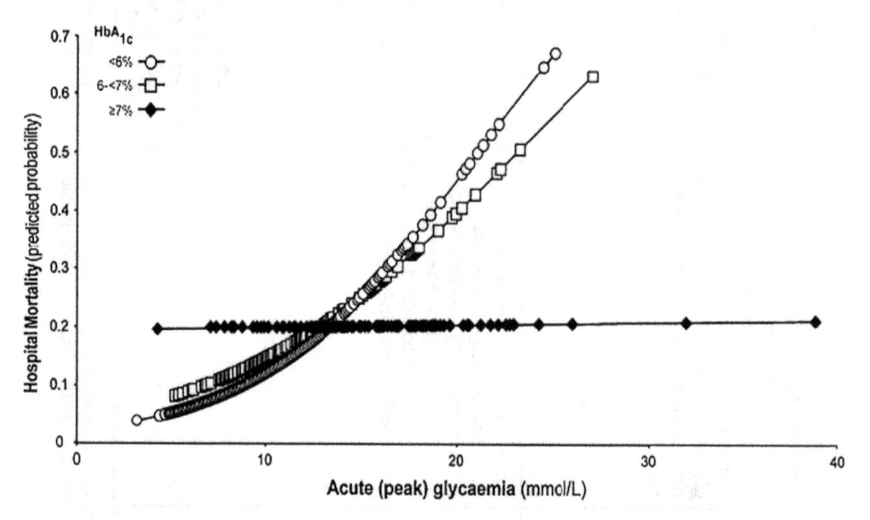

Figure 3.3—Hospital mortality versus acute glycemia according to preadmission HbA_{1c} in critically ill patients. Open circles, no diabetes or stringently controlled (HbA_{1c} <6%); open squares, diabetes (HbA_{1c} 6–<7%); closed diamonds, (HbA_{1c} ≥7%).

Source: From Plummer et al.[67]

population of 4,691 admissions of adult nonobstetric patients, in a multivariable analysis containing glucose, SHR, and other defined variables, higher values for the SHR, but not for glucose, were found to be independently associated with critical illness (either in-hospital death or admission to the ICU). From the finding of a single elevation of admission HbA_{1c}, the authors did not diagnose diabetes but rather identified patients as having background hyperglycemia.[68] None of these studies attempted to infer the likely presence of stress-induced exacerbation of hyperglycemia by the company it might keep, such as increased lactate levels.

Attempts have been made to infer the prevalence of diabetes from sampling of HbA_{1c} upon admission to the hospital.[69] Even in the ambulatory setting, many intercurrent conditions may affect the HbA_{1c}, so as to invalidate its utility in diagnosing diabetes or assessing glycemic control. Factors such as anemia, transfusions, renal disease with or without use of erythropoietin, and other conditions may be even more prevalent among hospitalized patients. Although we believe it is premature to embrace specific targets based on the absence of diabetes or admission HbA_{1c} in the presence of diabetes, it is noted that Marik and Egi have suggested a spectrum of therapeutic targets for each of six categories of ICU patients.[1,70]

The Paradox of the Protective Effect of Diabetes: Fact or Artifact?

When the evidence is considered that diabetes may be a risk factor for some adverse outcomes, but that a given level of hyperglycemia is more strongly associated with harms for patients not having diabetes than for those with diabetes, then a paradox would appear to be presented.[38,71] The paradox arises from comparison of outcomes at comparable bands of hyperglycemia between those hyperglycemic patients with or without diabetes. Kotagal et al. examined possible explanations for the seeming paradox and have suggested that one likely contributing factor, among several suggested explanations, could be that insulin therapy is more consistently and better delivered in patients with a known diagnosis of diabetes and that insulin therapy is less well tolerated when delivered to those not having diabetes.[38,57] Another interpretation acknowledged by Kotagal et al.[38] and others[9,67] deserving consideration here could be that habituation to and tolerance of chronic

Table 3.4

Patient group	Therapeutic blood glucose target, mg/dL
Without diabetes	140–200
With diabetes, HbA_{1c} <7%	140–200
With diabetes, HbA_{1c} ≥7%	160–220
Cardiac surgery, without diabetes	140–180
Cardiac surgery, with diabetes, HbA_{1c} <7%	140–180
Cardiac surgery, with diabetes, HbA_{1c} ≥7%	160–200

hyperglycemia may occur for patients with diabetes, in contrast to intolerance that may be experienced by patients rendered acutely hyperglycemic who formerly did not have diabetes.[47] Another highly plausible possibility could be that a given level of hyperglycemia for a patient not having diabetes may signify greater physiologic stress than for a patient with diabetes. In fact, some of the hyperglycemic group members cataloged as not having diabetes may in fact have had unrecognized diabetes.[38] HbA_{1c}, for example, is often falsely low in patients who have chronic illness and it may be impossible to have an accurate glycemic history for those patients.[72]

In describing the effect of hyperglycemia upon outcomes among patients with diabetes, we are reluctant to accept the terms "paradox" or "protective," because we lack knowledge of the appropriate comparative groups of patients. Those who would advocate more lenient targets for patients who have diabetes with hyperglycemia generally have argued that the hyperglycemia may be protective or that acute reduction may be poorly tolerated. Given that stress hyperglycemia is recognized to have prognostic significance among people who do not have diabetes, it seems desirable to recognize stress-induced exacerbation of hyperglycemia among patients with diabetes. We suggest that outcomes for the following groups be considered separately, not only looking at observational studies but also, using effective technologies, eventually randomizing with the intent to treat to specific targets:

- No diabetes, no stress hyperglycemia
- No diabetes, stress hyperglycemia
- Diabetes, lacking stress-induced exacerbation of hyperglycemia, or lacking physiology of stress hyperglycemia
- Diabetes, having stress-induced exacerbation of chronic hyperglycemia, or having physiology of stress hyperglycemia

Additionally, it is important to recognize other physiologic markers such as lactate elevation and to include adjustment for severity of illness such as the Apache II score in comparative analyses. It is conceivable, although not specifically suggested by the evidence, that some form of "early worsening" could result from overly aggressive correction. Randomized trials would be needed to attempt to discern optimal levels of glycemia in relation to preadmission glycemic control of diabetes, according to comorbidities.

We believe that advances in technology for monitoring and treatment may improve our ability to achieve and maintain specific targets, permitting effective randomization in clinical trials that are designed to test hypotheses related to condition-specific assignment of glycemic targets.[1,73] After further study, if the impression that hyperglycemia should be approached cautiously according to preadmission HbA_{1c} elevations is upheld, then one approach would be that hospitalized patients with uncontrolled diabetes should have higher glycemic targets for the short term than other patients hospitalized with the same conditions. An alternative approach would be that the universal targets, if applicable, should be approached more slowly for patients with uncontrolled diabetes. On the other hand, a strong case can be made that before elective surgery, glycemic control should be optimized safely, in the ambulatory setting.

CONCLUSION

Observational data suggest that glycemic variability may be an independent predictor of adverse hospital outcomes. To confirm a causal relationship between variability and outcomes, interventional trials are required that have the capability of randomizing patients to greater or lesser variability while maintaining similar mean glycemia. Methods for future research and treatment might include improvements in glycemic monitoring and insulin delivery algorithms, as well as non-insulin-based therapeutic interventions, including incretin-based therapies. It is hoped that improvement in therapeutic regulation of glycemic control will be capable of reducing glycemic variability. Importantly, at the present time, providers may have relatively little control over glycemic variability.

In contrast, the actions of providers may determine whether or not patients experience acute correction of chronic hyperglycemia. In the presence of diabetes, chronic hyperglycemia may increase the risk for adverse outcomes, especially for patients considering elective surgery. For some outcomes among critically ill populations, however, the impact of chronic hyperglycemia in the presence of diabetes may be less than the impact of stress hyperglycemia of comparable magnitude among patients without diabetes. Any mechanisms of harms from rapid correction are unknown at this time, but they would not necessarily be limited to harms of the concomitant risk of hypoglycemia. Harms from rapid correction of chronic hyperglycemia are not yet proven to outweigh potential benefits. The balance between harms (if any) and benefits of rapid correction of chronic hyperglycemia are likely to differ according to comorbidities, concomitant therapies, site of care, and the underlying reasons for admission.

We conclude that it is premature to establish specific cautionary guidelines about the correction of chronic hyperglycemia for hospitalized patients with diabetes, but acknowledge evidence suggestive that these guidelines could differ from recommendations for the general population. Analysis will be complex, with due consideration for the importance of glycemic control to concomitant medical conditions, in the presence of diabetes. A take-home message may be that caregivers should "stay tuned" to personalized glycemic targets in the hospital and, for now, should ascertain the HbA_{1c} or indicators of preadmission glycemic control and at least consider the results when individualizing patient care plans.

REFERENCES

1. Krinsley JS. Glycemic control in the critically ill—3 domains and diabetic status means one size does not fit all! *Crit Care* 2013;17(2):131

2. Egi M, Bellomo R, Stachowski E, French CJ, Hart G. Variability of blood glucose concentration and short-term mortality in critically ill patients. *Anesthesiology* 2006;105(2):244–252

3. Krinsley JS. Glycemic variability: a strong independent predictor of mortality in critically ill patients. *Crit Care Med* 2008;36(11):3008–3013

4. Krinsley JS. Glycemic variability and mortality in critically ill patients: the impact of diabetes. *J Diabetes Sci Technol* 2009;3(6):1292–1301

5. Hermanides J, Vriesendorp TM, Bosman RJ, Zandstra DF, Hoekstra JB, DeVries JH. Glucose variability is associated with intensive care unit mortality. *Crit Care Med* 2010;38(3):838–842

6. Mackenzie IM, Whitehouse T, Nightingale PG. The metrics of glycaemic control in critical care. *Intensive Care Med* 2011;37(3):435–443

7. Lipska KJ, Venkitachalam L, Gosch K, Kovatchev B, Van den Berghe G, Meyfroidt G, et al. Glucose variability and mortality in patients hospitalized with acute myocardial infarction. *Circ Cardiovasc Qual Outcomes* 2012;5(4):550–557

8. Meynaar IA, Eslami S, Abu-Hanna A, van der Voort P, de Lange DW, de Keizer N. Blood glucose amplitude variability as predictor for mortality in surgical and medical intensive care unit patients: a multicenter cohort study. *J Crit Care* 2012;27(2):119–124

9. Krinsley JS, Egi M, Kiss A, Devendra AN, Schuetz P, Maurer PM, et al. Diabetic status and the relation of the three domains of glycemic control to mortality in critically ill patients: an international multicenter cohort study. *Crit Care* 2013;17(2):R37

10. Mendez CE, Mok KT, Ata A, Tanenberg RJ, Calles-Escandon J, Umpierrez GE. Increased glycemic variability is independently associated with length of stay and mortality in noncritically ill hospitalized patients. *Diabetes Care* 2013;36(12):4091–4097

11. Farrokhi F, Chandra P, Smiley D, Pasquel FJ, Peng L, Newton CA, et al. Glucose variability is an independent predictor of mortality in hospitalized patients treated with total parenteral nutrition. *Endocr Pract* 2014;20(1): 41–45

12. Braithwaite SS, Umpierrez GE, Chase JG. Multiplicative surrogate standard deviation: a group metric for the glycemic variability of individual hospitalized patients. *J Diabetes Sci Technol* 2013;7(5):1319–1327

13. Braithwaite SS. Glycemic variability in hospitalized patients: choosing metrics while awaiting the evidence. *Curr Diab Rep* 2013;13(1):138–154

14. Rodbard D. Clinical interpretation of indices of quality of glycemic control and glycemic variability. *Postgrad Med* 2011;123(4):107–118

15. Rodbard D. Hypo- and hyperglycemia in relation to the mean, standard deviation, coefficient of variation, and nature of the glucose distribution. *Diabetes Technol Ther* 2012;14(10):868–876

16. Rodbard D. The challenges of measuring glycemic variability. *J Diabetes Sci Technol* 2012;6(3):712–715

17. Kovatchev B, Clarke W. Peculiarities of the continuous glucose monitoring data stream and their impact on developing closed-loop control technology. *J Diabetes Sci Technol* 2008;2(1):158–163

18. Saur NM, Kongable GL, Holewinski S, O'Brien K, Nasraway SA, Jr. Software-guided insulin dosing: tight glycemic control and decreased glycemic derangements in critically ill patients. *Mayo Clin Proc* 2013;88(9):920–929

19. Umpierrez GE, Gianchandani R, Smiley D, Jacobs S, Wesorick DH, Newton C, et al. Safety and efficacy of sitagliptin therapy for the inpatient management of general medicine and surgery patients with type 2 diabetes: a pilot, randomized, controlled study. *Diabetes Care* 2013;36(11):3430–3435

20. Umpierrez GE, Schwartz S. Use of incretin-based therapy in hospitalized patients with hyperglycemia. *Endocr Pract* 2014;20(9):933–944

21. Arnold P, Paxton RA, McNorton K, Szpunar S, Edwin SB. The effect of a hypoglycemia treatment protocol on glycemic variability in critically ill patients. *J Intensive Care Med* 2015;30(3):156–160

22. Barassi A, Umbrello M, Ghilardi F, Damele CA, Massaccesi L, Iapichino G, et al. Evaluation of the performance of a new OptiScanner 5000 system for an intermittent glucose monitoring. *Clin Chim Acta* 2015;438:252–254

23. Schwartz SS, DeFronzo RA, Umpierrez GE. Practical implementation of incretin-based therapy in hospitalized patients with type 2 diabetes. *Postgrad Med* 2015;127(2):251–257

24. Diabetes Control and Complications Trial Research Group (DCCT). The effect of intensive treatment of diabetes on the development and progression of long-term complications in insulin-dependent diabetes mellitus. *N Engl J Med* 1993;329:977–986

25. UK Prospective Diabetes Study (UKPDS) Group. Intensive blood-glucose control with sulphonylureas or insulin compared with conventional treatment and risk of complications in patients with type 2 diabetes (UKPDS 33). *Lancet* 1998;352(9131):837–853

26. Ellenberg M. Diabetic neuropathy precipitating after institution of diabetic control. *Am J Med Sci* 1958;236(4):466–471

27. Oyibo SO, Prasad YD, Jackson NJ, Jude EB, Boulton AJ. The relationship between blood glucose excursions and painful diabetic peripheral neuropathy: a pilot study. *Diabet Med* 2002;19(10):870–873

28. Boulton AJ, Vinik AI, Arezzo JC, Bril V, Feldman EL, Freeman R, et al. Diabetic neuropathies: a statement by the American Diabetes Association. *Diabetes Care* 2005;28(4):956–962

29. Tesfaye S, Chaturvedi N, Eaton SE, Ward JD, Manes C, Ionescu-Tirgoviste C, et al. Vascular risk factors and diabetic neuropathy. *N Engl J Med* 2005;352(4):341–350

30. Gibbons CH, Freeman R. Treatment-induced diabetic neuropathy: a reversible painful autonomic neuropathy. *Ann Neurol* 2010;67(4):534–541

31. Diabetes Control and Complications Trial Research Group (DCCT). Early worsening of diabetic retinopathy in the Diabetes Control and Complications Trial. *Arch Ophthalmol* 1998;116(7):874–886

32. Aiello LP. Diabetic retinopathy and other ocular findings in the diabetes control and complications trial/epidemiology of diabetes interventions and complications study. *Diabetes Care* 2014;37(1):17–23

33. Gerstein HC, Miller ME, Byington RP, Goff DC, Jr., Bigger JT, Buse JB, et al. Effects of intensive glucose lowering in type 2 diabetes. *N Engl J Med* 2008;358(24):2545–2559

34. Riddle MC, Ambrosius WT, Brillon DJ, Buse JB, Byington RP, Cohen RM, et al. Epidemiologic relationships between A1C and all-cause mortality during a median 3.4-year follow-up of glycemic treatment in the ACCORD trial. *Diabetes Care* 2010;33(5):983–990

35. Inzucchi SE, Bergenstal RM, Buse JB, Diamant M, Ferrannini E, Nauck M, et al. Management of hyperglycemia in type 2 diabetes, 2015: a patient-centered approach: update to a position statement of the American Diabetes Association and the European Association for the Study of Diabetes. *Diabetes Care* 2015;38(1):140–149

36. Moghissi E, Inzucchi S. The Evolution of Glycemic Control in the Hospital Setting. In *Managing Diabetes and Hyperglycemia in the Hospital Setting*. Draznin, B, Ed. Alexandria, VA, American Diabetes Association, 2016, p. 1–10

37. Dungan KM, Braithwaite SS, Preiser JC. Stress hyperglycaemia. *Lancet* 2009;373(9677):1798–1807

38. Kotagal M, Symons RG, Hirsch IB, Umpierrez GE, Dellinger EP, Farrokhi ET, et al. Perioperative hyperglycemia and risk of adverse events among patients with and without diabetes. *Ann Surg* 2015;261(1):97–103

39. Dhatariya K, Levy N, Kilvert A, Watson B, Cousins D, Flanagan D, et al. NHS Diabetes guideline for the perioperative management of the adult patient with diabetes. *Diabet Med* 2012;29(4):420–433

40. Umpierrez GE, Smiley D, Jacobs S, Peng L, Temponi A, Mulligan P, et al. Randomized study of basal-bolus insulin therapy in the inpatient management of patients with type 2 diabetes undergoing general surgery (RABBIT 2 surgery). *Diabetes Care* 2011;34(2):256–261

41. Draznin B, Wang Y, Seggelke S, Hawkins RM, Gibbs J, Bridenstine M, et al. Glycemic control and outcomes of hospitalization in noncritically ill patients with type 2 diabetes admitted with cardiac problems or infections. *Endocr Pract* 2014;20(12):1303–1308

42. Murphy CV, Coffey R, Wisler J, Miller SF. The relationship between acute and chronic hyperglycemia and outcomes in burn injury. *J Burn Care Res* 2013;34(1):109–114

43. Siegelaar SE, Hickmann M, Hoekstra JB, Holleman F, DeVries JH. The effect of diabetes on mortality in critically ill patients: a systematic review and meta-analysis. *Crit Care* 2011;15(5):R205

44. Esper AM, Moss M, Martin GS. The effect of diabetes mellitus on organ dysfunction with sepsis: an epidemiological study. *Crit Care* 2009;13(1):R18

45. Stegenga ME, Vincent JL, Vail GM, Xie J, Haney DJ, Williams MD, et al. Diabetes does not alter mortality or hemostatic and inflammatory responses in patients with severe sepsis. *Crit Care Med* 2010;38(2):539–545

46. Vincent JL, Preiser JC, Sprung CL, Moreno R, Sakr Y. Insulin-treated diabetes is not associated with increased mortality in critically ill patients. *Crit Care* 2010;14(1):R12

47. Schlussel AT, Holt DB, Crawley EA, Lustik MB, Wade CE, Uyehara CF. Effect of diabetes mellitus on outcomes of hyperglycemia in a mixed medical surgical intensive care unit. *J Diabetes Sci Technol* 2011;5(3):731–740

48. Umpierrez GE, Isaacs SD, Bazargan N, You X, Thaler LM, Kitabchi AE. Hyperglycemia: an independent marker of in-hospital mortality in patients with undiagnosed diabetes. *J Clin Endocrinol Metab* 2002;87(3):978–982

49. Rady MY, Johnson DJ, Patel BM, Larson JS, Helmers RA. Influence of individual characteristics on outcome of glycemic control in intensive care unit patients with or without diabetes mellitus. *Mayo Clin Proc* 2005;80(12):1558–1567

50. Whitcomb BW, Pradhan EK, Pittas AG, Roghmann MC, Perencevich EN. Impact of admission hyperglycemia on hospital mortality in various intensive care unit populations. *Crit Care Med* 2005;33(12):2772–2777

51. Krinsley JS. Glycemic control, diabetic status, and mortality in a heterogeneous population of critically ill patients before and during the era of intensive glycemic management: six and one-half years experience at a university-affiliated community hospital. *Semin Thorac Cardiovasc Surg* 2006;18(4):317–325

52. Ascione R, Rogers CA, Rajakaruna C, Angelini GD. Inadequate blood glucose control is associated with in-hospital mortality and morbidity in diabetic and nondiabetic patients undergoing cardiac surgery. *Circulation* 2008;118(2):113–123

53. Egi M, Bellomo R, Stachowski E, French CJ, Hart GK, Hegarty C, et al. Blood glucose concentration and outcome of critical illness: the impact of diabetes. *Crit Care Med* 2008;36(8):2249–2255

54. Falciglia M, Freyberg RW, Almenoff PL, D'Alessio DA, Render ML. Hyperglycemia-related mortality in critically ill patients varies with admission diagnosis. *Crit Care Med* 2009;37(12):3001–3009

55. Frisch A, Chandra P, Smiley D, Peng L, Rizzo M, Gatcliffe C, et al. Prevalence and clinical outcome of hyperglycemia in the perioperative period in noncardiac surgery. *Diabetes Care* 2010;33(8):1783–1788

56. Abdelmalak BB, Knittel J, Abdelmalak JB, Dalton JE, Christiansen E, Foss J, et al. Preoperative blood glucose concentrations and postoperative outcomes after elective non-cardiac surgery: an observational study. *Br J Anaesth* 2014;112(1):79–88

57. Kwon S, Thompson R, Dellinger P, Yanez D, Farrohki E, Flum D. Importance of perioperative glycemic control in general surgery: a report from the

Surgical Care and Outcomes Assessment Program. *Ann Surg* 2013;257(1): 8–14

58. Marik PE, Bellomo R. Stress hyperglycemia: an essential survival response! *Crit Care* 2013;17(2):305

59. Revelly JP, Tappy L, Martinez A, Bollmann M, Cayeux MC, Berger MM, et al. Lactate and glucose metabolism in severe sepsis and cardiogenic shock. *Crit Care Med* 2005;33(10):2235–2240

60. Green JP, Berger T, Garg N, Horeczko T, Suarez A, Radeos MS, et al. Hyperlactatemia affects the association of hyperglycemia with mortality in nondiabetic adults with sepsis. *Acad Emerg Med* 2012;19(11):1268–1275

61. van Beest PA, Brander L, Jansen SP, Rommes JH, Kuiper MA, Spronk PE. Cumulative lactate and hospital mortality in ICU patients. *Ann Intensive Care* 2013;3(1):6

62. Kaukonen KM, Bailey M, Egi M, Orford N, Glassford NJ, Marik PE, et al. Stress hyperlactatemia modifies the relationship between stress hyperglycemia and outcome: a retrospective observational study. *Crit Care Med* 2014;42(6):1379–1385

63. Van den Berghe G, Wilmer A, Milants I, Wouters PJ, Bouckaert B, Bruyninckx F, et al. Intensive insulin therapy in mixed medical/surgical intensive care units: benefit versus harm. *Diabetes* 2006;55(11):3151–3159

64. Egi M, Bellomo R, Stachowski E, French CJ, Hart GK, Taori G, et al. The interaction of chronic and acute glycemia with mortality in critically ill patients with diabetes. *Crit Care Med* 2011;39(1):105–111

65. Hirata Y, Tomioka H, Sekiya R, Yamashita S, Kaneda T, Kida Y, et al. Association of hyperglycemia on admission and during hospitalization with mortality in diabetic patients admitted for pneumonia. *Intern Med* 2013; 52(21):2431–2438

66. Liao WI, Sheu WH, Chang WC, Hsu CW, Chen YL, Tsai SH. An elevated gap between admission and A1C-derived average glucose levels is associated with adverse outcomes in diabetic patients with pyogenic liver abscess. *PLoS One* 2013;8(5):e64476

67. Plummer MP, Bellomo R, Cousins CE, Annink CE, Sundararajan K, Reddi BA, et al. Dysglycaemia in the critically ill and the interaction of chronic and acute glycaemia with mortality. *Intensive Care Med* 2014;40(7):973–980

68. Roberts GW, Quinn SJ, Valentine N, Alhawassi T, O'Dea H, Stranks SN, et al. Relative hyperglycemia, a marker of critical illness: introducing the stress hyperglycemia ratio. *J Clin Endocrinol Metab* 2015:jc20152660

69. Carpenter DL, Gregg SR, Xu K, Buchman TG, Coopersmith CM. Prevalence and impact of unknown diabetes in the ICU. *Crit Care Med* 2015;43(12):e541–e550

70. Marik PE, Egi M. Treatment thresholds for hyperglycemia in critically ill patients with and without diabetes. *Intensive Care Med* 2014;40(7):1049–1051

71. Krinsley JS, Fisher M. The diabetes paradox: diabetes is not independently associated with mortality in critically ill patients. *Hosp Pract (1995)* 2012;40(2):31–35

72. Rubinow KB, Hirsch IB. Reexamining metrics for glucose control. *JAMA* 2011;305(11):1132–1133

73. Devi R, Zohra T, Howard BS, Braithwaite SS. Target attainment through algorithm design during intravenous insulin infusion. *Diabetes Technol Ther* 2014;16(4):208–218

Chapter 4

Insulin Errors in the Inpatient Setting

Richard Hellman, MD, FACP, FACE[1]

INTRODUCTION

Insulin therapy is the best and most powerful tool at our disposal for the control of glucose levels in the inpatient setting, but errors in providing this crucial therapy not only diminish the effectiveness of this therapy, but also, in some cases, cause in-hospital morbidity and even mortality. It is for this reason that the Joint Commission on Hospital Accreditations (JCOHA) considers insulin one of the five "high-alert" medicines that are most commonly associated with serious injury or death.[1] Numerous studies have shown that errors in insulin therapy are a frequent cause of excessive morbidity and mortality.[2] In one study, in the inpatient setting, one-third of the deaths of patients with diabetes resulting from a catastrophic error were due to errors in insulin therapy.[3]

This chapter offers explanations for why errors in insulin therapy occur, discusses the types of errors, and provides a practical guide to strategies that have been shown to be useful to both reduce the frequency of errors and prevent injuries resulting from errors related to insulin therapy in the inpatient setting.

The chapter looks at the problems from three different, but overlapping, perspectives. The first perspective takes a systemic approach—looking at the dominant role that organizational and systems issues play in the development and continuation of higher rates of errors in insulin therapy. The second perspective follows the individual providers of health care, the physicians and nurses and other key hospital personnel, and pays special attention to a relatively underdiscussed but crucial aspect: diagnostic errors and their role in injurious errors in insulin therapy. The third perspective examines the prevention of specific types of errors, looking at the type of medication errors in insulin therapy described in a recent publication by the American Society of Health-System Pharmacists (ASHP).[4] The chapter concludes with a list of proposals to reduce the frequency of errors in insulin therapy and to reduce risk of any morbidity and mortality from such errors.

[1]Clinical Professor of Medicine, University of Missouri-Kansas City School of Medicine; Medical Director, Heart of America Diabetes Research Foundation, North Kansas City, MO.

DOI: 10.2337/9781580406086.04

BACKGROUND

Despite overwhelming evidence of the need to reduce significant hyperglycemia and avoid hypoglycemia during the routine use of insulin in hospitals,[5,6] glycemic control remains suboptimal in many inpatient settings. In some cases, as a result of errors in insulin therapy, glycemic control deteriorates during a hospital stay. For example, in 2007, the Centers for Medicare and Medicaid Services (CMS) reported data on so-called never events related to glycemic control, that is, disorders of glycemic control that should never have their onset in a hospital. They identified three such events: hospital-acquired diabetic ketoacidosis (DKA), hyperosmolar hyperglycemic syndrome (HHS), and severe hypoglycemia. They reported that during a one-year period there were 15,848 documented such events. Of these, 72.4% were episodes of DKA that began during an inpatient stay, 20.5% were significant cases of HHS, and 7.1% were cases of severe hypoglycemia resulting in coma. In 2008, CMS announced it would not pay for hospital stays in which those never events occurred. Yet, some data from several states show that these never events in glycemic management are still occurring in U.S. hospitals at a rate of close to half of the 2007 rates.[7]

Few experts in hospital medicine were surprised that the threat of nonpayment by CMS did not have a greater effect on reducing the frequency of these so-called never events. Hospitals are extraordinarily complex structures, and the complexity of care needed for patients who need improvement of their glycemic control often stresses the systems of care present in the hospitals and reveals their shortcomings.[8] Changes in the present hospital systems of care will be needed if we are to make in-hospital care safe for the patient with diabetes.

SYSTEMIC ISSUES IN THE DEVELOPMENT OF ERRORS IN INSULIN THERAPY

To understand why some of the errors occur so often and why it is so hard to prevent them, it is important to look at systemic issues that play an important role in the development and persistence of errors in insulin therapy over time. It may seem counterintuitive, but some decisions made far from the bedside, often termed the "blunt end of care," have a profound effect on the chance that errors will occur. The shortage of nursing personnel is one such example. Errors involving nurses at the point of care, also termed the "sharp end of care,"[9] are more likely to occur when shortages in nurses result in the individual nurse being overworked,[10] and spending too little time focusing on the many crucial tasks involved in accurate use of insulin therapy. These include (1) assessing whether the order for insulin is reasonable and appropriate for the patient at that point in time; (2) checking to ensure that the appropriate insulin dose of the correct type of insulin is administered to the right patient by the right route at the right time; and (3) verifying that the patient's blood glucose and clinical status are being monitored sufficiently so the effect of the insulin can be measured and, if needed, the therapy can be altered. The support staff responsible for glucose monitoring also need to have an appropriate workload and training to provide reliable and timely glucose testing. In addition, it is important for all care providers to listen to the patient's perspective and to use that information to ensure that the care being given is patient centered, effective, efficient, equitable, timely, and safe.

ELECTRONIC HEALTH RECORDS

Many hospitals are moving from the traditional paper-based hospital charts to fully operative electronic health records (EHR). This key system change has many benefits, including the ability to share information more rapidly and widely among members of the health-care teams.[11] As a systems tool, EHRs have great potential. The clarity and lack of ambiguity of data sources, particularly physician and nursing notes and orders, reduces the chance for medical errors.[12] If properly designed, the EHR can provide decision support and forcing functions that may reduce certain types of errors of insulin therapy. But flaws in any electronic record can introduce other errors—for example, if the screen routinely accessed by the providers does not contain crucial information needed at the time they are ordering insulin therapy, or when the decision support tools are judged to be unhelpful or burdensome and, as a result, are routinely bypassed by the user of the EHR.

Computerized Physician Order Entry (CPOE) systems are extremely important[12] and have great value in the care of the patient with diabetes, particularly when the algorithms used for specific insulin orders can be reduced to a validated, evidence-based order set and provided to the user of the CPOE system. Examples of these widely used types of order sets are shown in Table 4.1.

The more often a validated and complete set of tasks can be put into an order set that is available to the physician and hospital staff, preferably in a CPOE set but alternatively in a paper-based order set, the easier it is to administer therapy with fewer errors, to monitor the quality of the work that has been done, and to identify opportunities for improvement. It would be a mistake to believe that a set of often-complex orders for insulin therapy will improve care by itself. The process of introducing it and teaching health-care providers and staff how and when it should be used is key. Subsequent proficiency testing is central to the success of any new CPOE, particularly in the case of insulin therapy, in which the effects of a momentary slip or omission in an order sequence can result in harm to the patient.

Table 4.1—Examples of Order Sets Widely Used in CPOE Systems

- Intravenous (IV) insulin infusion
- Subcutaneous (SQ) basal-bolus insulin
- Hypoglycemia recognition and treatment
- Treatment of diabetic ketoacidosis
- Treatment of hyperosmolar hyperglycemic syndromes
- Discharge insulin therapy
- Transition from IV to SQ insulin therapy
- Insulin therapy for patients on IV hyperalimentation
- Insulin therapy for patients on high-dose corticosteroids
- Insulin when there is an interruption of nutritional therapy (IV or oral)
- Consideration of patient self-use of SQ insulin pumps in the hospital setting
- Criteria for continuing or discontinuing patient self-use of their insulin pumps.

CULTURE OF SAFETY

Many experts in the area of patient safety believe that sponsoring a culture of safety is important for nearly any institution involved in patient care, and mandatory for a high-alert therapy, such as insulin therapy. A culture of safety is created when a collection of individuals decide that they will work together in a collaborative way to eliminate injurious errors and to promote patient safety.[8] A culture of safety in hospitals is much more effective when the hospital leadership is strongly supportive. The group engaged in the culture of safety should develop a nonhierarchical approach, which includes checking not only their own work, but also that of others. Back-up checks should be routine. The entire group must focus on and measure their performance and use nonpunitive methods to improve performance. A successful team strives to work in collaboration and to develop a sense of both collective and individual mindfulness.[13] Organizations that adopt such a philosophy are typically ones that value education and quality improvement, including constant measurement of relevant metrics, examination of their own performance, and continued collaboration to reduce the errors in care.[4,14–16] Human error is part of the human condition and is to be expected, but injury to patients can and should be prevented.

Both the patient and their family as well as other key supportive figures should be included in the culture of safety. In the inpatient setting, an engaged patient and family can be an important set of observers of the patient's clinical status, and a highly motivated group of helpers to prevent errors in insulin therapy.

EDUCATION

Education is often overshadowed by the acute medical need and not a priority in the inpatient setting. From a systems perspective, however, education is an important tool in the prevention of insulin errors.[17,18] For example, recent data show that the faculty caring for patients in academic centers may not be up to speed when queried about their knowledge of basic principles of modern management of insulin in the inpatient setting.[19,20] Several organizations have developed excellent tools to educate health-care providers and patient care teams involved in the care of patients with diabetes regarding necessary information to deliver appropriate insulin therapy, reduce insulin errors, and provide quality care.

There is a misconception that the most important aspect of education is the content of the education. Although content is crucial, data suggest that attention to the preferred style of learning of the health-care providers can greatly increase retention and understanding of the insulin safety principles.[21] Flexibility of the education style and format may pay great dividends in patient education as well.

The education should be first targeted at the areas of highest frequency of errors, such as choosing the appropriate types, dosing, and route of insulin therapy; administering the insulin safely and accurately; and timely and accurate monitoring of the glucose levels. Other targets should include the development of the health-care provider's understanding of how insulin therapy affects the patient's clinical outcomes and how the clinical status of the patient in turn affects the decisions for their insulin therapy.

SCOPE OF EDUCATION OF HOSPITAL STAFF

All staff involved in the care of the patient with diabetes require education and training in the tasks needed to safely use insulin therapy. Too often, the as-needed (or per diem nurse, PRN) nursing staff and the evening or night shifts receive little training and education. A common cause of inpatient hypoglycemia is when insulin is given before a meal, but the patient is then transported to another part of the hospital and unable to eat the planned meal, resulting in hypoglycemia. Ideally, the hospital will have a comprehensive, in-depth resource and training available for the entire hospital staff, but this is a labor-intensive project, which so far has been done by only a few.[16,22] The use of diabetes teams throughout the hospital is a useful tool,[15,16] as is the development of preferred areas for more complex glycemic control. The use of online resources, especially for education modules or for reference, is also useful.

GLUCOSE MONITORING

In the hospital setting, glucose monitoring is sometimes done by the central hospital laboratory, but the majority of the glucose monitoring is done with the use of point-of-care (POC) glucose monitors. A few centers are using POC blood-gas analyzers to measure glucose in critical care units, and a small but slowly growing number of centers are using continuous glucose monitoring systems (CGMS) in specific settings.[23–25] At present, most inpatient centers rely heavily on POC glucose monitors for the vast majority of their glucose measurements, in large part because of the ease of use and timeliness. It should be remembered, however, that the central hospital laboratory method is highly accurate and relatively free of interfering substances, and should always be used when a POC glucose level needs confirmation or when the accuracy of the POC meter is in question.

From a systems perspective (see Figure 4.1), several key aspects of POC glucose monitoring should be evaluated constantly:

1. The choice of a POC glucose monitoring system;
2. The frequency of validation of the glucose strips and the monitors;
3. The robustness of the staff education programs and proficiency testing; and
4. The degree to which glucometrics are used to improve in-hospital glycemic control and to reduce errors in insulin therapy.

These systemic issues are key because a significantly inaccurate glucose level may lead to relatively large insulin dosing errors. Additionally, the vulnerability of the particular POC glucose meter may make it unsafe in selected circumstances, and no POC glucose meter should be used without a clear understanding of its limitations and when it is unsafe to use that meter to monitor glucose levels.

GLUCOSE MONITORING ERRORS

When insulin is to be administered, the glucose level at that time point is important data needed to select the correct dose and the optimal route of administration, and

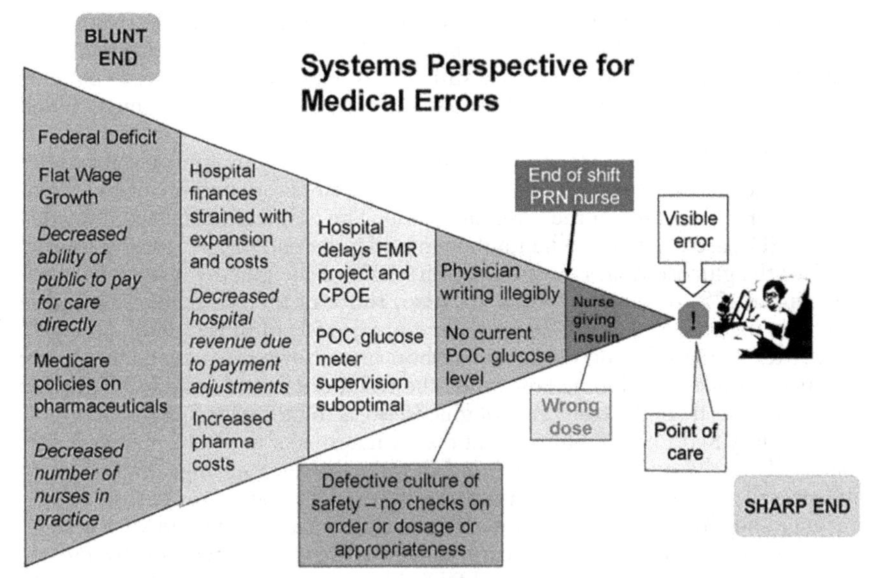

Figure 4.1—Systems perspective for medical errors.

an important safety check to avoid iatrogenic hypoglycemia. Other factors that should be considered to avoid hypoglycemia include the clinical context of the patient and the factors that can be expected to influence insulin resistance of the patient and the expected effect of the dose of insulin. The patient's vulnerability to hypoglycemia also needs to be considered. For example, an 80-year-old patient with chronic renal failure and hypoglycemic unawareness will be extremely vulnerable to fasting hypoglycemia.[26] This patient requires careful and conservative insulin dosing and frequent glucose monitoring. To do otherwise would be an error. Likewise, if a patient receives intravenous (IV) insulin, but the frequency of glucose monitoring is every 6 h, the infrequent monitoring is an error, because the change in glucose levels after IV insulin can be rapid. In this case, the probability of harm increases greatly when the glucose measurements are too far apart.

Often the health-care team uncritically assumes that the monitoring method is accurate. In 2009, the U.S. Food and Drug Administration (FDA) reported the death of 13 patients with diabetes on peritoneal dialysis who were being monitored with a widely used glucose meter that followed a glucose dehydrogenase method, using a pyrrolo-quinoline quinone (PQQ) coenzyme to measure glucose concentrations. This method is less sensitive to ambient oxygen levels and some other interfering substances and will falsely measure maltose as glucose. Because patients who receive icodextrin in their peritoneal infusate will slowly metabolize the icodextrin to maltose, this process can lead to high maltose levels in the patient's blood up to 2 weeks after the last peritoneal dialysate. In each of the cases reported by the FDA, the health-care providers used a POC glucose meter of the PQQ type, resulting in an erroneously measured and markedly elevated POC glucose, which was used to order inappropriately large doses of insulin and resulted in severe hypoglycemia, coma, seizures, and ultimately death. Despite the 2009 FDA report, however, a recently published report indicates patients in some hospitals and outpatient centers are still using meters of this type with patients who either are or recently have been on peritoneal dialysis with similar lethal outcomes.

The FDA, in response to strong concerns presented by multiple organizations and individuals, most recently tightened the standards for accuracy of POC glucose meters being used in the hospital setting. The new standards recommended by the FDA are expected to be implemented by the end of 2015, and state that 99% of the glucose values must be within ±10% of the glucose levels ≥70 mg/L and within ±7% of values <70 mg/dL. Also, 100% of the values must be within ±20% of the glucose levels ≥70mg/dL or within ±15% of those values <70mg/L. The latter standard is crucial, as other authors have shown the potential for severe errors in clinical decision making when the result obtained by the POC glucose meter is so far from the true value of glucose so as to be misleading.[27]

Recently Scott et al.[28] pointed out the weaknesses of the POC meters in use, especially in the operating room[29] and in intensive care settings. Variations in hematocrit, blood pH, oxygen saturation, fever, dehydration, or ketosis all had varying and sometimes significant effects on the results obtained with a POC glucose meter,[30] and in critical care, most POC glucose meters were clearly inferior in accuracy to the results obtained by intra-arterial samples tested for glucose levels on POC blood-gas analyzers. Arterial samples are used in preference to fingerstick glucose samples in patients who have circulatory compromise, and the capillary values of glucose may diverge significantly from the arterial values when acidosis or circulatory collapse alters the capillary blood flow.

Errors in monitoring may be due to sampling errors when the site from which the blood sample is obtained does not accurately represent the true blood glucose value. In the operating room, severe hypoglycemia has resulted when the anesthesiologist did not realize the arterial line that they were sampling from was being flushed with 5% glucose solution.[31] As a result, insulin was given in error to a hypoglycemic patient. Similar errors can occur when the line from which the specimen is being drawn has "dead space" and that line cannot be flushed adequately, diluting the sample and giving an erroneous result.[31]

Each hospital must be aware of the strengths and the weaknesses of the POC meters used in their institution. POC meters that use a glucose-oxidase method will tend to give falsely elevated glucose values when the patient is hypoxic, and lower glucose levels when high levels of acetaminophen are present. Glucose-dehydrogenase meters will give more accurate levels in the presence of hypoxia, but falsely lower results in the presence of dopamine infusions and falsely higher glucose levels when higher levels of acetaminophen are present.

In addition, the storing and the care of the glucose monitoring strips are crucial. If the bottle containing the strips is left open, the strips may deteriorate rapidly. If the strips are stored at a temperature ≥39.2°C, the strips may give falsely low blood glucose values, and when the strips are stored <20°C, the strips may give falsely high values. Strips also may be destroyed by extremes in temperature or humidity.

Some of the strips hospitals now use do not have good corrections for hematocrit levels. This is particularly crucial in intensive care and operating room suites, where wide variations of hematocrit are common. Falsely elevated glucose levels in POC meters when patients are anemic occur and most meters do not have a specific method to deal with hematocrit variation. Cembrowski, a NICE-SUGAR investigator,[32] found that some of the batches of his POC glucose meter strips did not correct for hematocrit variations as claimed by the manufacturer. He concluded that the error due to the faulty strips may have misled his team and caused the diagnosis of hypoglycemia to be either delayed or missed entirely.[32]

In addition, proper training of staff on the proper technique of performing POC glucose monitoring is crucial. Too often, POC glucose monitoring is done in hospitals by the most poorly trained and poorly supervised staff. The resultant errors can be quite large. For example, if a person fails to clean the finger properly before obtaining a glucose sample, the result may be as much as 35% or more above the true glucose level, while failure to adequately dry the finger can dilute the sample and give a falsely low value that may be as much as 25% below the true glucose level. Such large deviations from the true blood glucose may cause an outlier that can mislead the prescribing health-care provider.[33]

GLUCOMETRICS

Evidence-based metrics can be used to evaluate not only the harmful errors but also noninjurious errors and latent errors. A latent error occurs when a deviation from optimal care occurs that, although not directly causing harm, increases the probability that an important error will occur later. Some latent errors include systemic issues that create recurrent vulnerability of the health-care system, such as excessively high patient-to-nurse ratios, a situation in which the nurses have more to do than they can safely perform. Another common example of a latent error is leaving a vial of U-500 amid a number of U-100 vials. This can be reliably expected to increase the risk of vial confusion, potentially resulting in an overdose of insulin. Another example of a latent error that is a systemic error at the so-called blunt end of care is allowing inadequate lighting in an area of the hospital where staff must read labels on vials, syringes, and infusion sets.

Both latent errors and noninjurious errors are important to identify and correct, as these ultimately may lead to patient injury. It is imperative to educate the caregivers and to give them feedback, if we are to reduce the total number of errors. Moreover, because injurious errors usually involve multiple errors, often by multiple caregivers, the chain of undetected errors and the sequence of errors may result in an injurious error. Medicine is a high-risk endeavor and errors are frequent. Although most errors are corrected by the person who made them, multiple errors often include some that escape detection and cause harm. As an example, the development of DKA de novo in a hospital setting, still a far-too-common event, usually involves multiple people and multiple errors of omission and may result in an injurious or even lethal event.

DIAGNOSTIC ERRORS

No discussion of errors in insulin therapy is complete without discussing the role of the individual and the human factor in errors in insulin therapy. Although defective systems may create potential for "error traps" or situations in which different individuals make the same error, the role of the individual at the POC is key to understanding how to prevent injurious errors.

Humans frequently make errors and, when candid, most people will admit that they frequently have slips and lapses that, for the most part, they correct themselves. Not only do people have different cognitive abilities, but most people have two distinct mental processes active at any time, often termed by cognitive psychologists as type 1 and type 2 thinking.[34] Type 1 is intuitive, rapid, and almost automatic, relying upon a vast warehouse of experience and knowledge. Many people use this method of thinking much of the time because of its ease and speed. Examples of this type of thinking include what we do when driving a car or when a jazz musician is playing with their fellow musicians. This type of thinking, however, although blindingly fast and intuitive, is still error prone, subject to cognitive biases, and not at all quantitative. Type 2 thinking, by contrast, is slow, deliberative, and analytic. This form of thinking is more likely to be useful in quantitating risk, but may be just as prone to some cognitive biases as type 1 thinking. We would prefer our accountant to use type 2 thinking. But when it comes to the formulation of a medical diagnosis, particularly when the diagnostician feels confident or is working quickly, pattern recognition, which is usually a function of type 1 mental processes, is the predominant pattern. Although the experienced diagnostician may be correct, the pattern of thinking they most often use is particularly prone to overconfidence and a premature closing of the possibility that the diagnosis may either be incorrect or incomplete.

In a seminal study of the causes and frequency of diagnostic errors, Graber et al.[35] looked at 100 cases of diagnostic error. These resulted in 90 injuries and 33 deaths. Of the 100 cases, seven were due to no-fault errors alone. Of the remaining 93 cases, many had system-related factors (63%) and cognitive errors. The system-related factors were most often organizational problems (94.3%). Only 5.6% of the system-related factors were the result of technical and equipment problems.

In 74 cases of diagnostic errors resulting from faulty cognition, cognitive factors were noted 320 times (4.3/case). The most common problems were faulty synthesis (82.8%) or faulty data gathering (14.6%). Surprisingly, inadequate knowledge or skill accounted for only 3.4% of the diagnostic errors resulting from faulty cognition. Put another way, it wasn't common that the errors occurred because of a lack of knowledge, but rather because of how the clinician collected and put together the data to formulate a diagnosis.

Certain cognitive and system-related factors co-occur commonly, such as an inadequate history leading to misinterpretation of lab results. In general, faulty information gathering greatly increased the risk that there would be a faulty synthesis of data and premature closure, as for example, "it can only be this." Faulty data gathering was identified in 45 instances by Graber et al.,[35] but they identified inadequate or faulty knowledge or skills least often, in only 11 cases overall in the study. The researchers also identified failure to consult an expert as a significant cause of diagnostic error (15 cases), as well as failure to periodically review the situation (10 cases) or failure to gather other important information to verify the diagnosis.

Medical diagnostic errors are common when the presentation of the patient is atypical, as for example if a young woman appears in the emergency room with right lower quadrant pain that in actuality is due to undiagnosed DKA and not appendicitis. If therapy for DKA is delayed or even not done, the results may be catastrophic. It is likely that many of the so-called never events noted by CMS were due to diagnostic errors early in the development of DKA, HHS, or severe hypoglycemia.

Another not uncommon example of a diagnostic error that may occur is in the elderly patient with diabetes with HHS. The patient may present with focal signs of limb weakness that mimic a cerebro-vascular accident (CVA), but the real diagnosis is severe HHS, and if care is delayed the risk for mortality is very high.

The routine checking of other providers' work and conclusions in real-time is crucial in preventing such diagnostic errors. It is always useful for the diagnostician to ask whether there is some other explanation for what they see than the diagnosis they have decided on. It is also useful to provide feedback to all members of the diabetes care team. Often the feedback of relevant data will allow people to revise their initial impression and protect the patient from serious errors in insulin therapy.

It is surprising that rule-based errors are often difficult to correct. The presence of a rule that is easy to use, but incorrect, often generates resistance to change. Probably the best known example is sliding-scale insulin (SSI). It is an example of a simple, clear rule of giving insulin that is "strong, but wrong." Because of the simplicity of such rules, there is often resistance to discontinue using these, even when people know that the rule does not work well. Ideally, SSI as monotherapy should not be allowed to be part of a computerized insulin order set, and basal-bolus insulin orders promoted as the alternative.

TYPES OF INSULIN ERRORS

In 2013, the ASHP convened a panel of experts to focus on the goal of enhancing the safety of insulin use in hospitals. They began by grouping the types of errors in insulin therapy into six categories: prescribing, transcribing, dispensing, storage, administering, and monitoring. Their nomenclature is a useful place to begin.[4]

PRESCRIBING ERRORS

These errors are among the most common and the most important. Among the common examples is when the prescriber chooses an incorrect dosage or a method of insulin dosing that is irrational, as for example, SSI as monotherapy. More variables should affect the choice of insulin dosage than just the immediate glucose result. SSI monotherapy is both a rule-based error and also a knowledge-based error, because it indicates both an illogical belief and a lack of understanding of insulin therapy. The evidence shows that it is an inferior method of prescribing insulin at best, and at worst, it has resulted in severe morbidity and even mortality when prescribed to a patient with DKA or HHS.

During insulin prescribing in hospitals, the prescriber needs to provide for both basal and bolus insulin requirements, the bolus doses used to balance nutritional intake, and correction doses when the glucose is outside of the optimal glycemic range. The basal needs may be highly variable, affected by the underlying comorbid conditions and by concurrent medications, which may increase or decrease insulin resistance, or by other mechanisms increasing the risk for hyper- or hypoglycemia. Some examples are shown in Tables 4.2 and 4.3.

The nutritional needs of the patient need to be coordinated with a coherent plan for insulin therapy, and the prescription for insulin therapy must reflect the current nutritional therapy and route, as well as provide for a change in insulin therapy if nutritional intake is reduced or stopped. Different methods of nutrition require different types of insulin, and sometimes different routes. For example, basal insulin dosing twice daily may be optimal for enteral feedings, but IV insulin is best when oral intake is uncertain and the expected insulin requirements may decrease rapidly. Orders for varying contingencies, such as what to do if oral intake is suddenly interrupted, will reduce errors.

Table 4.2—Comorbid Conditions

Increasing hyperglycemia risk	Increasing hypoglycemia risk
Infections	Weight loss
Myocardial infarction	Renal failure
Metabolic acidosis	Advanced age
Severe pain or anxiety	Adrenal insufficiency
Pregnancy	Liver failure
Surgery	Heart failure
Acute asthma	Alcoholism

Table 4.3—Medications

Increasing hyperglycemia risk	Increasing hypoglycemia risk
Corticosteroids	β-blockers
β-agonists	Incretins (when used with insulin, sulfonylureas)
Protease inhibitors	Sulfonylureas
Sirolimus	Haloperidol
L-asparagine	Pentamidine
Atypical antipsychotics	Tramadol

Poor communication between the prescribing and treating health-care providers can result in an error of inadequate insulin dosage. For example, if a pulmonary intensivist adds β-agonists and corticosteroids for the respiratory needs of the patient, but the prescriber of insulin is unaware that the consultant, in effect, has increased the insulin resistance, the prescriber will choose inadequate insulin doses that will result in severe hyperglycemia.

The route of insulin administration is a key consideration. A patient with shock and hypotension or severe dehydration may be highly likely to have delayed and erratic absorption from subcutaneous (SQ) sites. An IV approach for insulin therapy would be much more effective. Alternately, in another scenario, the rapidity of the change in insulin resistance may be so fast that only an IV use of insulin therapy will be able to match the rapidity of the change in insulin needs.

The type of medical record, either paper-based or electronic, may affect the type and frequency of prescription errors. In paper-based hospital records, the errors may occur when prescribers write down what they believe to be the correct insulin type, but instead list an incorrect type of insulin because the insulin they chose had a similar sounding, but incorrect, type (short-acting versus long, or vice-versa). This kind of error is often termed an intentional error. In contrast, an example of a so-called unintentional error is a misspelling or error in the prescriber's penmanship, which makes the result ambiguous in appearance. The most common error is using a "U" to depict units, which, if not written clearly, may be read as a zero. Another common error is to have a trailing zero after a decimal point, as for example, an IV insulin rate of 1.0 units/h, which, if the decimal point is not easily visible, may be seen as 10 units/h. Other examples of prescribing errors occur when the orders are verbal and may not be clearly understood by the transcriber, who is not familiar with the plan. These common errors can be reduced with the use of evidence-based order sets, preferably in an EHR.

TRANSCRIBING ERRORS

Transcription errors, while much more common when paper charts are used or a verbal order is transcribed, also may occur whenever there is a transition of care and a new set of orders is used. In many hospitals, a reconciliation of medication is done on a transfer from one care unit to another, and a new set of orders for insulin is generated. The person who performs the reconciliation is the one who may cause a transcription error and it is particularly common upon discharge in cases in which new orders are generated for post-hospital care. As an example, in one recent study, 18% of all patients who were discharged after an acute myocardial infarction (MI) did not receive their medications to control blood glucose levels upon discharge.[36] Sixty-seven percent of the time, one of the omitted medications was insulin.[36] Their retrospective review confirmed that 81% of the time, the omission of the medication for glycemic control upon discharge was the result of medical error. The frequency of readmission postdischarge is directly related to such errors upon discharge. The "hand-offs" in care transitions are among the events at highest risk for errors.

DISPENSING ERRORS

Dispensing insulin can be a complex process and can vary widely from one institution to another. The trend, correctly so, is to have the hospital pharmacy solely responsible for the labeling, storage, and dispensing of the insulin to the nurse who is to administer the dose, whether it be IV or SQ. The pharmacist usually has the responsibility of being sure that the correct insulin dose is in the IV solution that is to be administered, and in the single dose pen or syringe that is to be sent to the floor, but the accuracy of the dispensing process is not guaranteed. As with all aspects of the processes of care, it is helpful to keep metrics on the performance in the pharmacy regarding errors of all types and to provide timely feedback so workflows can be changed to improve performance.

STORAGE ERRORS

Storage of insulin is an issue in the hospital setting and can be the source of serious errors. There are many types of these errors. Some hospitals, for example, may use U-500 insulin as well as the standard concentration, U-100 insulin, and may store the U-500 insulin vials in the clinical area, at the nurses' station, for the convenience of the staff. This error type can be remedied by storing U-500 insulin in the hospital pharmacy and dispensing it only with bar-code labeling that is specific for a patient on the clinical unit. Some insulin pens and vials, however, may be stored on the unit in a secure drawer, for the individual patient. The use of double-checks and bar coding of all insulin-containing pens or vials or syringes is highly recommended to reduce risk of patient injury.

ADMINISTERING ERRORS

After prescribing and transcribing errors, the administration of insulin is perhaps the next most frequent type of error, and it is certainly the one that is most visible. Unfortunately, in many hospitals, the important function of administering the dose of insulin is not done without frequent errors. A recent review of insulin therapy error data from the British National Patient Safety Agency showed the high frequency in which patients received a wrong dose, strength, or frequency of insulin.[2] They also found that insulin doses were commonly omitted or the wrong insulin product was used.

Prefilled insulin IV containers and insulin syringes prepared by the pharmacy may reduce the burden somewhat, but there are many potential sources of error. The nurse needs to double-check to ensure that the ordered insulin dosage is correct. In addition to checking the insulin type, route, and dose, time may have elapsed since the order was given, and understanding whether the order for this dose of insulin is still appropriate for the patient is important. Communication between nurses and physicians is essential to the safety of insulin administration. In many discussions on errors of insulin therapy, the role of the nurse in catching errors or potential errors made by others is overlooked, but in one study, 86% of the errors that were avoided were found by the nurses.[37]

New technologies may present special challenges as well. Although insulin pens have been widely used in hospital settings, the accuracy of pen delivery depends on the use of proper technique.[38] For example, some pens will not deliver the full dose of insulin unless the needle is held in place for 6 sec after administering the dose. If the pen is removed before 6 sec has elapsed, the full dose is not injected into the site. Likewise, although needle guards are designed to prevent needle-stick injuries, when unfamiliar with the type of insulin pen, nurses not infrequently suffer needle-stick injuries despite these guards.

Smart IV pumps are IV infusion pumps designed not to allow infusion errors by prohibiting rates of infusion outside of what the pump memory has programmed to be the limits of safe infusion for that individual drug. They are a technological advance and have been shown to reduce some types of errors, but even these smart pumps may present complexities for the health-care provider unfamiliar with their proper function and errors may result.

GLUCOSE MONITORING ERRORS

The ASHP recommendations regarding glucose monitoring emphasize the training of those who perform the glucose monitoring and the establishment of minimum frequencies of glucose monitoring: no less than every 4–6 h if a patient is on insulin but as often as hourly with insulin infusions. These recommendations focus on the need to document and communicate the results of glucose monitoring to the clinical team and to provide both critical values on an urgent basis and alerts to notify appropriate caregivers when there is an increased risk for hypoglycemia. The ASHP also emphasizes the need to verify POC glucose values when a critical result is noted. They also recommend the need for observation of the patient if self-monitoring is allowed. These are all sound recommendations.[39]

RECOMMENDATIONS FOR CHANGE

SYSTEMIC RECOMMENDATIONS

- Establish a culture of safety with specific attention to assuring patient safety throughout insulin therapy. The need for timely and effective communication, coordination, and teamwork is key. The environment should promote a nonpunitive learning environment.
- A multidisciplinary management team should be formed and given authority to manage or comanage critical clinical problems or emergencies in glycemic control. They should have an ability to provide education and consultation for hospital staff, health-care providers, and patients as resources allow, and to advise the hospital administrator on suggested improvements in glycemic control.
- The hospital administrator should seek input from the glucose management team and other relevant people or groups regarding the need for additional staffing or training or other resources relevant to improving diabetes care and reducing errors in insulin administration. The hospital administrator should strongly support a culture of safety at the institution and focus care staff on clinical goals, not on nonclinical goals.

- The ASHP professional practice recommendations for the safe use of insulin in hospitals should be incorporated into the hospital's policies and procedures. Double checks should be the norm for each of the steps in insulin therapy.
- An EHR with capabilities of CPOE should be instituted hospital-wide and all parts of the hospital should use either the same system or one that communicates transparently with the main EHR. Decision support tools and forcing functions, if carefully validated, may be used to improve safety of insulin therapy.
- Hospital-wide insulin order sets should be made available for each of the clinical situations in which errors in insulin use may occur.
- Processes of care for each step in the provision of insulin therapy, from prescription to administration and monitoring, should be written unambiguously in preprinted, approved, evidence-based orders and should be reviewed at least annually to ensure that they are being used correctly and remain valid.
- The quality of POC glucose monitoring should be a high priority. The POC glucose meter performance should be tested at regular intervals under the direction of the hospital clinical laboratory. All users of the POC glucose monitors should receive thorough education and must regularly pass proficiency testing. POC meters or strips that do not meet the new FDA standards for POC meters used in clinical units should be replaced.
- The hospital should provide guidelines delineating the strengths and weaknesses of the POC meters, and only POC meters that can demonstrate accuracy at the new FDA standard should be allowed in operating rooms or intensive care units. The hospital should consider whether a POC blood-gas analyzer using arterial blood samples for more optimal POC glucose measurement should be made available for use in critical care areas.
- Metrics for glycemic control should be obtained on a periodic, regular basis, and feedback should be provided to the clinical care areas. Benchmarking to national standards should be performed and a continuous quality improvement strategy followed. When problem areas emerge, nonpunitive steps to remedy the problem should be provided.
- Extensive education programs that provide a general understanding of diabetes care standards in the inpatient setting and specific staff responsibilities should be provided. Proficiency standards should be established. Health-care providers and staff should be tested initially and annually to ensure continued proficiency. Education programs should be tailored to the learning styles and strengths of the intended audience.
- All never-events should be given a root-cause analysis and efforts to educate and correct the errors should be undertaken.
- Encourage education of all staff, including ancillary staff such as transportation staff, on safety in insulin therapy.
- Educate nurses on the new technologies they will be responsible for, particularly POC glucose monitoring systems, smart pumps, and other new technologies used in the care of the patient with diabetes.

- Perform studies on a regular basis to ensure that the interventions to improve insulin safety are working as expected. Use objective metrics such as test scores and timely feedback of near misses and errors to obtain a more complete assessment of what is actually taking place in the hospital.
- Checklists should be developed for each provider or specialized care unit so the key steps in their tasks in insulin therapy can be clearly noted and always performed in the correct sequence.

RECOMMENDATIONS TO REDUCE THE FREQUENCY OF DIAGNOSTIC ERRORS

- Utilize system-related factors to decrease diagnostic errors, as for example, to provide timely feedback on diagnostic studies that are needed to verify a diagnosis, both radiologic, laboratory, and other consultant-generated studies.
- Educate clinicians as to common pitfalls of clinical reasoning and provide back-up checks on their own diagnoses and real-time team discussions of the patient's clinical status.
- Encourage clinicians to consider whether their initial diagnoses are correct or whether new information will alter their initial judgment. Premature closure is the most common cognitive error that leads to faulty diagnoses.
- Provide timely consultative expertise to the responsible provider of the diabetes care.
- Encourage the use of diagnostic simulations and case studies to provide training and education and review to improve diagnostic accuracy.
- Transitions of care must be done with the highest level of mindfulness because of the high error rates, particularly with insulin therapy.
- Errors that cause injury should be studied in depth to learn where processes of care and education need to be modified.
- Encourage feedback from patients and families regarding insulin therapy and errors, and incorporate that data in reports.

CONCLUSION

This chapter discussed different types of errors in insulin therapy and provided examples of each category. Unfortunately, prescribing errors, transcribing errors, dispensing errors, storage errors, administration errors, and monitoring errors are still far too common. The systemic causes of error are most important, because many of the remedies that can be done at this level are much more likely to have the largest impact on making insulin therapy safer. It is also important to look at the performance of individuals involved in the care of the patient receiving the insulin therapy, if we are to create an environment that will always protect the patient from harm and also reduce the number of noninjurious and latent errors. Cognitive psychology helps us better understand the different ways in which our cognitive processes make us vulnerable to error and to help us avoid our own diagnostic errors—the kinds of errors most difficult for the individual to discover and most likely to cause an injurious error. One of the strengths of a culture-of-safety approach is the constant back-up checks and feedback provided to the clinicians, which greatly reduces the risk that a diagnostic error will go undetected. Involvement of the patient and their family in their care is crucial in reducing insulin errors. A culture of safety should strive to always include an informed patient and their family as a central aspect of a team approach in the provision of insulin therapy in the inpatient setting.

Human factors are important to consider in the effort to reduce errors in insulin therapy. Even a highly skilled and knowledgeable provider of care may make a serious error if their sequence of steps during clinical care is interrupted, and these errors often are not noticed when rushed. Yet, along with a propensity for cognitive errors, humans have remarkable cognitive flexibility. A successful culture of safety must include back-up checks to discover these human errors and use the cognitive flexibility of the team members to create an environment that has patient safety as the highest priority.

Finally, the best institutions will need to consider the danger of burdening the clinical team with nonclinical priorities. The more the clinical team is rewarded primarily for nonclinical priorities, the harder the task becomes for making insulin therapy safe for every patient.

REFERENCES

1. "High-alert" medications and patient safety (Patient safety alert). *Int J Qual Health Care* 2001;13(4):339–340

2. Cousins D, Rosario C, Scarpello J. Insulin, hospitals and harm: a review of patient safety incidents reported to the National Patient Safety Agency. *Clin Med* 2011;11(1):28-30

3. Hellman R. A systems approach to reducing errors in insulin therapy in the inpatient setting. *Endocr Pract* 2004;10(Suppl. 2):100–108

4. Cobaugh DJ, Maynard G, Cooper L, Kienle PC, Vigersky R, Childers D, Weber R, Carson SL, Mabrey ME, Roderman N, Blum F, Burkholder R, Dortch M, Grunberger G, Hays D, Henderson R, Ketz J, Lemke T, Varma SK, Cohen M. Enhancing insulin-use safety in hospitals: practical recommendations from a ASHP Foundation expert consensus panel. *Am J Health-Syst Pharm* 2013;70:e18–27

5. Umpierrez GE, Hellman R, Korytkowski MT, Kosiborod M, Maynard GA, Montor VM, Seley JJ, Van den Berghe G. Management of hyperglycemia in hospitalized patients in non-critical care setting: an Endocrine Society clinical practice guideline. *J Clin Endocrinol Metab* 2012;97:16–38

6. Moghissi ES, Korytkowski MT, DiNardo M, Einhorn D, Hellman R, Hirsch IB, Inzucchi SE, Ismail-Beigi F, Kirkman MS, Umpierrez GE. American Association of Clinical Endocrinologists and American Diabetes Association consensus statement on inpatient glycemic control. *Diabetes Care* 2009;32: 1119–1131

7. Healy D, Cromwell J. Hospital-acquired conditions–present on admission: examination of spillover effects and unintended consequences. Final Report. RTI International CMS Contract No: HHSM-500-2005-00029I, September 2012, Accessed Jan 2016. https://www.cms.gov/Medicare/Medicare-Fee-for-Service-Payment/HospitalAcqCond/index.html?redirect=/hospitalacqcond/06_hospital-acquired_conditions.asp

8. Kohn LT, Corrigan JM, Donaldson MS (Eds.); Committee on Quality of Health Care in America, Institute of Medicine. *To Err Is Human: Building a Safer Health System.* Washington, DC, National Academies Press, 2000

9. Reason J. *Human Error.* Cambridge, UK, Cambridge University Press, 1990

10. Hughes RG (Ed.). Nurses at the "sharp end" of patient care. In *Patient Safety and Quality: An Evidence-Based Handbook for Nurses.* Rockville, MD, Agency for Healthcare Research and Quality, 2008, chap. 2

11. Hellman R. Patient safety and inpatient glycemic control: translating concepts into action. *Endocr Pract* 2006;12(Suppl. 3):49–55

12. Bates D, Clark NG, Cook RI, Garber JR, Hellman R, Jellinger PS, Kukora JS, Petak SM, Reason JT, Tourtelot JB. American College of Endocrinology and American Association of Clinical Endocrinologists position statement on patient safety and medical system errors in diabetes and endocrinology. *Endocr Pract* 2005;11(3):197–202

13. Bogner, MS. *Human Error in Medicine.* Hillsdale, NJ, Erlbaum, 1994

14. Korytkowski M, DiNardo M, Donihi AC, Bigi L, DeVita M. Evolution of a diabetes inpatient safety committee. *Endocr Pract* 2006;12(Suppl. 3):91–99

15. Maynard G, Kulaza K, Ramos P, Childers D, Clay B, Sebasky M, Fink E, Field A, Renvall M, Juang PS, Choe C, Pearson D, Serences B, Lohnes S. Impact of a hypoglycemia reduction bundle and a systems approach to inpatient glycemic management. *Endocr Pract* 2014;Dec 22:1–34 [Epub ahead of print]

16. Draznin B, Gilden J, Golden S, Inzucchi SE, for the PRIDE investigators. Pathways to quality inpatient management of hyperglycemia and diabetes: a call to action. *Diabetes Care* 2013;36:1807–1814

17. Dungan K, Lyons S, Manu K, Kulkarni M, Ebrahim K, Grantier C, Harris C, Black D, Schuster D. An individualized inpatient diabetes education and hospital transition program for poorly controlled hospitalized patients with diabetes. *Endocr Pract* 2014;20(12):1265–1273

18. Hellman R. An individualized inpatient diabetes education and hospital transition program for poorly controlled hospitalized patients with diabetes. *Endocr Pract* 2014;20(10):1097–1099

19. Pichardo-Lowden AR, Kong L, Haidet PM. Knowledge, attitudes and decision-making in hospital glycemic management: are faculty up to speed? *Endocr Pract* 2015;21(4):307–322. doi:10.4158/EP14246.OR

20. Hellman R, Draznin B. Do we need to broaden the scope of inpatient diabetes education to include our faculty? *Endocr Pract* 2015;21(4):448–449

21. Goldman E, Shah K, Greenberg L, Cogen FR. A pediatric resident diabetes curriculum targeting different learning styles. *Diabetes Spectr* 2012;25(1):45–48

22. Maynard G, Schnipper JL, Messler J, Ramos P, Kulasa K, Nolan A, Rogers K. Design and implementation of a web-based reporting and benchmarking center for inpatient geriatrics. *J Diabetes Sci Technol* 2014;8(4):630–640

23. Schuster KM, Barre K, Inzucchi SE, Udelsman R, Davis KA. Continuous glucose monitoring in the surgical intensive care unit: concordance with capillary glucose. *J Trauma Acute Care Surg* 2014;76(3):798–803

24. Joseph J, Torjman MC, Strasma PJ. Vascular glucose sensor symposium: continuous glucose monitoring systems (CGMS) for hospitalized and ambulatory patients at risk for hyperglycemia, hypoglycemia, and glycemic variability. *J Diabetes Sci Technol* 2015;9(4):725–738

25. Poljakova I, Elsikove E, Chlup R, Kalabus S, Hasala P, Zapletalova J. Glucose sensing module—is it time to integrate it into real-time perioperative monitoring? An observational pilot study with subcutaneous sensors. *BiomedPap Med Fac Univ Palacky Olomouc Czech Repub* 2013;157:1–12

26. Maynard G, O'Malley CW, Kirsh SR. Perioperative care of the geriatric patient with diabetes or hyperglycemia. *Clin Geriatr Med* 2008;24:649–665

27. Blood glucose monitoring test systems for prescription point-of-care use. Draft guidance for industry and Food and Drug Administration Staff. Washington, DC, US Department of Health and Human Services, Food and Drug Administration, Center for Devices and Radiological Health, Office of In Vitro Diagnostic Device Evaluation and Radiological Health, Division of Chemistry and Toxicology Devices, 2014

28. Scott MG, Bruns DE, Boyd JC, Sacks DB. Tight glucose control in the intensive care unit: are glucose meters up to the task? *Clin Chem* 2009;55:18–20

29. Rice MJ, Pitkin AD, Coursin DB. Glucose measurement in the operating room: more complicated than it seems. *Anesth Analg* 2010;110:1056–1065

30. Dungan K, Chapman J, Braithwaite SS, Buse J. Glucose measurements: confounding issues in setting targets for inpatient management. *Diabetes Care* 2007;30:403–409

31. Woodcock TE, Cook TM, Gupta KJ, Hartle A, for the Association of Anaesthetists of Great Britain and Ireland. Guidelines: arterial line blood sampling: preventing hypoglycaemic brain injury 2014. *Anaethesia* 2014;69:380–385

32. Cembrowski GS, Tran DV, Slater-Maclean L, Chin D, Gibney RTN, Jacka M. Could susceptibility to low hematocrit interference have compromised the results of the NICE-SUGAR trial? *Clin Chem* 2010;56:1193–1195

33. Hellman R. Interfering factors in quality of glucose management: technological advances in the treatment of type 1 diabetes. In *Frontiers in Diabetes.* Vol. 24. Bruttomesso D, Grassi G, Eds. Basel, Karger, 2015, p. 63–80

34. Kahneman, Daniel. *Thinking, fast and slow.* New York, Farrar, Straus and Giroux, 2011

35. Graber ML, Franklin N, Gordon R. Diagnostic error in internal medicine. *Arch Intern Med* 2005;165:1493–1499
36. Lovig KO, Horwitz L, Lipska K, Kosiborod M, Krumholz HM, Inzucchi SE. Discontinuation of antihyperglycemic therapy after AMI: medical necessity or medical error? *Jt Comm J Qual Patient Saf* 2012;38(9):403-407
37. Leape LL, Berwick DM, Bates DW. What practices will most improve safety? Evidence-based medicine meets patient safety. *JAMA*. 2002;288(4): 501–507
38. Davis EM, Foral PA, Dull RB, Smith AN. Review of insulin therapy and pen use in hospitalized patients. *Hosp Pharm* 2013;48(5):396–405
39. American Society of Health-System Pharmacists and the Hospital and Health System Association of Pennsylvania. Professional practice recommendations for safe use of insulin in hospitals. 2004. Accessed Jan 2016. https://www.google.com/url?sa=t&rct=j&q=&esrc=s&source=web&cd=7&cad=rja&uact=8&ved=0ahUKEwjflK2dgZHKAhUDPT4KHXXBDXgQFghCMAY&url=http%3A%2F%2Fpicsolution.ir%2Fwp-content%2Fuploads%2F2013%2F04%2FSafe-Use-of-Insulin-in-Hospitals.pdf&usg=AFQjCNE-cZolHpD6raqQDrAo41FqYe0imA&sig2=Hzy6i_LcN5fo4naGLOcTPg&bvm=bv.110151844,d.cWw

Chapter 5

Food, Fasting, Insulin, and Glycemic Control in the Hospital

Mary Korytkowski, MD,[1] Boris Draznin, MD, PhD,[2] and Andjela Drincic, MD[3]

INTRODUCTION

Diabetes treatment in the hospital poses unique challenges that differ from those encountered in the outpatient setting.[1–5] These challenges arise from patient factors that include illness-related variability in insulin sensitivity, as well as system factors related to inconsistency in hospital procedures for insulin dosing and meal delivery, complicating the ability to achieve and maintain desired glycemic goals.[3–7] Despite the demonstrated superiority of scheduled insulin therapy over sliding-scale insulin (SSI) regimens, the latter persists as a fallback strategy for many providers who may be unfamiliar or uncomfortable with basal-plus or basal-bolus insulin (BBI) regimens.[8–13]

A major challenge to insulin use in the hospital is related to variability in food intake and carbohydrate exposure, with associated concerns for hypoglycemia when patients are not eating regular meals.[14–16] Appropriate timing of prandial insulin administration can be complicated by lack of coordination in the timing of food tray delivery with point-of-care (POC) measures of capillary blood glucose (BG) and insulin administration, tasks that are performed by personnel from different departments in the hospital setting. Some patients are unable to ingest prescribed calories because of lack of appetite or dislike of hospital meals. Other patients may skip meals and instead consume snacks and meals brought to the hospital by friends or family members without informing nursing personnel of the need for prandial insulin.[14]

One of the most frequently encountered scenarios in the care of individuals with diabetes treated with noninsulin or insulin therapy in the hospital is what to do during periods of fasting or inability to take oral nutrition.[3,4,15] Scheduled periods of fasting for diagnostic testing or surgical procedures are frequent occurrences in the inpatient setting. Although there is a general awareness of the need for continuation of some form of glucose-lowering therapy during periods of fasting in patients with diabetes, there is uncertainty about how to modify therapy in a way that prevents both hyperglycemia and hypoglycemia.[7,15,17] Many patients are admitted through same-day surgery units for short outpatient procedures as well

[1]Division of Endocrinology and Metabolism, University of Pittsburgh, Pittsburgh, PA. [2]Division of Endocrinology, Diabetes, and Metabolism, University of Colorado School of Medicine, Aurora, CO. [3]Division of Diabetes, Endocrinology and Metabolism, Medical Director, The Nebraska Medical Center Diabetes Center, Omaha, NE.

DOI: 10.2337/9781580406086.05

as complicated prolonged procedures that require postoperative hospitalization. Therefore, recommendations for adjustments to a glycemic management regimen often begin at home.[15]

This chapter will review an approach to adjustments in noninsulin and insulin therapies during periods of fasting and will address the issue of timing of insulin therapy with meals. This section starts with a patient case followed by a discussion of how to modify BBI therapy during a 2-day period of consumption of only clear liquids before a planned surgical procedure. For purposes of this discussion, NPO (*nil per os*: nothing by mouth) will be used whenever a patient is placed in a fasted state.

ISSUES TO CONSIDER WHEN WRITING CONSULT NOTES AND MAKING RECOMMENDATIONS

Patient Case

A 64-year-old woman with insulin-treated type 2 diabetes (T2D) is admitted to the hospital for aortic valve replacement. She will be receiving only clear liquids for 2 days before the procedure and will remain NPO after midnight before the procedure. Her admission weight is 76 kg (167 lbs). Her HbA1c 1 month before admission was 8.7%. Her home insulin regimen consists of detemir insulin 40 units at 8 P.M. with fixed doses of 14 units of insulin aspart prior to each meal. She reports home fasting glucose levels of 130–150 mg/dL with daytime values that range between 120 and 260 mg/dL. You are asked to make recommendations regarding her insulin regimen.

INSULIN MODIFICATIONS FOR PATIENTS ON CLEAR LIQUID DIETS

Clear liquid diets include the use of fruit juices, sodas (lemon-lime soda and ginger ale), gelatin, popsicles, and broth. Many of these foods are caloric beverages with high sugar content that require doses of nutritional insulin to maintain glycemic control (Table 5.1).

Similar to insulin glargine, detemir is a basal insulin, ideally covering insulin needs in the absence of any food intake.[18,19] In the majority of instances, there is no need to reduce the dose of the basal insulin for a clear liquid diet. The patient in this case was on fixed doses of premeal insulin with wide variability in her glycemic control at home, likely representing variability in her caloric consumption at home.

To determine a premeal insulin dose for a clear liquid diet, calculate the prandial insulin dose according to planned carbohydrate intake (Table 5.1).[16,20] For example, 4 ounces of apple juice or lemon-lime soda contains ~15 g of carbohydrate. The ratio of insulin-to-carbohydrate intake (insulin-to-carbohydrate ratio [ICR]) could be based on the total daily dose (TDD) of basal insulin using one of several published formulas. Of these, the following formulas are the easiest to use:[21]

$$400/\text{TDD basal insulin} \quad (5.1)$$

$$2.8 \times \text{weight (lb)}/\text{TDD basal insulin} \quad (5.2)$$

Table 5.1—Caloric Content of Selected Clear Liquid Beverages/Foods*

	Volume	Grams of carbohydrate
Lemon-lime soda	12 ounces	39
Ginger ale	12 ounces	32
Apple juice	8 ounces	29
Beef or chicken broth	8 ounces	1
Lemon gelatin	1 serving	19

*Caloric and carbohydrate content can vary according to brand.

Although these formulas have been accepted and used in many clinical trials, other authors have proposed dosing formulas that call for higher mealtime insulin delivery.[20,22–26] Caution is advised in using any formula because of differences in patient populations (type 1 diabetes [T1D] vs. type 2 diabetes [T2D]) and insulin delivery devices (subcutaneous injections vs. insulin pumps) used in these prior studies, with some including lean patients with T1D using insulin pump therapy.[26]

For the patient in this case, consumption of 12 ounces of ginger ale (32 g), 1 cup of gelatin (19 g), and 1 popsicle (17 g) at a meal provides a total carbohydrate intake of 68 g (Table 5.1). Using the first formula (i.e., 400/TDD detemir), her prandial insulin dose would be based on an ICR of 1 unit for each 10 g of carbohydrate or 7 units of insulin aspart. Using the second formula (2.8 × 167 lbs/TDD detemir), her ICR would be 1 unit for each 12 g of carbohydrate or 6 units of aspart. Both methods provide a dose of aspart that is roughly equivalent to what would be achieved by reducing the current dose of 14 units by 50%. Correction insulin can be used to provide additional aspart insulin for premeal blood glucose above the desired range, with the majority of correction scales beginning at blood glucose levels >140 mg/dL.[20,27]

Another option for this patient would be to use a basal-plus-insulin regimen.[28,29] This option continues her current dose of detemir insulin once daily in combination with correction insulin before meals. In one study, this type of regimen was found to have a similar efficacy to BBI in hospitalized patients with T2D.[29] Correction insulin can be calculated using a formula of 1,700/TDD of insulin, which would calculate to a correction factor of 21 for the patient in this case.[21] In the inpatient setting, standardization of correction insulin scales can help prevent errors that occur when too many different algorithms are used.[30] Although the calculated correction insulin dose[21] for this patient is >40 mg/dL, incremental dosing that is made available on many published correction insulin scales, it would be reasonable to use one of the standardized correction scales to avoid confusion and potential medication errors.[30,31] An argument against using a basal-plus regimen for the patient in this case is her requirement for fairly high doses of prandial insulin as an outpatient. This indicates the patient is likely to experience significant hyperglycemia following ingestion of moderate amounts of simple carbohydrates available on a clear liquid diet.

INSULIN REGIMEN MODIFICATIONS RECOMMENDED FOR PATIENTS WHO BECOME NPO

Once a patient is no longer consuming any caloric foods or liquids, there is no need to provide scheduled nutritional or prandial doses of insulin. Continuation of the basal insulin in combination with correctional insulin for glycemic excursions outside of established goal ranges (i.e., basal plus) is required. Although there is no consensus regarding what percentage of basal insulin to administer to patients who are in the fasting state, there is consensus that insulin-treated patients will require continuation of some portion of basal insulin, often in combination with periodic doses of correctional short- or rapid-acting insulin during a surgical procedure to avoid hyperglycemia.[3–5,7] Withholding insulin in patients with T1D or insulin-treated T2D increases risk for diabetic ketoacidosis (DKA) or hyperosmolar hyperglycemic state (HHS) with high risk for perioperative complications.[15]

To calculate the percentage of basal insulin to be administered to patients during periods of fasting, consider the degree of preoperative glycemic control as determined from measures of HbA_{1c} and results of bedside BG monitoring, patient characteristics, type of diabetes, and analysis of their home regimen (physiologic vs. basal heavy). In one study, patients with T1D were given their full dose of basal insulin (glargine) on a day when they were maintained in a fasting state with a low incidence of hypoglycemia.[32] Similar studies with detemir or NPH insulin have not been performed. The pharmacokinetics of NPH insulin with a peak time of action at 6–10 h following administration would support reductions in dose of 25–50% of usual doses.[33,34] The pharmacokinetics of detemir can vary from a flat profile at lower doses (<0.3 units/kg/day) to a more pronounced peak action time at higher doses, again supporting recommendations for dose modifications in some patients during periods of fasting.[35]

One general guideline is to provide 50–75% of the usual basal insulin dose before a surgical procedure.[3–5,7,15,17] In one study that employed this recommendation in 585 patients with diabetes admitted to a same-day surgical center, 21% of patients arrived at the center with BG >200 mg/dL and 2% had BG <70 mg/dL.[15] This study reveals the wide variability in insulin requirements in patients during periods of fasting. Patients who are under what is considered "tight" glycemic control may require reductions in their doses of basal insulin to avoid hypoglycemia, whereas those who are under fair or poor control may require the full dose to avoid significant hyperglycemia.

Given that the patient in this case was under suboptimal control with BBI as an outpatient, she likely will require the full dose of detemir insulin before surgery. It also is likely that administration of detemir 40 units will not be sufficient to maintain glycemic control during this surgical procedure for which she will receive general anesthesia. General anesthesia is associated with increases in counterregulatory hormones and insulin resistance, often increasing insulin requirements.[7,36,37] This differs from regional or spinal anesthesia in which insulin requirements often remain unchanged.[7,36,37] The responsibility for glucose monitoring with administration of subcutaneous or intravenous (IV), which is preferred, doses of regular or rapid-acting insulin analogs will fall to the anesthesiologist.[15,37,38]

Basal-heavy insulin refers to the (usually inappropriate) use of high doses of a single daily injection of basal insulin (glargine, detemir, or NPH) to cover both prandial and basal insulin requirements. Patients on these regimens often receive >0.6 to >1 unit/kg/day of basal insulin each day. Although not recommended by endocrinologists, in reality, this is a fairly common practice. When carbohydrate intake is decreased or eliminated in the NPO state, more aggressive decreases in basal insulin doses of ≥50% are required.

PERIOPERATIVE MANAGEMENT OF PATIENTS RECEIVING NONINSULIN DIABETES THERAPY

Evidence is insufficient regarding the best ways to manage patients receiving noninsulin diabetes therapy.[7,15,17] It is generally accepted that on the morning before surgery, although patients are consuming a normal diet, all usual diabetes medications should be continued. For patients on a clear liquid diet such as the patient in this case, or those who are receiving dietary preparation for a colonoscopy, we recommend holding sulfonylurea agents because of the risk of hypoglycemia.[39] Short-acting insulin secretogogues such as repaglinide and nateglinide can be continued in reduced doses. Other noninsulin therapies usually can be continued until a patient is in the fasted (NPO) state. On the morning of surgery, we recommend holding all oral and injectable noninsulin diabetes medications.[15]

SUBOPTIMAL HBA_{1C} AND HIGH-RISK FOR POSTOPERATIVE COMPLICATIONS

Although some evidence links preoperative glycemic control with the risk for postoperative complications, available evidence is more suggestive than absolute.[40,41] In the patient in this case, there is no need to delay surgery based on her HbA_{1c}. Two days in the hospital preoperatively allows time for insulin adjustments and for the institution of a reasonable level of glycemic control, defined as maintaining BG values between 140 and 180 mg/dL.[6,7]

For elective procedures (e.g., joint replacement surgery, hernia repair), patients with previous poor diabetes control can be encouraged to improve their metabolic status with the motivating factor being that this will reduce risk for postoperative complications.[40,42] The optimal level of "improved control" is not defined, but the authors of this chapter recommend HbA_{1c} values of <8.5%, which correspond to a mean BG of <200 mg/dL, the level at which risk for perioperative complications increases most significantly.[43–46]

Not all patients will have the ability to achieve this level of glycemic control. In these situations, personal experience and judgment are important. For example, a patient with chronically uncontrolled insulin requiring T2D with HbA_{1c} values >12% resulting from personal chaos and stress may be encouraged to reduce their HbA_{1c} to <10% in preparation for elective surgery, but they may have difficulty getting to lower values. In some cases, allowing an elective surgical procedure to take place has the potential to contribute to improved glycemic control by addressing issues such as chronic pain that interfere with self-management. For patients who are unable to achieve desired levels of glycemic control or for whom a procedure is urgent, glycemic control can be achieved rapidly with the use of an IV insulin infusion before, during, and following the surgical procedure.[15,47]

METABOLIC EFFECTS ASSOCIATED WITH NPO STATUS

Prolonged fasting is associated with reductions in insulin sensitivity in patients with and without diabetes.[48,49] In the absence of diabetes, fasting is associated with a decline in insulin levels and an increase in glucagon, with associated increases in circulating free fatty acids that further impair insulin sensitivity.[49] Although it is beyond the scope of this chapter, the reader is referred to several recent publications that explore the continued administration of carbohydrates in preparation for surgical procedures as a way to avoid potentially harmful increases in counter-regulatory hormones.[49–52]

For prolonged procedures, the IV administration of glucose- or dextrose-containing IV fluids may help to limit perioperative changes in insulin sensitivity. Administration of glucose-containing IV fluids contributes to elevated BG. One liter of D5%-containing IV fluid has 50 g of glucose or ~200 calories. If this is infused at a rate of 100 cc/h, this provides 5 g of glucose or 20 calories/h. This calculates to ~1.2 mg/kg/min for an individual who wieghts 70 kg. Although this amount may seem trivial, personal experience indicates that in some cases, this is sufficient to contribute to mild elevations in BG that prompt administration of additional insulin. No published studies have investigated the effect of these low glucose infusion rates on hyperglycemia in hospitalized patients. In one study, glucose infusion rates of ≤4 mg/kg/min were not associated with hyperglycemia in patients without diabetes receiving total parenteral nutrition.[53]

PREVENTING HYPOGLYCEMIA WHEN NPO STATUS IS IMPOSED ABRUPTLY

Some patients may be abruptly placed in the fasting state after full doses of a weight-based BBI regimen has been administered, placing patients at increased risk for hypoglycemia.[39] We generally recommend that infusions of D5% or D10% be initiated with more frequent glucose monitoring as a way to reduce this risk.[54]

PATIENTS WHO EXPERIENCE HYPOGLYCEMIA WHILE NPO FOR A PROCEDURE

Little data have addressed the issue of patients who experience hypoglycemia while NPO.[7] Studies that discuss the benefit of preoperative carbohydrate loading can provide a guide to the safety of ingesting carbohydrate-containing liquids in the event of a hypoglycemic event.[55,56] Our recommendation to patients is to consume 4 ounces of a caloric clear liquid beverage in the event of a hypoglycemic event during the fasting period (Table 5.1).[15] If hypoglycemia persists, this can be repeated as necessary. Patients need to inform personnel in the same-day surgical suite that that this occurred.

TIMING OF INSULIN AND MEALS

Patient Case

The patient in this case eventually will resume eating regular meals within 24–36 h of a surgical procedure. Although food intake may begin while she is in a surgical intensive care unit, she eventually will be transferred to a nursing unit where they will need to coordinate insulin dosing and meal administration.

Hospitalized patients with diabetes depend on hospital personnel to monitor blood glucose levels, administer diabetes medications, and deliver meals in a timely and coordinated manner.[14,16,57] This is a challenge to personnel providing care to inpatients with diabetes in the best of circumstances. This has become even more difficult following the introduction of "meals on demand" or "room service" as part of routine care in many hospitals.[16]

Hospitals have responded to the introduction of meals on demand in one of several ways. Some have tried unsuccessfully to disallow this practice in insulin-treated patients, resulting in patient and therefore administrative dissatisfaction. Others have implemented guidelines to help minimize the chaos that leads to poor coordination of the components of administering meal-related insulin (Table 5.2).[57] One institution introduced a procedure that included posting of signs on the doors of patients scheduled to receive nutritional insulin with the following statement: "Before you eat, please call your nurse for your premeal medication." Meal servers remove the sign at the time of meal tray delivery and give this to the patient who then calls the nurse to bring their insulin. This resulted in a significant improvement in the percentage of patients receiving meal insulin in a timely manner.[58]

The most important component of promoting the glycemic success (i.e., avoiding hypoglycemia and hyperglycemia) is the need to establish communication among the patient, nurse, and nutrition services. This can be achieved by providing education to nursing and nutrition services personnel regarding the pharmacokinetics of insulin preparations as this relates to meal ingestion.[16] Engaging patients, dietary, and nursing personnel in ensuring timely administration of

Table 5.2—Guideline for Promoting Appropriate Insulin Administration for Meals on Demand

- Patients are able to order meals within regularly scheduled time intervals
- Nutrition services will call patient for any orders not placed with these intervals
- Personnel distributing meals alert the RN that a meal has been delivered to patient to prompt a BG check and insulin administration
- Prominent note is provided with meal to remind a patient to request a BG check and insulin dose before ingesting a meal
- Avoid administration of meal insulin at intervals of <4 h to avoid insulin stacking

premeal insulin can facilitate the coordination of activities that promote patient safety in the hospital setting.

CARBOHYDRATE COUNTING IN THE HOSPITAL

Even patients with a good appetite who are eating regular meals pose a challenge to diabetes management in the hospital. The decisions as to how and when to cover carbohydrate content of patient meals usually fall under the direction of hospital personnel rather than the patient, even for patients who self-managed their diabetes before admission.[1,3–5] Some hospitals use carbohydrate-controlled diets for all patients with diabetes, which provide a fixed amount of carbohydrate with each meal allowing for more accurate prandial insulin administration.

As outlined previously, many hospitals have introduced programs that allow patients more flexibility in the timing and content of their meals. One justification for this approach is an improvement in patient satisfaction with their care while hospitalized, which has increased their popularity among hospital administrators who are concerned with hospital rankings. As a way to adjust to this variability in the timing of meal delivery for individual patients, some hospitals have adopted the practice of administrating prandial insulin based on carbohydrate intake. This practice requires extensive training and education of nutrition and nursing personnel.

These meal-on-demand practices, in association with insulin dosing based on carbohydrate counting and insulin sensitivity, can allow for more accurate prandial insulin coverage. To date, only one relatively small study had formally examined this issue and has found that a fixed meal dosing strategy provided similar glucose control as flexible meal dosing.[20] There were no group differences in mean carbohydrate intake per meal consumed, frequency of hypoglycemia, or overall patient satisfaction. In this study, an inpatient diabetes team provided all diabetes treatment with expertise in glycemic management, a service that is not available in most hospitals. This raises questions about the safety of this practice in hospitals where these teams may not be available.

TIMING OF PRANDIAL INSULIN ADMINISTRATION

There are varying opinions as to the optimal timing of insulin administration in the hospital setting. Some clinicians prefer that insulin be given about 15 min before the meal, which is similar to recommendations for the outpatient setting for rapid-acting insulin administration. Others feel that it is safer to administer prandial doses of insulin following a meal, particularly when there is uncertainty regarding how much food a patient will consume. This latter approach may help reduce risk for hypoglycemia in patients who have a variable appetite or who have difficulty with hospital diets. In these cases, it may be appropriate to administer insulin immediately after each meal. A usual approach is to administer half the dose when a patient consumes half of the meal and to withhold the dose if less than half of the meal is consumed. Although adequate inpatient-based studies on postprandial administration of rapid-acting insulin are lacking, this practice has been evaluated in other patient populations and found to provide satisfactory glycemic control.[59,60]

CONCLUSION

There is an underappreciation of the contribution of nutritional intake, or lack thereof, to glycemic management in the hospital setting. This chapter has provided an approach to the management of patients on clear liquid and regular diets, in which case the issue of matching insulin dosing to the number of carbohydrates consumed is identical. In addition, we have provided a review of the currently available literature describing approaches to use of pharmacologic glycemic-lowering therapy in patients who are in the fasting state in preparation for surgery or other medical procedures. We described the difficulty in making one recommendation for all insulin-treated patients given the number of different regimens that are prescribed in the greater medical community, with some basal-heavy regimens requiring more significant reductions and some basal-appropriate regimens requiring minimal reductions in dosing. Little data have been published to guide the management of these patients. This means that many of the recommendations reflect consensus opinion that incorporates knowledge of the pharmacokinetics of different insulin and oral preparations, published literature, and extensive personal clinical experience.

REFERENCES

1. Korytkowski M, Dinardo M, Donihi AC, Bigi L, Devita M. Evolution of a diabetes inpatient safety committee. *Endocr Pract* 2006;12(Suppl. 3):91–99

2. Draznin B, Gilden J, Golden SH, Inzucchi SE. Pathways to quality inpatient management of hyperglycemia and diabetes: a call to action. *Diabetes Care* 2013;36:1807–1814

3. Moghissi ES, Korytkowski MT, DiNardo M, Einhorn D, Hellman R, Hirsch IB, Inzucchi SE, Ismail-Beigi F, Kirkman MS, Umpierrez GE. American Association of Clinical Endocrinologists and American Diabetes Association consensus statement on inpatient glycemic control. *Endocr Pract* 2009;15:353–369

4. Moghissi ES, Korytkowski MT, DiNardo MM, Einhorn D, Hellman R, Hirsch IB, Inzucchi SE, Ismail-Beigi F, Kirkman MS, Umpierrez GE. American Association of Clinical Endocrinologists and American Diabetes Association consensus statement on inpatient glycemic control. *Diabetes Care* 2009;32:1119–1131

5. Umpierrez GE, Hellman R, Korytkowski MT, Kosiborod M, Maynard GA, Montori VM, Seley JJ, Van den Berghe G. Management of hyperglycemia in hospitalized patients in non-critical care setting: an Endocrine Society clinical practice guideline. *J Clin Endocrinol Metab* 2012;97:16–38

6. American Diabetes Association. Diabetes care in the hospital, nursing home, and skilled nursing facility. *Diabetes Care* 2015;38(Suppl.):S80–S85

7. Joshi GP, Chung F, Vann MA, Ahmad S, Gan TJ, Goulson DT, Merrill DG, Twersky R. Society for Ambulatory Anesthesia consensus statement on

perioperative blood glucose management in diabetic patients undergoing ambulatory surgery. *Anesth Angalg* 2010;111:1378–1387

8. Hirsch IB. Sliding scale insulin—time to stop sliding. *JAMA* 2009;301: 213–214
9. Desimone ME, Blank GE, Virji M, Donihi A, DiNardo M, Simak DM, Buranosky R, Korytkowski MT. Effect of an educational inpatient diabetes management program on medical resident knowledge and measures of glycemic control: A randomized controlled trial. *Endocr Pract* 2012;18:238–243
10. Cheekati V OR, Jameson KA, Cook CB. Perceptions of resident physicians about management of inpatient hyperglycemia in an urban hospital. *J Hosp Med* 2009;4:E1–E8
11. Cook CB, Jameson KA, Hartsell ZC, Boyle ME, Leonhardi BJ, Farquhar-Snow M, Beer KA. Beliefs about hospital diabetes and perceived barriers to glucose management among inpatient midlevel practitioners. *Diabetes Educ* 2008;34:75–83
12. Trujillo JM, Barsky EE, Greenwood BC, Wahlstrom SA, Shaykevich S, Pendergrass ML, Schnipper JL. Improving glycemic control in medical inpatients: a pilot study. *J Hosp Med* 2008;3:55–63
13. Wexler DJ, Shrader P, Burns SM, Cagliero E. Effectiveness of a computerized insulin order template in general medical inpatients with type 2 diabetes: a cluster randomized trial. *Diabetes Care* 2010;33:2181–2183
14. Curll M, DiNardo M, Noschese M, Korytkowski MT. Menu selection, glycaemic control, and satisfaction with standard and patient-controlled consistent carbohydrate diet meal plans in hospitalised patients with diabetes. *Qual Saf Health Care* 2010;19:355
15. DiNardo M, Donihi AC, Forte P, Gieraltowski L, Korytkowski M. Standardized glycemic management and perioperative glycemic outcomes in patients with diabetes mellitus who undergo same-day surgery. *Endocr Pract* 2011;17:404
16. Ryan DB, Swift CS. The mealtime challenge: nutrition and glycemic control in the hospital. *Diabetes Spect* 2014;27:163–168
17. DiNardo M, Griffin C, Curll M. Outpatient surgery. A guide for people with diabetes. *Diabetes Forecast* 2005;58:50–54
18. Holman RR, Farmer AJ, Davies MJ, Levy JC, Darbyshire JL, Keenan JF, Paul SK, Group TS. Three-year efficacy of complex insulin regimens in type 2 diabetes. *New Engl J Med* 2009;361:1736–1747
19. Wallia A, Molitch ME. Insulin therapy for type 2 diabetes mellitus. *JAMA* 2014;311:2315–2325
20. Dungan KM, Sagrilla C, Abdel-Rasoul M, Osei K. Prandial insulin dosing using the carbohydrate counting technique in hospitalized patients with type 2 diabetes. *Diabetes Care* 2013;36:3476–3482

21. Davidson PC, Hebblewhite HR, Steed RD, Bode BW. Analysis of guidelines for basal-bolus insulin dosing: basal insulin, correction factor, and carbohydrate-to-insulin ratio. *Endocr Pract* 2008;14:1095–1101

22. Walsh J, Roberts R, Bailey T. Guidelines for optimal bolus calculator settings in adults. *J Diabetes Sci Technol* 2011;5:129–135

23. Kuroda A, Yasuda T, Takahara M, Sakamoto F, Kasami R, Miyashita K, Yoshida S, Kondo E, Aihara K, Endo I, Matsuoka TA, Kaneto H, Matsumoto T, Shimomura I, Matsuhisa M. Carbohydrate-to-insulin ratio is estimated from 300-400 divided by total daily insulin dose in type 1 diabetes patients who use the insulin pump. *Diabetes Technol Therap* 2012;14:1077–1080

24. Noh YH, Lee WJ, Kim KA, Lim I, Lee JH, Lee JH, Kim S, Choi SB. Insulin requirement profiles of patients with type 2 diabetes after achieving stabilized glycemic control with short-term continuous subcutaneous insulin infusion. *Diabetes Technol Therap* 2010;12:271–281

25. Pelzer R, Mathews EH, Liebenberg L. Preliminary application of a new bolus insulin model for type 1 diabetes. *Diabetes Technol Therap* 2011;13:527–535

26. King AB, Armstrong DU. A prospective evaluation of insulin dosing recommendations in patients with type 1 diabetes at near normal glucose control: bolus dosing. *J Diabetes Sci Technol* 2007;1:42–46

27. Noschese M, Donihi AC, Koerbel G, Karslioglu E, DiNardo M, Curll M, Korytkowski MT: Effect of a Diabetes Order Set on glycaemic management and control in the hospital. *Qual Saf Health Care* 2008;17:464–468

28. Ampudia-Blasco FJ, Rossetti P, Ascaso JF. Basal plus basal-bolus approach in type 2 diabetes. *Diabetes Technol Therap* 2011;13(Suppl. 1):S75–S83

29. Umpierrez GE, Smiley D, Hermayer K, Khan A, Olson DE, Newton C, Jacobs S, Rizzo M, Peng L, Reyes D, Pinzon I, Fereira ME, Hunt V, Gore A, Toyoshima MT, Fonseca VA. Randomized study comparing a basal bolus with a basal plus correction insulin regimen for the hospital management of medical and surgical patients with type 2 diabetes: basal plus trial. *Diabetes Care* 2013;36:2169–2174

30. Donihi AC, DiNardo MM, DeVita MA, Korytkowski MT. Use of a standardized protocol to decrease medication errors and adverse events related to sliding scale insulin. *Qual Saf Health Care* 2006;15:89–91

31. Umpierrez GE, Smiley D, Zisman A, Prieto LM, Palacio A, Ceron M, Puig A, Mejia R. Randomized study of basal-bolus insulin therapy in the inpatient management of patients with type 2 diabetes (RABBIT 2 trial). *Diabetes Care* 2007;30:2181–2186

32. Mucha GT, Merkel S, Thomas W, Bantle JP. Fasting and insulin glargine in individuals with type 1 diabetes. *Diabetes Care* 2004;27:1209–1210

33. Krug EI, DeRiso L, Tedesco MB, Rao H, Korytkowski MT. Glucodynamics and pharmacokinetics of 70/30 vs. 50/50 NPH/regular insulin mixtures after subcutaneous injection. *Diabetes Care* 2001;24:1694–1695

34. Heinemann L, Linkeschova R, Rave K, Hompesch B, Sedlak M, Heise T. Time-action profile of the long-acting insulin analog insulin glargine (HOE901) in comparison with those of NPH insulin and placebo. *Diabetes Care* 2000;23:644–649

35. Plank J, Bodenlenz M, Sinner F, Magnes C, Gorzer E, Regittnig W, Endahl LA, Draeger E, Zdravkovic M, Pieber TR. A double-blind, randomized, dose-response study investigating the pharmacodynamic and pharmacokinetic properties of the long-acting insulin analog detemir. *Diabetes Care* 2005;28:1107–1112

36. Bromage PR, Shibata HR, Willoughby HW. Influence of prolonged epidural blockade on blood sugar and cortisol responses to operations upon the upper part of the abdomen and the thorax. *Surg Gyn Obst* 1971;132:1051–1056

37. Akhtar S, Barash PG, Inzucchi SE. Scientific principles and clinical implications of perioperative glucose regulation and control. *Anesthes Analges* 2010;110:478–497

38. Third-party reimbursement for diabetes care, self-management education, and supplies. *Diabetes Care* 2003;26(Suppl. 1):S143–144

39. Eiland L, Goldner W, Drincic A, Desouza C. Inpatient hypoglycemia: a challenge that must be addressed. *Curr Diabetes Rep* 2014;14:445

40. Frisch A, Chandra P, Smiley D, Peng L, Rizzo M, Gatcliffe C, Hudson M, Mendoza J, Johnson R, Lin E, Umpierrez GE. Prevalence and clinical outcome of hyperglycemia in the perioperative period in noncardiac surgery. *Diabetes Care* 2010;33:1783–1788

41. Umpierrez GE, Smiley D, Jacobs S, Peng L, Temponi A, Mulligan P, Umpierrez D, Newton C, Olson D, Rizzo M. Randomized study of basal-bolus insulin therapy in the inpatient management of patients with type 2 diabetes undergoing general surgery (RABBIT 2 surgery). *Diabetes Care* 2011;34: 256–261

42. Halkos ME, Puskas JD, Lattouf OM, Kilgo P, Kerendi F, Song HK, Guyton RA, Thourani VH. Elevated preoperative hemoglobin A1c level is predictive of adverse events after coronary artery bypass surgery. *J Thoracic Cardio Surg* 2008;136:631–640

43. Furnary AP, Wu Y, Bookin SO. Effect of hyperglycemia and continuous intravenous insulin infusions on outcomes of cardiac surgical procedures: the Portland Diabetic Project. *Endocr Pract* 2004;10(Suppl. 2):21–33

44. Golden SH, Peart-Vigilance C, Kao WH, Brancati FL. Perioperative glycemic control and the risk of infectious complications in a cohort of adults with diabetes. *Diabetes Care* 1999;22:1408–1414

45. Lazar HL, Chipkin SR, Fitzgerald CA, Bao Y, Cabral H, Apstein CS. Tight glycemic control in diabetic coronary artery bypass graft patients improves perioperative outcomes and decreases recurrent ischemic events. *Circulation* 2004;109:1497–1502

46. Lipshutz AKM, Gropper MA. Perioperative glycemic control: an evidence-based review. *Anesthesiology* 2009;110:408–421

47. Gandhi GY, Nuttall GA, Abel MD, Mullany CJ, Schaff HV, O'Brien PC, Johnson MG, Williams AR, Cutshall SM, Mundy LM, Rizza RA, McMahon MM. Intensive intraoperative insulin therapy versus conventional glucose management during cardiac surgery: a randomized trial. *Ann Intern Med* 2007;146:233–243

48. Ljungqvist O. Insulin resistance and outcomes in surgery. *J Clin Endocr Metab* 2010;95:4217–4219

49. Brown L, Heuberger R. Nothing by mouth at midnight: saving or starving? A literature review. *Gastroenterol Nurs* 2014;37:14–23

50. Crenshaw JT. Preoperative fasting: will the evidence ever be put into practice? *Am J Nurs* 2011;111:38–43

51. Gustafsson UO, Scott MJ, Schwenk W, Demartines N, Roulin D, Francis N, McNaught CE, MacFie J, Liberman AS, Soop M, Hill A, Kennedy RH, Lobo DN, Fearon K, Ljungqvist O. Guidelines for perioperative care in elective colonic surgery: Enhanced Recovery After Surgery (ERAS) Society recommendations. *Clin Nurt* 2012;31:783–800

52. Wang ZG, Wang Q, Wang WJ, Qin HL. Randomized clinical trial to compare the effects of preoperative oral carbohydrate versus placebo on insulin resistance after colorectal surgery. *Br J Surg* 2010;97:317–327

53. Rosmarin DK, Wardlaw GM, Mirtallo J. Hyperglycemia associated with high, continuous infusion rates of total parenteral nutrition dextrose. *Nutrit Clin Pract* 1996;11:151–156

54. Korytkowski MT, Salata RJ, Koerbel GL, Selzer F, Karslioglu E, Idriss AM, Lee KKW, Moser AJ, Toledo FGS. Insulin therapy and glycemic control in hospitalized patients with diabetes during enteral nutrition therapy: a randomized controlled clinical trial. *Diabetes Care* 2009;32:594–596

55. Noblett SE, Watson DS, Huong H, Davison B, Hainsworth PJ, Horgan AF. Pre-operative oral carbohydrate loading in colorectal surgery: a randomized controlled trial. *Colorectal Disease* 2006;8:563–569

56. Svanfeldt M, Thorell A, Hausel J, Soop M, Rooyackers O, Nygren J, Ljungqvist O. Randomized clinical trial of the effect of preoperative oral carbohydrate treatment on postoperative whole-body protein and glucose kinetics. *Br J Surg* 2007;94:1342–1350

57. Cohen LS, Sedhom L, Salifu M, Friedman EA. Inpatient diabetes management: examining morning practice in an acute care setting. *Diabetes Educ* 2007;33:483–492

58. Donihi AC, Abriola C, Hall R, Korytkowski MT. Getting the timing right in the hospital: Synching insulin administration with meal tray arrival. *Diabetes* 2010;59:1028–P

59. Jovanovic L, Giammattei J, Acquistapace M, Bornstein K, Sommermann E, Pettitt DJ. Efficacy comparison between preprandial and postprandial insulin aspart administration with dose adjustment for unpredictable meal size. *Clin Therap* 2004;26:1492–1497

60. Ratner R, Wynne A, Nakhle S, Brusco O, Vlajnic A, Rendell M. Influence of preprandial vs. postprandial insulin glulisine on weight and glycaemic control in patients initiating basal-bolus regimen for type 2 diabetes: a multicenter, randomized, parallel, open-label study (NCT00135096). *Diabetes Obes Metab* 2011;13:1142–1148

Chapter 6

Glycemic Control in the Setting of Parenteral Nutrition or Enteral Nutrition via Tube Feeding

Cecilia C. Low Wang, MD,[1] R. Matthew Hawkins, PA-C, MMSc,[2] Roma Gianchandani, MD,[3] and Kathleen Dungan, MD[4]

INTRODUCTION

Parenteral nutrition (PN) and enteral nutrition (EN) via tube feeding (TF) are used both within and outside the hospital setting to provide nutrition in individuals who are not able to eat via the traditional oral route because of various factors, including recovery from major abdominal surgery, critical illness, malabsorption, dysphagia, decreased level of consciousness, oropharyngeal processes, and esophageal dysmotility. The incidence of hyperglycemia with or without diagnosed diabetes in patients receiving EN via TF is unclear, but it may range from 34 to 50%.[1] For hospitalized patients receiving PN, the prevalence of hyperglycemia ranges from 28 to 44% when a glucose threshold of 200 mg/dL is used,[2,3] and up to 90% with a lower glucose threshold of 150 mg/dL.[3,4] In another study, 51% of patients on PN were found to have at least one blood glucose (BG) measurement >140 mg/dL.[5]

The development of hyperglycemia during EN via TF/PN increases the risk of complications and mortality. Adverse consequences may include cardiac complications, infections, sepsis, acute kidney injury, and increased mortality. Pasquel et al. found an increased risk of pneumonia (odds ratio [OR] 3.1, 95% confidence interval [CI] 1.4–7.1), acute renal failure (OR 2.3, 95% CI 1.1–5.0), and mortality (OR 2.8, 95% CI 1.2–6.8, $P = 0.02$) for patients on total parenteral nutrition (TPN) with a BG >180 mg/dL within 24 h of starting PN.[4] A multicenter study in Spain reported a 5.6-fold risk of mortality after adjusting for multiple factors in patients with a mean BG >180 mg/dL during PN infusion as compared with a mean BG of <140 mg/dL.[6]

The Endocrine Society's clinical practice guidelines for the management of hyperglycemia in the non-critical-care inpatient setting include the following

[1]Associate Professor of Medicine/Director, Glucose Management Team University of Colorado School of Medicine/University of Colorado Hospital Aurora, CO. [2]Physician Assistant/Instructor, Department of Endocrinology, Diabetes, and Metabolism, University of Colorado School of Medicine Anschutz Medial Campus, Aurora CO. [3]Associate Professor, Department of Internal medicine/Metabolism, Endocrinology and Diabetes Director, Hospital Hyperglycemia Program University of Michigan Medical Center, Ann Arbor, MI. [4]Ohio State University, Wexner Medical Center, Columbus, OH.

 DOI: 10.2337/9781580406086.06

recommendations for patients receiving EN or PN, with or without a history of diabetes:[7]

1. All patients on EN or PN should be monitored with bedside point-of-care (POC) glucose testing every 4–6 h for at least 24–48 h after initiation of the therapy.
2. POC glucose testing can be discontinued in patients without a prior history of diabetes if BG values are <7.8 mmol/L (140 mg/dL) without insulin therapy for 24–48 h after achievement of desired caloric intake.
3. Scheduled insulin therapy should be initiated in patients receiving EN or PN who have hyperglycemia (i.e., BG >7.8 mmol/L (140 mg/dL), with and without known diabetes, and who demonstrate a persistent requirement (i.e., 12–24 h) for correction insulin.

Unfortunately, strong evidence for the effects of good glycemic control on clinical outcomes or for specific glucose-lowering regimens in patients on EN or PN is lacking; well-designed research studies are needed to close these gaps and improve clinical care.

BLOOD GLUCOSE TARGETS IN EN AND PN

A recently published systematic review and meta-analysis of randomized control trials comparing intensive insulin therapy (IIT) versus control in an intensive care unit (ICU) setting is relevant to this discussion because a significant proportion of these patients received PN or EN.[8] The mean BG of patients on IIT was 112 mg/dL, whereas the mean BG on control therapy was 151 mg/dL. Overall, there was no reduction in mortality with IIT at 28 days, and no decrease in incidence of bloodstream infection or need for renal replacement therapy. Unfortunately there was a higher odds ratio for hypoglycemia (OR 7.7). Because of the difference in 28-day mortality between the Leuven IIT Trials and subsequent trials, a metaregression analysis was performed, which showed a significant difference between 28-day mortality and the proportion of calories provided parenterally ($P = 0.005$). This suggested that the difference in outcome between the two Leuven IIT Trials and the subsequent trials could be related to the use of PN. After excluding the two Leuven trials that included patients receiving a high percentage of calories from PN, the authors found lower mortality in the control group patients. In general, there was less mortality with IIT in PN patients, but increased mortality with IIT in EN patients. No data support the use of an intensive insulin target in patients receiving EN, and a BG target of 150 mg/dL was considered reasonable for patients being fed enterally.

The American Society for Parenteral and Enteral Nutrition (ASPEN) recently reviewed available trials comparing tight versus standard glycemic control and mortality.[9] Five retrospective reviews were included in the analysis that found harm associated with PN-associated hyperglycemia. Tight control resulted in lower mortality in one randomized controlled trial (RCT) and two historical control trials, but there was no difference between tight versus standard control in five other RCTs. The largest RCT[10] demonstrated higher mortality with tight glycemic control. Overall, the ASPEN group found strong evidence for the recommendation of a BG target of 140–180 mg/dL in patients receiving nutritional support and strong evidence for defining hypoglycemia in this setting as a BG of <70 mg/dL.

The authors suggest that patients receiving artificial nutrition in the form of PN or EN are in a postprandial state, and the previous evidence supports a BG target of 140–180 mg/dL in this setting.

PARENTERAL NUTRITION

EVIDENCE FOR GLYCEMIC CONTROL IN PATIENTS ON PN

A number of studies have examined the effect of glycemic control on clinical outcomes in patients receiving PN. A few of these studies are summarized in this section.

In a single-center retrospective analysis of 109 patients receiving TPN, the odds ratio in relation to BG level of developing a number of different complications ranged from 1.36 to 1.77, all of which were statistically significant.[11] Patients in the highest quartile of BG level had an odds ratio of 10.9 for mortality or for acute renal failure, and an odds ratio of 4.3 for developing any complication as compared with patients in the lowest quartile of mean BG level, independent of age, sex, or prior diabetes status.

Another single-center retrospective study of 276 medical and surgical patients receiving TPN examined the likelihood of death and BG levels on admission, pre-TPN, within 24 h of starting TPN, and 2–10 days after starting TPN.[4] In multiple regression models adjusted for age, sex, and history of diabetes, the likelihood of death was independently predicted by an elevated pre-TPN BG between 121 and 150 mg/dL (OR 2.2, 95% CI 1.1–4.4, $P = 0.030$), 151 and 180 mg/dL (OR 3.41, 95% CI 1.3–8.7, $P = 0.010$), >180 mg/dL (OR 2.2, 95% CI 0.9–5.2, $P = 0.077$), or >180 mg/dL within 24 h of starting TPN, as compared with patients with a mean BG <120 mg/dL. Patients with higher BG levels during TPN had a longer hospital ($P = 0.011$) and ICU ($P = 0.008$) length of stay.

A prospective multicenter study of 605 noncritically ill patients receiving PN in Spain with 58 deaths (9.6%) revealed a 5.6-fold higher risk of mortality for patients with a mean BG >180 mg/dL during TPN infusion after multiple logistic regression analysis.[6] The total number of grams of carbohydrates infused was associated with risk of in-hospital death. However, the presence of diabetes was not significant. Approximately half of these patients had normal glucose tolerance (mean HbA_{1c} 5.3%, $n = 308$, 50.9% of patients), 27.4% of patients had hyperglycemia without diabetes (mean HbA_{1c} 5.7%, $n = 166$), 17.9% of patients had known diabetes (mean HbA_{1c} 6.6%, $n = 108$), and the remainder had "unknown," or previously undiagnosed diabetes (mean HbA_{1c} 7.2%, $n = 23$). Forty-one (6.9%) patients had at least one episode of hypoglycemia <70 mg/dL at some time during PN administration.

Hyperglycemia before and during PN is associated with an increased risk for complications and mortality in patients receiving PN. No published RCT data, however, show that glycemic control reduces the risk for complications or mortality in this setting.

Table 6.1—Selected Studies of Glucose-Lowering Strategies for Patients on PN

First author	Year	Study design	Regimens compared	Population	Setting	Diabetes status	Results and conclusions
Sajbel	1987	Retrospective chart review	Safety, efficacy, and cost effectiveness of a separate continuous insulin infusion	Patients with serum glucose (SG) >200 mg/dL at a TPN rate of <75% of their calculated caloric requirement. *N* = 16 (5 known to have diabetes)	ICU and non-ICU	With and without diabetes	■ In critically ill or hemodynamically compromised patients, treatment with IV insulin is preferred (allows for frequent dose adjustments). ■ 73% of serum glucose (SG) on IV were 100-250 mg/dL. No SG < 50 mg/dL. ■ Average time to caloric goal was 2.7 days
Hongsermeier	1993	Prospective cohort and retrospective record review	Safety and applicability of an algorithm using prehospitalization insulin dose (PHI) to calculate the initial amount of regular insulin to be included in PN. Subsequent titration based on the amount of subcutaneous (SQ) correction insulin given per 24-h period.	Patients on insulin before hospitalization, on PN for ≥5 days including 3 days receiving stable caloric content in PN. Divided into infected and noninfected groups. *N* = 20 (16 retrospective, 4 prospective)	Hospital patients (acuity not specified)	All patients had known T1D or T2D	■ An algorithm for determining starting dose of insulin based on the pre-hospitalization insulin dose (PHI) plus sliding-scale insulin for fine tuning can be a safe and effective way to provide TPN to diabetic patients. ■ Infected patients received 217% +/– 144% of PHI plus 10.6 +/– 7.0 units sliding-scale insulin in 3 days ■ Noninfected patients received 199% +/– 78% of PHI plus 2.3 +/– 3.4 units sliding-scale insulin in 3 days ■ No significant hypoglycemia (<60 mg/dL) in either group

continued

Table 6.1—Selected Studies of Glucose-Lowering Strategies for Patients on PN *(continued)*

First author	Year	Study design	Regimens compared	Population	Setting	Diabetes status	Results and conclusions
Jakoby	2012	Prospective cohort with historical controls	Protocol using IV regular insulin PN plus SQ NPH versus standard-of-care insulin regimen	Adults at a large county hospital on PN with >50% of capillary BG (CBG) >140 mg/dL with or without steroids. Control data were from patients meeting same criteria before the study. *N* = 55 (*n* = 25 on protocol, *n* = 30 control)	Hospital patients (acuity not specified)	With and without diabetes	■ Protocol linking insulin to carbohydrate in PN improves glycemic control ■ Mean CBG protocol group 138 +/− 37 ■ Mean CBG control group 159 +/− 46 ■ TDD of insulin same for both groups but 93% given as scheduled in protocol group versus 43% in in controls ■ Protocol directed management on PN induced hyperglycemia is superior to ad hoc dosing
Neff	2014	Retrospective record review	Protocol-based IV insulin delivery vs. SQ insulin prescribed individually	Patients with PN-associated hyperglycemia (>10 mmol/L on two or more occasions) who had received either IV or SQ insulin therapy. *N* = 53	Non-ICU	With and without diabetes	■ IV insulin group had lower daily mean capillary glucose level: IV 9.6 +/− 2.6 mmol/L versus SQ 11.2 +/− 2.6 mmol/L ■ Time in target range (4.0–10.0 mmol/L): IV 62% versus SQ 43% ■ No significant difference in hypoglycemia: IV 1% versus SQ 2%

EVIDENCE FOR GLUCOSE-LOWERING STRATEGIES IN PATIENTS RECEIVING PN

Despite the lack of RCT data showing that glycemic control reduces the risk for complications or mortality in patients receiving PN, the available data show significant harm associated with uncontrolled hyperglycemia in this population. Therefore, clinicians must anticipate and manage hyperglycemia in their patients on PN while avoiding hypoglycemia.

In the multicenter prospective cohort described earlier, 71% of patients received insulin along with PN, with 55% receiving this as subcutaneous (SQ) insulin only, 36% as a combination of insulin in the PN bag along with SQ insulin, and 9% as an insulin infusion independent of the PN.[6] Table 6.1 lists selected studies examining specific glucose-lowering regimens for PN. Standard strategies include (1) using a separate intravenous (IV) insulin infusion of regular insulin with an IV insulin protocol, (2) using subcutaneously administered long- or intermediate-acting insulin with correctional insulin, with or without scheduled prandial insulin, and (3) adding regular insulin to the PN bag in combination with subcutaneously administered basal or correctional insulin. Details of a few studies are outlined in the following paragraphs.

A prospective cohort study examining the use of an insulin therapy protocol for patients on TPN compared with historical controls was performed by Jakoby and Nannapaneni.[12] The protocol was rather complex and utilized a combination of NPH insulin only (for total daily insulin dose <14 units), or regular insulin in the TPN bag plus NPH insulin given subcutaneously. BG was monitored every 4 h, and patients were initially monitored for 24 h without initiation of therapy. Patients were placed on the insulin protocol if more than half of the BG values were >140 mg/dL. Regular insulin in the TPN bag was started using a ratio of 1 unit for every 20 g carbohydrate. Patients with diabetes or on glucocorticoids with capillary BG <209 mg/dL were started on 1 unit of insulin for every 10 g carbohydrate (with two-thirds of this given as regular insulin in the PN bag and one-third as NPH added to the following) plus 0.15 units/kg/day of NPH insulin. If the capillary BG was >209 mg/dL, patients with diabetes or on glucocorticoids were given 1 unit of regular insulin for every 5 g carbohydrate (with two-thirds of this given as regular insulin in the PN bag and one-third as NPH added to the following) plus 0.25 units/kg/day of NPH insulin. The NPH insulin was given in three or four equally divided doses every 6–8 h. Insulin doses were adjusted daily according to an algorithm. Patients in the intervention group had a mean capillary BG of 138 ± 37 mg/dL compared to 159 ± 46 mg/dL in the control group. Both groups received about the same total daily dose of insulin, but patients on the protocol received scheduled insulin predominantly (93% of total daily dose), whereas those in the control group received more of their total daily dose as supplemental insulin (66% of total daily dose). Hypoglycemia occurred more frequently in the intervention group than in the control group (3% vs. 1%, $P = 0.12$).

Neff et al. compared SQ- and IV-administered insulin in a retrospective single-center review of patients receiving TPN.[13] A hospital-wide practice change involving IV insulin and a dose adjustment algorithm was instituted for patients with

BG >10 mmol/L (180 mg/dL). Before this, patients were managed with SQ insulin using a nonstandardized approach. The authors analyzed data for patients admitted before and after the hospital-wide protocol was initiated. Patients admitted to the ICU were excluded. Only 53 patients were included in the study, 32 in the IV protocol group and 21 in the SQ group. The IV insulin group had significantly lower daily mean capillary BG (9.6 +/− 2.1 mmol/L vs. 11.2 +/− 2.6 mmol/L) and spent a greater proportion of time in the glycemic target range (63% vs. 43%). There was no significant difference in hypoglycemia rates (1% vs. 2%).

An interesting RCT comparing lower calorie PN to standard PN was published by Ahrens et al.[14] The low-calorie PN consisted of 20 nonprotein kcal/kg/day versus 30 nonprotein kcal/kg/day in the standard PN. Lipids were included in 1,000 kcal increments, three times per week. The number of total calories varied only by the carbohydrate content administered, and hyperglycemia was defined as BG >200 mg/dL. The incidence of hyperglycemia was 0% versus 33.1% ($P = 0.001$) in the low-calorie group versus the standard calorie group, and the mean glucose area under the curve (AUC) was 118 +/− 22 mg-h/dL versus 172 ± 44 (mg-h)/dL, ($P < 0.001$), respectively, and the insulin requirement was 0 units versus 10.9 units ($P < 0.001$). A dextrose infusion rate of >4 mg/kg/min predicted hyperglycemia. Although this approach controls hyperglycemia while minimizing hypoglycemia, clinical outcomes and potential adverse effects of administering fewer calories were not explored.

PRACTICAL APPROACHES TO CONTROL HYPERGLYCEMIA IN PATIENTS ON PN

A combination of regular insulin added to the PN bag and correctional insulin administered subcutaneously is an effective method for controlling hyperglycemia in patients on PN without diabetes.[15] An initial insulin to dextrose ratio of 1:15–1:20 may be used, depending on whether the patient is more insulin resistant (obese, high insulin requirements) or more insulin sensitive (lean, renal insufficiency), respectively. POC glucose should be checked every 6 h, and a correctional dose of rapid-acting SQ insulin injection can be administered in a 1:50 ratio (1 unit for every 50 mg/dL above 150 mg/dL) as needed. The BG pattern and correctional insulin doses administered should be reviewed daily and the ratio adjusted as needed to maintain BG within the target range of 140–180 mg/dL. A hypoglycemia protocol should be used for BG <70 mg/dL.

For patients with known diabetes, an effective strategy for maintaining glycemic control includes regular insulin added to the PN bag, basal insulin, and correctional doses of rapid-acting insulin administered subcutaneously as needed to maintain BG within the target range of 140–180 mg/dL. The starting dose for insulin in the PN bag should be higher, with 1 unit for every 12–15 g of dextrose. Patients should receive (1) their usual basal dose of insulin, or (2) long-acting insulin (glargine or detemir) using 0.2 units/kg/day if renal function is not compromised, or (3) 0.1 unit/kg/day in the setting of renal dysfunction or insulin sensitivity. The blood glucose pattern and correction insulin doses administered should be reviewed daily, and the ratio should be adjusted as needed to maintain

BG within the target range of 140–180 mg/dL. A hypoglycemia protocol should be used for BG <70 mg/dL.

Figure 6.1 illustrates a recommended flowchart for clinical decision making and management of hyperglycemia in patients on PN.

ENTERAL NUTRITION VIA TUBE FEEDING

TF is given either by continuous infusion over 24 h, in boluses to mimic meals, or nocturnal infusions overnight (typically 8–12 h) with patients who are NPO or eating during the day; the latter is usually temporary. Bolus TF are more physiologic and may be preferred for patients with diabetes. For bolus feeding, the total daily volume is divided into four to six separate feedings. Because TF often causes diarrhea or nausea initially, it usually is initiated at a low rate with a diluted preparation and is increased as tolerated. Diabetes-specific TF formulas have

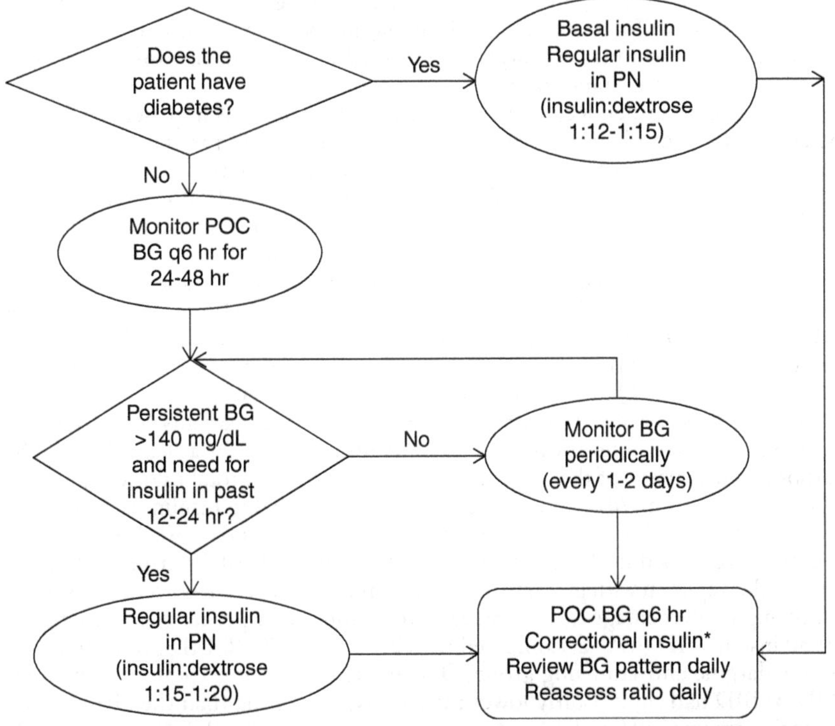

Figure 6.1—Algorithm for clinical decision making and glycemic management of patients on parenteral nutrition. *Correctional rapid-acting subcutaneous insulin as needed every 6 h for BG >150 mg/dL: 1 unit for every 50 mg/dL BG >150 mg/dL.

been developed that are carbohydrate-restricted and are discussed further in the following.

TF can cause hyperglycemia in a significant proportion of patients with or without a prior history of diabetes, as mentioned earlier in this chapter. On the other hand, patients on glucose-lowering therapies while on TF are at high risk for developing hypoglycemia with either planned or unintended interruption of TF. Interruption of TF may occur because of dislodgement of the tube, when thick feedings or pills block the lumen of the tube, or when patients are not able to tolerate the tube feeds and develop diarrhea (including osmotic diarrhea), GI discomfort, nausea, or vomiting. Planned interruption often occurs when TF infusion is stopped in preparation for planned radiological or surgical procedures.

EVIDENCE FOR STRATEGIES TO CONTROL HYPERGLYCEMIA IN TF

Key strategies for glucose control in patients on TF include using a particular insulin regimen, close BG monitoring, using a dextrose infusion (D10% or D5%) for interruption of TF to avoid hypoglycemia, and possibly modifying the composition of the TF formula by lowering carbohydrate content or using a diabetes-specific formula (see Figure 6.2).

Only one published RCT has examined insulin regimens in patients with diabetes on TF.[16] Korytkowski et al. studied 50 subjects randomized to sliding-scale regular insulin (SSRI) alone versus SSRI plus glargine. By the end of the insulin regimen titration, 48% of the subjects randomized to SSRI alone required the addition of NPH insulin. There were no differences between the two groups in terms of total daily dose of insulin, rate of hypoglycemia, or total adverse events. Another study consisted of a retrospective chart review of 159 patients on TF who were on sliding-scale NPH insulin versus aspart (n = 76 for NPH Q6 h, n = 52 for NPH Q4 h, and n = 31 for aspart).[17] Both groups on sliding-scale NPH had lower mean BG and BG within the target range than the aspart group ($P < 0.001$), but the group on NPH Q4 h experienced more hypoglycemia.

Hsia et al. performed a retrospective chart review of 22 patients with diagnosed diabetes who were noncritically ill and on continuous TF for at least 72 h.[18] The carbohydrate content of the TF ranged from 45 to 65% of total calories. The goal BG was 140–180 mg/dL, and correction doses of Humalog insulin were used for BG >180 mg/dL. The correction factor varied from 1:20 to 1:50. Three insulin regimens were used in these patients: 70/30 insulin BID, 70/30 insulin TID, or a basal-bolus regimen with glargine daily and Humalog every 4 h as needed. A significantly higher percentage of BG values were within the target range in patients on 70/30 insulin TID (69% as compared with 22% in the 70/30 BID group and 24% in the glargine and Humalog group). The patients receiving 70/30 insulin either TID or BID had significantly lower rates of hypoglycemia than the glargine and Humalog group (1.4% and 2.1%, respectively, as compared with 5.4%), presumably because of the longer duration of action of glargine and the higher potential for hypoglycemia with interruption of TF. The 70/30 insulin regimen order sets incorporated safety features, including instructions to hold the 70/30 insulin dose for BG <100 mg/dL, and to start a D10% infusion for interruption of TF at the same infusion rate as the tube feeds, along with a hypoglycemia protocol for BG <70 mg/dL.

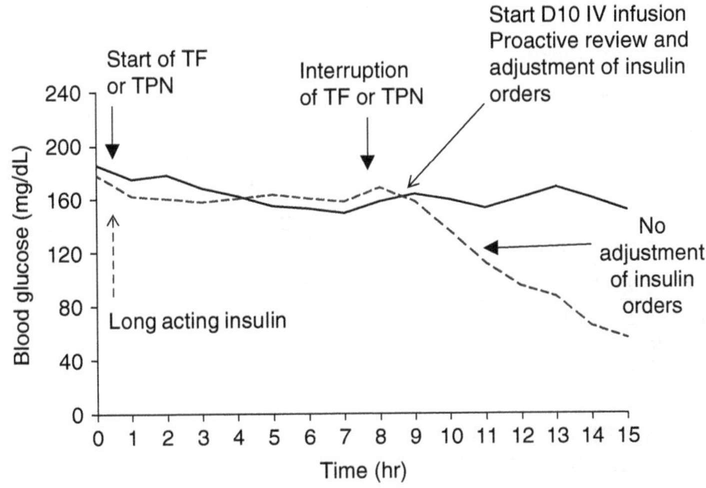

Figure 6.2—Graphic display of blood glucose (BG) response with interruption of tube feeding (TF) or parenteral nutrition (PN) in the presence or absence of appropriate interventions. Within the expected duration of action of the last insulin dose, interruption of EN or PN is highly likely to result in hypoglycemia unless a dextrose 10% (D10%) infusion is initiated and continued for the length of time that the insulin is "on board" or artificial nutrition is restarted. The D10% infusion can be initiated at the same IV rate as the artificial nutrition. TPN, total parenteral nutrition; D10%, dextrose 10%; IV, intravenous.

Source: Adapted with permission from Figure 4 of Low Wang et al.[15]

DIABETES-SPECIFIC FORMULAS FOR TF

The key differences between diabetes-specific formulas for TF versus standard formulas are a lower percentage of calories from carbohydrates and a higher percentage of calories from monounsaturated fatty acids. A meta-analysis of diabetes-specific formulas revealed lower postprandial rise in glucose, lower peak BG and lower BG AUC with the use of diabetes-specific formulas, but the differences were relatively small.[19] Furthermore, the postprandial increment in BG was reduced by only 18–29 mg/dL. Table 6.2 outlines key end points from this meta-analysis.

The ASPEN group reviewed two RCTs examining glycemic control and insulin requirements in patients receiving diabetes-specific formulas for TF: one showed improvement in both outcomes, and one showed no difference.[9] Therefore, their clinical guidelines conclude that evidence is insufficient for the use of diabetes-specific enteral formulas and recommend more research in this area (see Table 6.2).

Table 6.2—Key Findings from Meta-analysis of Studies Examining Diabetes-Specific Enteral Formulas

Outcome	Standardized mean difference between diabetes-specific versus standard formula (mmol/L; 95% CI)
Postprandial rise in glucose	−0.52 (−0.81 to −0.24)
Peak blood glucose	−1.28 (−1.94 to −0.63)
Change in blood glucose area under the curve	−1.19 (−1.69 to −0.7)

PRACTICAL STRATEGIES FOR HYPERGLYCEMIA IN TUBE FEEDING OR ENTERAL NUTRITION

A number of approaches can be used to manage hyperglycemia in patients on EN via tube feeding. The Endocrine Society clinical practice guidelines outline various methods depending on what type of EN is being administered (see Table 6.3). The co-authors use different strategies at their respective institutions. For example, at the University of Colorado Hospital, the inpatient Glucose Management Team advocates the use of 70/30 (NPH/regular) insulin TID for continuous EN via tube feeding. A 1:12–1:20 ratio of insulin:carbohydrate is used to calculate a total daily dose of 70/30 insulin, which then is divided into three doses and administered Q8 h. This dose is adjusted at least once daily based on the previous day's BG and need for correctional insulin. POC glucose is checked every 4 h, and correction doses of Humalog insulin are administered as needed using a 1:50 scale (1 unit for every 50 mg/dL) for BG >150 mg/dL. The 70/30 insulin

Table 6.3—Regimens for Glycemic Control in Patients on Enteral Nutrition (EN).

Method of EN administration	Potential approach to insulin therapy
Continuous EN	■ Basal insulin QD (glargine or detemir) or BID (detemir or NPH) ■ Short- or rapid-acting insulin Q4 h (rapid) or Q6 h (regular)
Cycled feeding	■ Basal insulin (G, D, or NPH) with short- or rapid-acting insulin at start of EN ■ Repeat rapid-acting insulin Q4 h or short-acting Q6 h*
Bolus feeding	■ Short- or rapid-acting insulin before each bolus

QD, daily; BID, twice daily; G, glargine; D, detemir.
*Last dose 4–6 h before discontinuation of EN.
Source: Adapted with permission from Umpierrez et al.[7]

is held for BG <100 mg/dL. An as-needed order is included in the electronic order set for a D10% infusion to be initiated if TF is interrupted, but unfortunately clinical staff often miss this order. Basal insulin (using a dose derived from the patients' home dose, or a weight-based starting dose of 0.2 units/kg/day) is continued in many patients with diabetes.

For patients receiving bolus TF, a dose of rapid-acting insulin is administered at the start of each bolus because the TF usually is administered one can at a time with approximately 4 h between boluses; basal insulin is continued for many patients with diabetes. Correction dose insulin is administered as needed QID to maintain BG within the 140–180 mg/dL range.

Nocturnal TF is often administered between 8 p.m. and 6 or 8 a.m. NPH or 70/30 insulin is administered at the start of TF, and a second dose of NPH or 70/30 insulin may be administered halfway through the TF administration. For patients who are eating in addition to receiving TF, rapid-acting insulin analogue is provided and POC glucose checks can be performed QAC and QHS, with an overnight POC check.

At the Ohio State University and the University of Michigan, continuous TF typically are covered with set-dose regular insulin Q6 h plus basal insulin analogue if needed at no more than 20–30% of the total daily dose. Hold parameters are in place if TF is not at goal. If there is unexpected TF interruption, dextrose is administered. At the University of Michigan, in patients with percutaneous endoscopic gastrostomy tubes, TF interruption is less of an issue and longer acting insulins may be used, such as NPH and 70/30 insulin for continuous or cyclic TF.

CHALLENGES

EN and PN via TF present the following challenges:

- Unanticipated or planned interruption of EN resulting from intolerance, medication administration, procedures, and cycling with oral intake, or discontinuation of PN.
- Insulin orders should specify that they are intended for EN coverage and should be held in case of anticipated EN interruption.
- The order set should include an IV dextrose infusion to be continued for a duration of action of the longest injected insulin dose. Many institutions use D10%, although some use D5 in this situation.
- The dextrose infusion should be initiated at the same infusion rate as the prior TF infusion rate.
- Close monitoring of BG is needed to prevent hypoglycemia and control hyperglycemia.

GAPS IN KNOWLEDGE/RESEARCH NEEDED

As alluded to earlier, more well-designed research studies are needed in a number of topics in the field of TF- or PN-associated hyperglycemia: comparative effectiveness trials comparing management approaches, such as scheduled basal and short-acting insulin versus premixed insulin, IV insulin infusion versus the addition of regular insulin to the PN bag versus a combination of basal insulin with regular insulin in the PN bag to cover nutritional requirements, and trials comparing insulin-based to incretin-based therapies in this specific patient population.[20]

CONCLUSION

Hyperglycemia in those found to have EN- or PN-associated hyperglycemia and in patients with diabetes on EN/PN can be managed effectively and potential complications can be minimized when clinicians are aware of the high risk for hyperglycemia in this setting even without a prior diagnosis of diabetes. This chapter outlined evidence for complications of untreated hyperglycemia in this population, and some of the available evidence for glycemic control and management strategies. A BG target of 140–180 mg/dL should be used in patients on PN or EN via TF. More studies are needed to determine which glucose-management approaches are best suited for which subsets of patients receiving PN or EN via TF, and more definitive studies are needed to address these gaps in clinical management.

REFERENCES

1. Olveira G, Garcia-Luna PP, Pereira JL, Rebollo I, Garcia-Almeida JM, Serrano P, Irles JA, Munoz-Aguilar A, Molina MJ, Tapia MJ. Recommendations of the GARIN group for managing non-critically ill patients with diabetes or stress hyperglycaemia and artificial nutrition. *Nutr Hosp* 2012;27:1837–1849

2. Marti-Bonmati E, Ortega-Garcia MP, Cervera-Casino P, Lacasa C, Llop JL, Villalobos JL, de la Morena L. Multicenter study on the prevalence of hyperglycemia among hospitalized patients with parenteral nutrition. *Farm Hosp* 2006;30:12–19

3. Pleva M, Mirtallo JM, Steinberg SM. Hyperglycemic events in non-intensive care unit patients receiving parenteral nutrition. *Nutr Clin Pract* 2009;24:626–634

4. Pasquel FJ, Spiegelman R, McCauley M, Smiley D, Umpierrez D, Johnson R, Rhee M, Gatcliffe C, Lin E, Umpierrez E, Peng L, Umpierrez GE. Hyperglycemia during total parenteral nutrition: an important marker of poor outcome and mortality in hospitalized patients. *Diabetes Care* 2010;33:739–741

5. Tapia MJ, Ocon J, Cabrejas-Gomez C, Ballesteros-Pomar MD, Vidal-Casariego A, Arraiza-Irigoyen C, Olivares J, Conde-Garcia MC, Garcia-Manzanares A, Botella-Romero F, Quilez-Toboso RP, Cabrerizo L, Rubio MA, Chicharro L, Burgos R, Pujante P, Ferrer M, Zugasti A, Petrina E, Manjon L, Dieguez M, Carrera MJ, Vila-Bundo A, Urgeles JR, Aragon-Valera C, Sanchez-Vilar O, Breton I, Garcia-Peris P, Munoz-Garach A, Marquez E, Olmo DD, Pereira JL, Tous MC, Olveira G. Nutrition-related risk indexes and long-term mortality in noncritically ill inpatients who receive total parenteral nutrition (prospective multicenter study). *Clin Nutr* 2014;34(5): 962–967

6. Olveira G, Tapia MJ, Ocon J, Cabrejas-Gomez C, Ballesteros-Pomar MD, Vidal-Casariego A, Arraiza-Irigoyen C, Olivares J, Conde-Garcia MC, Garcia-Manzanares A, Botella-Romero F, Quilez-Toboso RP, Cabrerizo L, Matia P, Chicharro L, Burgos R, Pujante P, Ferrer M, Zugasti A, Prieto J, Dieguez M, Carrera MJ, Vila-Bundo A, Urgeles JR, Aragon-Valera C, Rovira A, Breton I, Garcia-Peris P, Munoz-Garach A, Marquez E, Del OD, Pereira JL, Tous MC. Parenteral nutrition-associated hyperglycemia in non-critically ill inpatients increases the risk of in-hospital mortality (multicenter study). *Diabetes Care* 2013;36:1061–1066

7. Umpierrez GE, Hellman R, Korytkowski MT, Kosiborod M, Maynard GA, Montori VM, Seley JJ, Van den Berghe G. Management of hyperglycemia in hospitalized patients in non-critical care setting: an Endocrine Society clinical practice guideline. *J Clin Endocrinol Metab* 2012;97:16–38

8. Marik PE, Preiser JC. Toward understanding tight glycemic control in the ICU: a systematic review and metaanalysis. *Chest* 2010;137:544–551

9. McMahon MM, Nystrom E, Braunschweig C, Miles J, Compher C. ASPEN clinical guidelines: nutrition support of adult patients with hyperglycemia. *JPEN J Parenter Enteral Nutr* 2013;37:23–36

10. Finfer S, Chittock DR, Su SY, Blair D, Foster D, Dhingra V, Bellomo R, Cook D, Dodek P, Henderson WR, Hebert PC, Heritier S, Heyland DK, McArthur C, McDonald E, Mitchell I, Myburgh JA, Norton R, Potter J, Robinson BG, Ronco JJ. Intensive versus conventional glucose control in critically ill patients. *N Engl J Med* 2009;360:1283–1297

11. Cheung NW, Napier B, Zaccaria C, Fletcher JP. Hyperglycemia is associated with adverse outcomes in patients receiving total parenteral nutrition. *Diabetes Care* 2005;28:2367–2371

12. Jakoby MG, Nannapaneni N. An insulin protocol for management of hyperglycemia in patients receiving parenteral nutrition is superior to ad hoc management. *JPEN J Parenter Enteral Nutr* 2012;36:183–188

13. Neff K, Donegan D, MacMahon J, O'Hanlon C, Keane N, Agha A, Thompson C, Smith D. Management of parenteral nutrition associated hyperglycaemia: a comparison of subcutaneous and intravenous insulin regimen. *Ir Med J* 2014;107:141–143

14. Ahrens CL, Barletta JF, Kanji S, Tyburski JG, Wilson RF, Janisse JJ, Devlin JW. Effect of low-calorie parenteral nutrition on the incidence and severity of hyperglycemia in surgical patients: a randomized, controlled trial. *Crit Care Med* 2005;33:2507–2512

15. Low Wang CC, Draznin B. Practical approach to management of inpatient hyperglycemia in select patient populations. *Hosp Pract* 2013;41:45–53

16. Korytkowski MT, Salata RJ, Koerbel GL, Selzer F, Karslioglu E, Idriss AM, Lee KK, Moser AJ, Toledo FG. Insulin therapy and glycemic control in hospitalized patients with diabetes during enteral nutrition therapy: a randomized controlled clinical trial. *Diabetes Care* 2009;32:594–596

17. Cook A, Burkitt D, McDonald L, Sublett L. Evaluation of glycemic control using NPH insulin sliding scale versus insulin aspart sliding scale in continuously tube-fed patients. *Nutr Clin Pract* 2009;24:718–722
18. Hsia E, Seggelke SA, Gibbs J, Rasouli N, Draznin B. Comparison of 70/30 biphasic insulin with glargine/lispro regimen in non-critically ill diabetic patients on continuous enteral nutrition therapy. *Nutr Clin Pract* 2011;26:714–717
19. Elia M, Ceriello A, Laube H, Sinclair AJ, Engfer M, Stratton RJ. Enteral nutritional support and use of diabetes-specific formulas for patients with diabetes: a systematic review and meta-analysis. *Diabetes Care* 2005;28:2267–2279
20. Draznin B, Gilden J, Golden SH, Inzucchi SE, Baldwin D, Bode BW, Boord JB, Braithwaite SS, Cagliero E, Dungan KM, Falciglia M, Figaro MK, Hirsch IB, Klonoff D, Korytkowski MT, Kosiborod M, Lien LF, Magee MF, Masharani U, Maynard G, McDonnell ME, Moghissi ES, Rasouli N, Rubin DJ, Rushakoff RJ, Sadhu AR, Schwartz S, Seley JJ, Umpierrez GE, Vigersky RA, Low CC, Wexler DJ. Pathways to quality inpatient management of hyperglycemia and diabetes: a call to action. *Diabetes Care* 2013;36:1807–1814

Chapter 7

Steroid-Associated Hyperglycemia

Nestoras Mathioudakis, MD,[1] Kathleen Dungan, MD,[2] David Baldwin, MD,[3] Mary Korytkowski, MD,[4] and Jodie Reider, MD[5]

Systemic steroids (glucocorticoids) are used ubiquitously in the hospital for a variety of indications. Although they have clear and wide-ranging benefits, they are also a major contributor to severe hyperglycemia. In patients with and without preexisting diabetes, steroids can exacerbate glycemic control and can make glucose management in the hospital challenging. Variability in steroid type, dose, and dosing schedules poses additional challenges to proactive adjustments in glycemic management strategies that promote safe blood glucose (BG) control and avoidance of hypoglycemia. Moreover, many patients receiving steroids have comorbid conditions or are receiving other medications that can affect glucose homeostasis. An understanding of the pathophysiology and pattern of steroid-associated hyperglycemia is necessary to guide management of hospitalized patients on steroids.

DEFINITIONS

The terms *steroid-induced hyperglycemia* and *steroid-induced diabetes* often are used interchangeably to refer to elevated BG in people without preexisting diabetes in the setting of steroid use. This chapter uses the term *steroid-associated hyperglycemia* to describe the phenomenon of hyperglycemia that occurs in patients with or without preexisting diabetes who are receiving steroids.

PREVALENCE

Most studies on the prevalence of steroid-associated hyperglycemia have relied on data from the outpatient setting. A meta-analysis of 13 studies found that patients receiving steroids (of varying doses and duration) developed hyperglycemia and diabetes at a rate of ~20% and ~30%, respectively.[1] In a study of 50 hospitalized patients on the medicine service, treatment with high-dose steroids (≥40 mg/day

[1]Assistant Professor of Medicine, Division of Endocrinology, Diabetes, & Metabolism, Associate Director, Inpatient Diabetes Management Service, Johns Hopkins School of Medicine, Baltimore, MD. [2]Ohio State University, Wexner Medical Center, Columbus, OH. [3]Rush University Medical School, Chicago, IL. [4]Division of Endocrinology and Metabolism, University of Pittsburgh, Pittsburgh, PA. [5]Director, Inpatient Diabetes/Endocrine Program, Clinical Assistant Professor of Medicine, Division of Endocrinology & Metabolism, University of Pittsburgh, Pittsburgh, PA.

DOI: 10.2337/9781580406086.07

of prednisone or equivalent) for at least 2 days resulted in steroid-associated hyperglycemia among 56% of patients without preexisting diabetes and 64% of patients overall (of whom approximately half had diabetes).[2] Multiple episodes of hyperglycemia were found to be associated with comorbid diseases, longer duration of steroid use, and longer hospital stay.[2] In another study of 80 hospitalized patients without preexisting diabetes receiving high-dose steroids (≥25 mg of prednisone or approximate equivalent) for at least 2 days, 70% had a BG >180 mg/dL, typically within the first 48 h of treatment.[3]

The main risk factors for steroid-associated hyperglycemia include the traditional risk factors for type 2 diabetes (T2D), such as age, body mass index (BMI), and impaired glucose tolerance[4]. Additional risk factors include concurrent immunosuppression, particularly calcineurin inhibitors (cyclosporine and tacrolimus). It is difficult, however, to predict which patients will and will not develop hyperglycemia in response to steroid therapy.[5]

PATTERN OF STEROID-ASSOCIATED HYPERGLYCEMIA

Steroids cause hyperglycemia through multiple mechanisms, including suppression of insulin secretion, increased gluconeogenesis, and decreased glucose uptake from blunted insulin sensitivity.[4] Prolonged use of glucocorticoids has been shown to cause β-cell dysfunction with impaired insulin release in a dose-dependent manner.[4,6,7] The glycemic effect of short-acting steroids is often exaggerated in the fed state compared with the fasting state, resulting in a pattern of marked postprandial hyperglycemia and less of an effect on fasting BG.[3,8,9] This effect, however is not the result of a defect in prandial glucose regulation, but rather reflects the time course of steroid action, which typically is dosed in the morning.[10] Therefore, steroid-associated hyperglycemia can be missed if only fasting BG levels are monitored. Figure 7.1*A* shows the typical pattern of steroid-associated hyperglycemia in diabetic patients following short-term prednisone treatment: marked postprandial hyperglycemia after breakfast and particularly lunch, with return to normal fasting BG the following morning.[11] A similar but less dramatic pattern is observed in patients with normal glucose tolerance and prediabetes.[11]

STEROID DOSE AND GLYCEMIC EFFECT

The hyperglycemic effect of steroids is influenced by the steroid potency, duration of action, route of administration, and duration of use. An early study in healthy subjects showed similar acute hyperglycemic effects following equipotent doses of hydrocortisone, dexamethasone, and prednisone, with a slightly higher postprandial BG effect from hydrocortisone and a more pronounced insulin resistance from dexamethasone.[12] Although this study showed a similar acute postprandial glycemic response, there are no studies comparing the long-term (i.e., 24-h or 48-h) glycemic effects of differing steroid types at equivalent doses. In a prospective study of hospitalized patients without diabetes receiving high-dose steroids, the prevalence of hyperglycemia was similar comparing prednisone to dexamethasone, but the mean BG values were higher in patients receiving dexamethasone (162 mg/dL vs. 138.6 mg/dL), likely related to its longer biological action.[3]

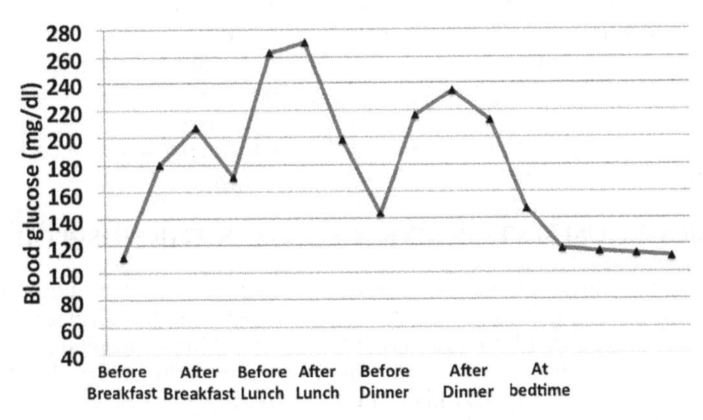

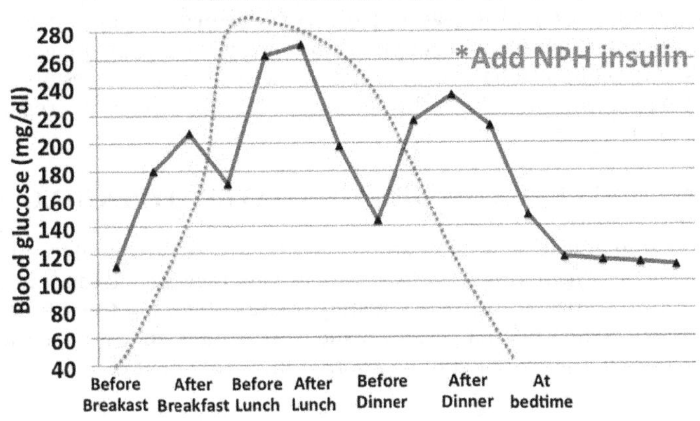

Figure 7.1—*A*: Pattern of steroid-associated hyperglycemia following 3-day course of morning prednisone 20 mg daily in patients with T2D. *B*: Dashed line shows pharmacodynamic profile of NPH insulin, which closely mirrors the hyperglycemic pattern following oral prednisone.

Source: Figure adapted from Yuen et al.[11]

Few studies have characterized the effect of steroid dose on changes in BG levels. In one study of healthy subjects, only the high doses of methylprednisolone (80 mg/day) or hydrocortisone (400 mg/day) resulted in impaired glucose tolerance (with a more dramatic effect resulting from methylprednisolone).[13] Similar findings were seen in a study of dexamethasone in healthy subjects, in which only high-dose dexamethasone (8 mg/day) resulted in significant postprandial hyperglycemia.[14] In this study, there was an ~20% increase in BG when the dose was escalated from medium dose (4 mg) to high dose (8 mg), which is important to bear in mind when considering the effects of a steroid taper on insulin requirements.[14] In another study, there was a similar 20% increase in the peak postprandial BG when prednisolone was increased from low dose (7.5 mg) to medium dose (30 mg).[7] Finally, in nondiabetic subjects receiving 1 g pulses of intravenous (IV) methylprednisolone, there was a steady 15% rise in fasting BG with each successive dose.[15]

COMMONLY USED STEROID REGIMENS IN THE HOSPITAL

Table 7.1 shows the relative potencies and duration of biological action of commonly used inpatient steroid regimens. Hydrocortisone has a relatively short duration of action of 8–12 hours and is most often used in the hospital at very high doses for acute conditions (i.e., septic shock or status asthmaticus). Prednisone, prednisolone, and methylprednisolone have similar potency and duration of action (12–16 h) and are used widely for chronic obstructive pulmonary disease (COPD) exacerbations, acute gout, immunosuppression after solid organ transplantation, autoimmune diseases, alcoholic hepatitis, and malignancy.[16] Dexamethasone is a potent, long-acting (20–36 h) steroid frequently used for neurological conditions or as an antiemetic following anesthesia or chemotherapy. Given its long biological half-life and high doses, it frequently results in severe inpatient hyperglycemia in both the fasting and postprandial state, regardless of the presence or absence of diabetes.

REASONS TO TREAT STEROID-ASSOCIATED HYPERGLYCEMIA

The main arguments in favor of treating steroid-associated hyperglycemia are the following: *1*) the glycemic effects of steroids are often severe and can lead to dehydration or even ketoacidosis if inadequately treated, *2*) failure to treat could lead to renal impairment from dehydration, and *3*) treatment may reduce the risk of infection and other potential complications. Once treatment commences, failure

Table 7.1—Comparison of Commonly Used Steroids

Steroid name	Equivalent dose (mg)	Estimated duration of biological action (h)
Hydrocortisone	20	8–12
Prednisone	5	12–16
Prednisolone	5	12–16
Methylprednisolone	4	12–16
Dexamethasone	0.75	20–36

Source: Perez et al.[30]

to adequately adjust insulin doses during a steroid taper can lead to hypoglycemia, which is associated with an increased risk of neurological complications, ischemic events, and in-hospital mortality.[16]

Few studies have explored the impact of intensive insulin therapy on clinical outcomes in patients with steroid-associated hyperglycemia. In one randomized study of 52 patients with acute lymphoblastic leukemia, basal-bolus insulin (BBI) therapy did not improve survival or clinical outcomes, and the study was terminated early because of medical futility.[17] Most patients, however, had glucose levels <200 mg/dL, and the separation of glucose levels between treatment arms may not have been adequate. In another study of patients with non-Hodgkin's lymphoma, hyperglycemia during chemotherapy was associated with increased chemotherapy-related toxicity.[18]

GENERAL MANAGEMENT RECOMMENDATIONS

No large randomized controlled trials have investigated the optimal management strategy for steroid-associated hyperglycemia.[19] The recommendations proposed in this chapter are derived from observational studies and expert opinion. Expert guidelines recommend the use of IV insulin for management of hyperglycemia, regardless of etiology, in most critically ill patients.[19] This section will focus on the use of subcutaneous (SQ) insulin injections in noncritically ill patients receiving steroids.

Because the extent of hyperglycemia can differ between patients with and without diabetes, we divide the management approach into two categories. Figure 7.2 shows the stepwise approach to initial management in patients with preexisting diabetes and Figure 7.3 shows the approach to steroid-associated hyperglycemia in patients without preexisting diabetes. In all patients, glucose monitoring should be conducted at least four times per day (premeal and at bedtime).

Three treatment approaches have been advocated for prevention and treatment of steroid-associated hyperglycemia in those with and without preexisisting diabetes in the hospital.

1. The first approach uses once- or twice-daily NPH insulin to "counteract" the hyperglycemic effect of steroids.[10,20] The rationale for this approach is that the pharmacodynamic profile of NPH, with a peak effect of 4–8 h and duration of action of 12–16 h, mirrors the pharmacodynamics of prednisone or prednisolone (Figure 7.1*B*). NPH should be dosed in the morning for patients receiving steroids once daily in the morning (e.g., prednisone or prednisolone) to avoid overnight hypoglycemia. NPH should be dosed twice daily for patients who are on a twice-daily steroid dosing schedule (e.g., prednisone or methylprednisolone). Typically, these patients also will need rapid-acting insulin with meals.
2. A second approach uses a BBI regimen using glargine or detemir once daily and rapid-acting insulin with meals. When facing the long biological half-life of dexamethasone and its "flatter" pharmacodynamic profile, a BBI regimen or twice-daily (BID) NPH are both effective approaches. In patients with severe hyperglycemia, it may be advantageous to use NPH

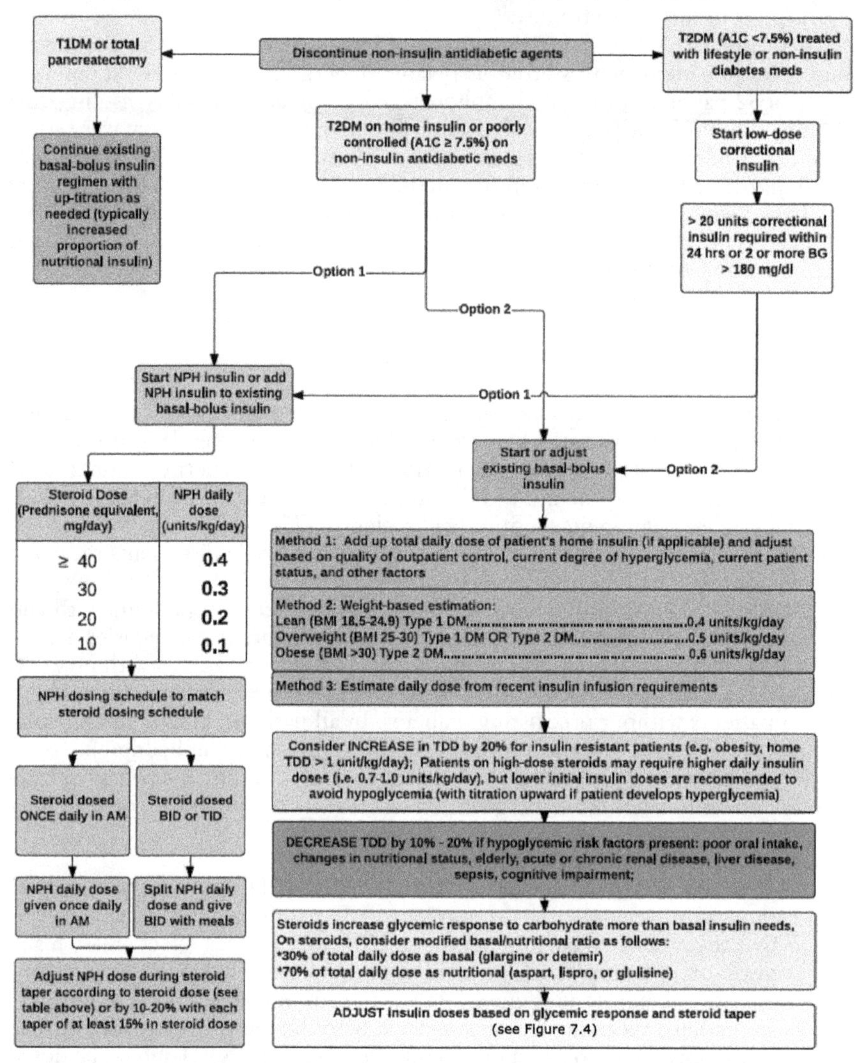

Figure 7.2—Suggested approach to initial management of steroid-associated hyperglycemia in patients with preexisting diabetes. BMI, body mass index; TDD, total daily dose; BID, twice daily; TID, three times daily.

because it can be uptitrated twice daily as compared with glargine or detemir.

3. The third treatment approach involves a modified BBI regimen containing a lower proportion of basal insulin (30%) and higher proportion of

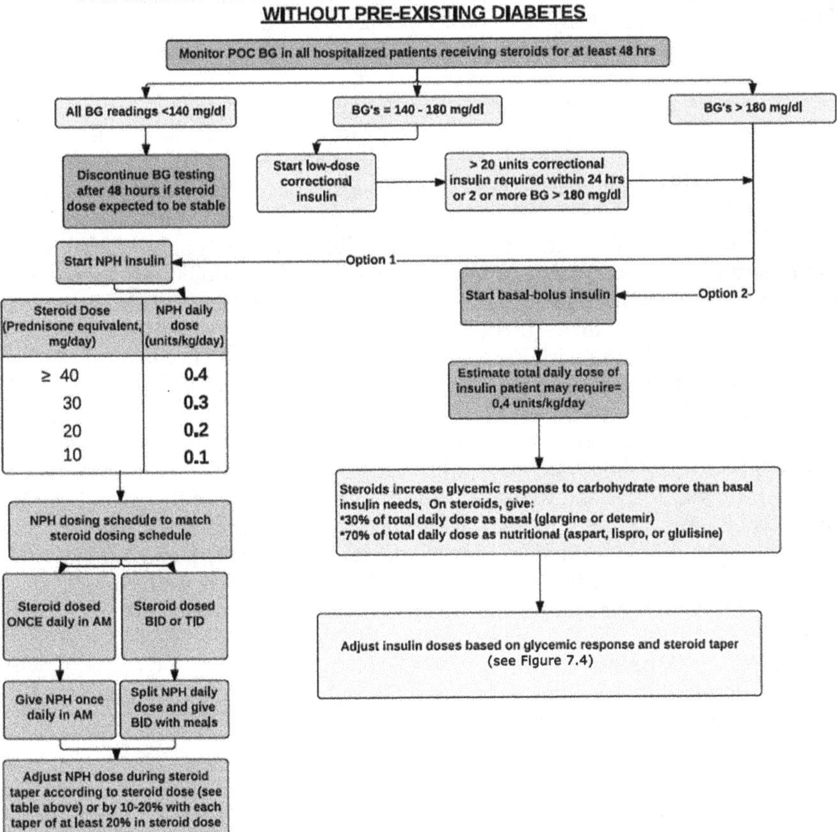

Figure 7.3—Suggested approach to initial management of steroid-induced hyperglycemia in patients without preexisting diabetes. BG, blood glucose; BID, twice daily; TID, three times daily.

nutritional insulin (70%), in contrast to the typical basal–nutritional ratio of 50/50 or 40/60. The rationale for this approach is the higher requirement for nutritional insulin observed with short-acting steroids. Providing a lower percentage of the total daily dose (TDD) as basal insulin reduces the potential for fasting hypoglycemia during a steroid taper.

Both NPH insulin and glargine have been shown to be equally effective in management of steroid-associated hyperglycemia. In a retrospective study of 120 patients with steroid-associated hyperglycemia (with and without preexisting diabetes), basal insulin provided either in the form of glargine or NPH insulin resulted in similar mean fasting BG concentrations with an average 30 mg daily dose of prednisone.[21] Total daily insulin requirements, however, were slightly lower in the NPH cohort compared with the glargine cohort. This is likely due to the fact that NPH provides some nutritional in addition to basal coverage.[21] Despite concerns about higher hypoglycemia risk with NPH, the rates of hypoglycemia were similar in both cohorts. In another study of patients with cystic fibrosis–related diabetes receiving methylprednisolone following transplantation, the addition of NPH to an existing BBI regimen with glargine and lispro insulin resulted in similar fasting BG readings but lower prelunch and predinner BG readings in the NPH cohort.[20] Limitations of this study were the lack of aggressive nutritional insulin titration in the BBI group, short duration of follow-up, and small sample size.[20]

The choice of NPH and rapid-acting insulin versus glargine or detemir and rapid-acting insulin may depend largely in part on institutional experience with either approach. Advantages of using NPH insulin include *1)* the ability to continue baseline insulin doses throughout the hospital stay while independently tapering the NPH dose with a steroid taper and *2)* possibly fewer insulin injections for patients who are not already on a BBI regimen at home.[10] This approach, however, has some recognized limitations. NPH will need to be dosed BID in patients taking dexamethasone or methylprednisolone/prednisone dosed BID. Nursing personnel should be made aware of the rationale for the timing of NPH and steroid administration to prevent mismatched delivery of these medications in a busy hospital setting. A limitation of the modified BBI approach is that changes in the dose of nutritional insulin during steroid tapers may not be intuitive, and it may not be effective in patients who are not eating well.[10]

Regardless of which scheduled insulin regimen is used, management with sliding-scale insulin (SSI) *alone* for patients with hyperglycemia is not recommended as it consistently has been shown to be inferior to BBI.[22] Compared with SSI, BBI resulted in 2.5 times more insulin being given, suggesting that SSI does not provide sufficient coverage for steroid-associated hyperglycemia.[22]

INITIAL MANAGEMENT

PATIENTS WITH PREEXISTING DIABETES

Discontinue Noninsulin Antidiabetic Medications

Noninsulin antidiabetic agents should be discontinued in the majority of hospitalized patients (including those receiving steroids) for several reasons. If steroids are used, it is difficult to adjust oral or noninsulin medications in parallel with steroid tapers, and there is the potential for hypoglycemia with agents that increase both basal and postprandial insulin secretion. Steroid-associated hyperglycemia can be significant and often is unlikely to be treated adequately with oral medications or the patient's usual diabetes regimen. Although some preliminary evidence suggests that glucagon-like peptide-1 receptor agonists have promise in the management of steroid-associated hyperglycemia, long-term studies are needed to evaluate their role in this clinical context.[23,24]

T1D or Total Pancreatectomy

For insulin-deficient patients with type 1 diabetes (T1D) or a history of total pancreatectomy, we generally recommend continuing the existing BBI regimen with uptitration as needed. These patients tend to be more insulin sensitive at baseline and may require only modest increases in their nutritional insulin dose to address the predominantly postprandial hyperglycemia from steroids. This applies to patients on insulin pumps, who may require more significant changes in their daytime insulin-to-carbohydrate ratio or insulin sensitivity (correction) factor compared with their basal rates.

Little data are available to guide insulin dose adjustments in patients with T1D receiving steroids. In a small study of 10 patients with T1D given a 3-day course of prednisone 60 mg daily, the mean total daily insulin dose increased from 0.5 units/kg/day to 0.9 units/kg/day during prednisone treatment and decreased to 0.6 units/kg/day the day following prednisone treatment.[25] In another study of pregnant women with T1D who received two daily intramuscular injections of betamethasone 12 mg, total daily insulin requirements increased by as much as 40%.[26]

T2D Treated with Insulin or Poorly Controlled on Oral Agents

For patients with T2D who are already taking insulin or who are uncontrolled ($HbA_{1c} \geq 7.5\%$) on noninsulin antidiabetic medications, we recommend scheduled insulin therapy with once- or twice-daily NPH or BBI. Beginning with weight-based insulin, dosing is appropriate for insulin-naïve patients. Substantial dose modifications typically are required on a daily basis for patients already taking insulin.

T2D Well-Controlled with Lifestyle or Noninsulin Medications

For patients with T2D who are fairly well controlled (HbA_{1c} <7.5%) as outpatients with lifestyle modification or noninsulin diabetes medications only, we recommend that noninsulin medications be discontinued and the patient be started initially on a low-dose correctional insulin. If more than 20 units of correctional insulin are required in a 24-h period to maintain BG within the desired range or the patient has two or more BG levels >180 mg/dL, we recommend that the patient receive scheduled therapy with either NPH or BBI.

NPH Insulin

NPH insulin can be given to supplement an existing basal insulin regimen or an existing BBI regimen,[20] or it can be given alone with a rapid-acting bolus insulin.[21] When used in this fashion, it can be thought of as providing predominantly prandial insulin coverage and offsetting any increase in bolus insulin. The dose of NPH can be determined using an estimate proposed by Clore and Thurby-Hay[10] (based largely on clinical experience) of 0.1 units of NPH per kg of body weight per 10 mg of prednisone equivalent to a maximum initial dose of 0.4 units/kg for doses ≥40 mg/day of prednisone.[10] The frequency of NPH (daily versus BID) dosing depends on the dosing schedule of the steroid. If morning NPH is given in combination with prandial insulin, prandial insulin may be required only before breakfast and dinner, because the NPH may provide sufficient nutritional coverage at lunch.

Modified (30/70) BBI Regimen

To start a BBI regimen, the first step is to estimate the TDD (Figure 7.2). For patients already on home insulin, the home TDD can be adjusted up or down based on the quality of outpatient glycemic control, patient's clinical status, and risk factors for hypoglycemia. As a rule of thumb, a total insulin dose of 0.4–0.5 units/kg/day is appropriate for many patients with T2D not on steroids, but a dose of 0.25 units/kg/day or lower may be required for elderly patients or people with chronic kidney disease.[27,28] For patients who are insulin resistant at baseline (i.e., home TDD >1 unit/kg/day) or obese, the glycemic effect of steroids is expected to be exaggerated, so an additional 20% increase in the TDD may be needed. Caution is necessary for patients who take higher home TDD insulin (i.e., >0.8 units/kg/day) particularly if the patient has tight outpatient glycemic control given the risk of hypoglycemia. Furthermore, adjustments should be made in the total insulin dose if hypoglycemic risk factors are present, such as poor oral intake, changes in nutritional status, acute or chronic renal disease (especially hemodialysis), liver disease, sepsis, and cognitive impairment. For patients transitioning from an IV insulin infusion, SQ insulin requirements can be inferred from stable insulin infusion rates.

Some patients with steroid-associated hyperglycemia may require a higher TDD of insulin (i.e., 0.7–1.0 units/kg/day or more), especially if their baseline insulin requirements are high. In a retrospective study of noncritically ill patients receiving an average daily dose of 30 mg of prednisone, an average TDD of insulin of nearly 0.8 units/kg/day was required to achieve glycemic control.[29] Because it is difficult to predict whether patients will develop steroid-associated hyperglycemia, we recommend conservative starting doses with uptitration using higher weight-based estimates or correctional insulin requirements.

After selecting a starting TDD, this should be divided into 30% basal insulin and 70% nutritional insulin for steroid-treated patients who are eating regular meals. These ratios were selected based on clinical experience and are supported by findings of a recent retrospective study of hospitalized noncritically ill patients with diabetes and steroid-associated hyperglycemia.[29] This study found that compared with patients on steroids who achieved normoglycemia, those who did not achieve glycemic targets had a higher ratio of basal:TDD and lower ratio of nutritional:TDD.[29] In this study, the basal:TDD ratio was 30% and the nutritional:TDD was ~60% (with remaining being correctional insulin) in the normoglycemic group.[29] This ratio may require modification in patients who are not eating or who are treated with long-acting glucocorticoids or glucocorticoids dosed multiple times per day.

PATIENTS WITHOUT PREEXISTING DIABETES

A suggested stepwise approach to initial management of steroid-induced hyperglycemia in patients without preexisting diabetes is shown in Figure 7.3. The management principles are similar to those for patients with diabetes, with the main exception being a more conservative initial starting TDD for insulin-naïve patients. All patients treated with steroids should have frequent point-of-care BG monitoring for at least 48 h. Given the rapid onset of steroid-induced hyperglycemia, if all BG readings are <140 mg/dL within the first 48 h, it is unlikely that hyperglycemia will develop and BG monitoring can be safely discontinued. For patients with mild hyperglycemia (BG 140–180 mg/dL), we recommend initiation of a low-dose correctional insulin; however, if more than 20 units of correctional insulin are required within 24 h, scheduled insulin therapy should be initiated.

Patients with two or more BG readings >180 mg/dL should be started directly on scheduled insulin therapy.

NPH monotherapy may be an attractive option for management of steroid-induced hyperglycemia in patients on once-daily prednisone or prednisolone, especially if the time course of treatment is expected to be short. The dosing principles for NPH insulin are the same as for patients with T2D, but the main difference is that NPH may be used alone in these cases rather than in conjunction with BBI.

If BBI is to be started, we recommend a conservative starting dose of 0.4 units/kg/day in insulin-naïve patients, with adjustment of the dose based on consideration of factors that can increase or decrease the BG. The TDD should be distributed as either a typical BBI or modified BBI regimen, as described previously.

For patients with steroid-induced hyperglycemia for whom steroids are expected to be discontinued shortly after discharge, it may be reasonable to stop insulin completely if BG readings are consistently <180 mg/dL before discharge. If insulin is continued, instructions should be provided to the patient on how to taper the insulin doses based on monitored BG readings at home. As a rule of thumb, we recommend decreasing the TDD or NPH dose by 10–20% for fasting BG <120 mg/dL. Close follow-up with a primary care physician or diabetes provider should be arranged following discharge for these patients. Alternatively, the dose can continue to be adjusted according to a weight-based algorithm for each 10 mg prednisone equivalent decrease in the dose of steroid.[10] For example, a patient receiving 0.4 units/kg of NPH insulin for prednisone 40 mg could be reduced to 0.3 units/kg of NPH when prednisone is decreased to 30 mg.[10]

ADJUSTING INSULIN

Given that steroid doses often are tapered over a period of several days to weeks, proactive adjustments in insulin doses are needed to maintain good glycemic control and avoid hypoglycemia. Figure 7.4 provides a suggested approach to adjusting insulin in patients receiving BBI. The approach to adjusting NPH insulin relies on the steroid dose conversion tables shown in Figure 7.2 and Figure 7.3.

The first step to adjusting insulin is to review the BG readings over the previous 24 h and to identify glycemic patterns. The main factor to consider when adjusting insulin doses is whether the steroid dose is expected to be reduced (by at least 15%) over the subsequent 24 h. In general, the extent of adjustment depends on the extent and consistency of hyperglycemia or hypoglycemia and consideration of other hypoglycemic risk factors.

Case Example 1: Obese Patient with Well-Controlled T2D Started on High-Dose Prednisone

A 62-year-old obese man with well-controlled T2D (HbA_{1c} 6.8%) is admitted to the hospital for a COPD exacerbation. At home, he takes glargine insulin 50 units at bedtime, metformin, and liraglutide. Prednisone 60 mg daily is prescribed. He weighs 100 kg with a BMI of 37.8 kg/m^2. Other than insulin therapy, he has no hypoglycemic risk factors. On hospital day 2, the patient's fasting BG is 176 mg/dL and daytime BG readings are 247–413 mg/dL. What are the possible treatment approaches?

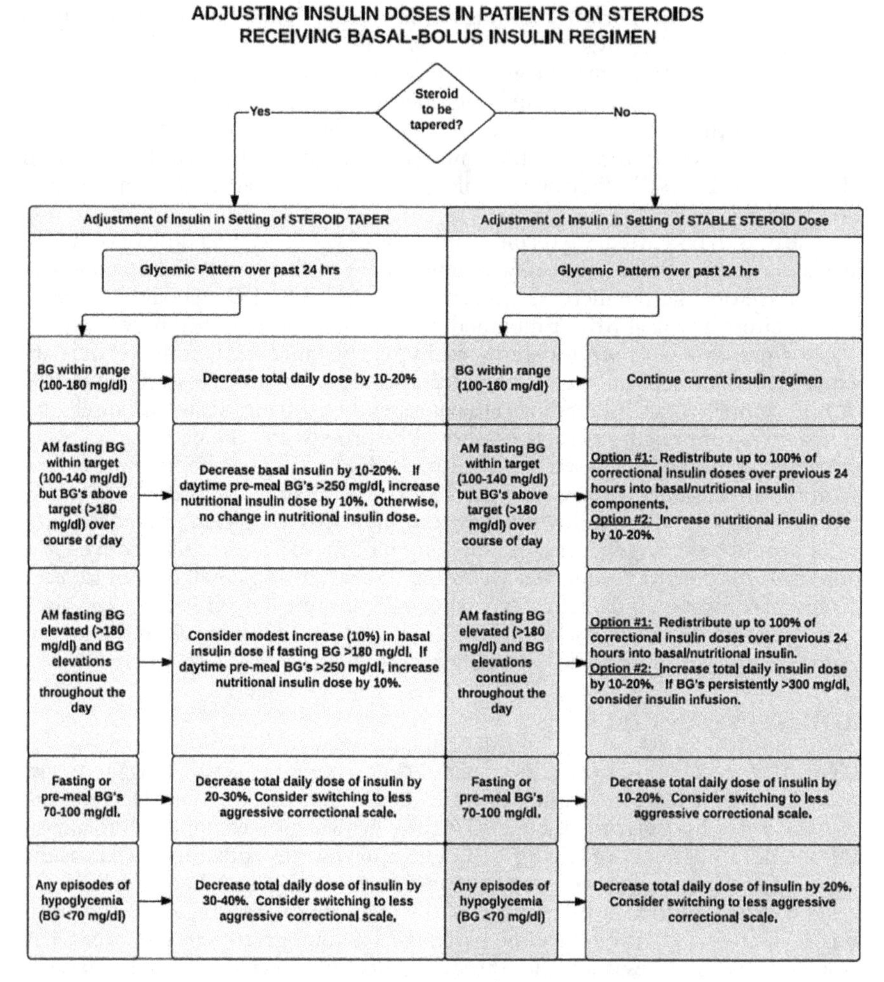

Figure 7.4—Suggested approach to adjusting basal-bolus insulin regimen in patients receiving steroids. BG, blood glucose.

One option is to continue glargine insulin 50 units at bedtime and add NPH 40 units with breakfast (0.4 units/kg/day) to be given concurrently with the prednisone dose, as well as a correctional insulin scale before meals and bedtime to determine the need for additional prandial insulin. Another option is to start a modified BBI insulin regimen. At 0.6 units/kg/day, a weight-based estimate of the TDD is 60 units. Because the patient is obese and likely to be insulin resistant, a 20% increase in this TDD could be made (i.e., 72 units/day). This dose would be divided into 30% basal/70% nutritional as follows: 22 units of glargine and 17 units of aspart with meals. Although the basal insulin dose in the hospital is lower than his home basal insulin, the initiation of standing nutritional insulin should target the largely postprandial hyperglycemic effect of prednisone. All doses would require daily titration based on frequent BG monitoring and steroid dosing.

Case Example 2: Lean Patient with Well-Controlled T2D on High-Dose Dexamethasone

A 68-year-old woman with T2D controlled on metformin and sitagliptin (HbA_{1c} 6.8%) is admitted to the hospital for an exacerbation of multiple sclerosis. Dexamethasone 4 mg every 6 h is started, with plans to reduce to 12 mg/day after 1 week. The patient has a BMI of 23.4 kg/m^2 and weighs 61 kg. The fasting BG on hospital day 2 is 204 mg/dL with later readings between 250–400 mg/dL. What are the possible options?

At 0.5 units/kg/day, this patient is expected to require at least 30 units of insulin daily. Because the patient is on a long-acting steroid, one option is to use a modified BBI partitioned into 30% basal insulin (glargine 10 units) and 70% nutritional insulin (rapid-acting 7 units with meals). On hospital day 3, the patient requires 12 units of correctional insulin, which you redistribute into basal and nutritional components. By hospital day 4, on a TDD of 42 units (0.7 units/kg/day), BG readings are largely between 140 and 180 mg/dL.

Another option is to start with NPH dosed twice daily. After converting the dose of dexamethasone to its prednisone equivalent, you determine a starting dose of NPH insulin of 0.4 units/kg/day (61 kg = 24 units). You divide this into 12 units of NPH twice daily and increase doses based on daily correctional insulin requirements.

Case Example 3: Patient with No History of Diabetes on High-Dose Methylprednisolone

A 58-year-old obese man with no prior history of diabetes is admitted for an episode of acute gout. He weighs 110 kg. He has stage III chronic kidney disease (CKD) with a glomerular filtration rate of 56 mL/min. Methylprednisolone 20 mg IV twice daily is started. The first three BG readings are 194, 218, and 235 mg/dL. What are the possible treatment approaches?

One approach is to start NPH insulin. After converting the dose of methylprednisolone to its prednisone equivalent, you determine a starting dose of NPH insulin of 0.4 units/kg/day (110 kg = 44 units). You divide this into 22 units twice daily timed with each methylprednisolone dose. You also start a medium-dose correctional insulin scale.

Another option is to start a modified BBI at a conservative dose of 0.4 units/kg/day (i.e., 44 units). Although the patient has mild CKD, you elect not to reduce his TDD because you suspect that the insulin resistance conferred by his obesity will offset any effect of mildly reduced renal function on insulin clearance. You divide 44 units into 30% basal (i.e., 13 units) and 70% nutritional (i.e., 10 units with meals). In this case, both methods yield similar TDDs of insulin.

CONCLUSION

Following are summary points:

- All hospitalized patients receiving steroids should have point-of-care BG monitoring for the first 24–48 h to determine whether hyperglycemia is present.
- Noninsulin medications should be discontinued for the majority of patients with preexisting diabetes.
- For patients with T1D or total pancreatectomy, we recommend continuing a BBI regimen either with multiple daily injections or insulin pump therapy. If uptitration in doses is needed, the focus initially should be on increasing bolus insulin doses (i.e., insulin:carbohydrate ratio, insulin sensitivity factor) with consideration of increasing basal insulin if overnight and fasting BG levels are high.
- Patients with preexisting T2D and steroid-associated hyperglycemia can be managed with NPH once or twice daily or glargine or detemir along with mealtime rapid-acting insulin. A combination of NPH and BBI regimen also may be used.
- A modified basal-bolus ratio of 30% to 70% is preferred for management of steroid-associated hyperglycemia to target the largely postprandial hyperglycemic effect of steroids.
- Patients without preexisting diabetes who develop steroid-induced hyperglycemia are treated the same as patients with preexisting diabetes.
- Estimates of total daily insulin requirements should be adjusted for hyperglycemia and hypoglycemic risk factors.
- Insulin doses require proactive reductions during steroid tapers according to the rapidity of the taper. As a rule of thumb, 10–20% reductions in insulin doses may be required per reduction in steroid dose.

REFERENCES

1. Liu XX, Zhu XM, Miao Q, Ye HY, Zhang ZY, Li YM. Hyperglycemia induced by glucocorticoids in nondiabetic patients: a meta-analysis. *Ann Nutr Metab* 2014;65:324–332
2. Donihi AC, Raval D, Saul M, Korytkowski MT, DeVita MA. Prevalence and predictors of corticosteroid-related hyperglycemia in hospitalized patients. *Endocr Pract* 2006;12:358–362
3. Fong AC, Cheung NW. The high incidence of steroid-induced hyperglycaemia in hospital. *Diabetes Res Clin Pract* 2013;99:277–280
4. Hwang JL, Weiss RE. Steroid-induced diabetes: a clinical and molecular approach to understanding and treatment. *Diabetes Metab Res Rev* 2014;30:96–102
5. Even JL, Crosby CG, Song Y, McGirt MJ, Devin CJ. Effects of epidural steroid injections on blood glucose levels in patients with diabetes mellitus. *Spine* 2012;37:E46–50
6. Ranta F, Avram D, Berchtold S, Dufer M, Drews G, Lang F, Ullrich S. Dexamethasone induces cell death in insulin-secreting cells, an effect reversed by exendin-4. *Diabetes* 2006;55:1380–1390

7. van Raalte DH, Kwa KA, van Genugten RE, Tushuizen ME, Holst JJ, Deacon CF, Karemaker JM, Heine RJ, Mari A, Diamant M. Islet-cell dysfunction induced by glucocorticoid treatment: potential role for altered sympathovagal balance? *Metab Clin Experiment Metabolism: clinical and experimental* 2013;62:568–577
8. Burt MG, Roberts GW, Aguilar-Loza NR, Frith P, Stranks SN. Continuous monitoring of circadian glycemic patterns in patients receiving prednisolone for COPD. *J Clin Endocr Metab* 2011;96:1789–1796
9. Uzu T, Harada T, Sakaguchi M, Kanasaki M, Isshiki K, Araki S, Sugiomoto T, Koya D, Haneda M, Kashiwagi A, Yamauchi A. Glucocorticoid-induced diabetes mellitus: prevalence and risk factors in primary renal diseases. *Nephron Clin Pract* 2007;105:c54–c57
10. Clore JN, Thurby-Hay L. Glucocorticoid-induced hyperglycemia. *Endocr Pract* 2009;15:469–474
11. Yuen KC, McDaniel PA, Riddle MC. Twenty-four-hour profiles of plasma glucose, insulin, C-peptide and free fatty acid in subjects with varying degrees of glucose tolerance following short-term, medium-dose prednisone (20 mg/day) treatment: evidence for differing effects on insulin secretion and action. *Clin Endocrinol* 2012;77:224–232
12. Yasuda K, Hines E, 3rd, Kitabchi AE. Hypercortisolism and insulin resistance: comparative effects of prednisone, hydrocortisone, and dexamethasone on insulin binding of human erythrocytes. *J Clin Endocrinol Metab* 1982;55:910–915
13. Bruno A, Carucci P, Cassader M, Cavallo-Perin P, Gruden G, Olivetti C, Pagano G. Serum glucose, insulin and C-peptide response to oral glucose after intravenous administration of hydrocortisone and methylprednisolone in man. *Europ J Clin Pharmacol* 1994;46:411–415
14. Abdelmannan D, Tahboub R, Genuth S, Ismail-Beigi F. Effect of dexamethasone on oral glucose tolerance in healthy adults. *Endocr Pract* 2010;16: 770–777
15. Tamez Perez HE, Gomez de Ossio MD, Quintanilla Flores DL, Hernandez Coria MI, Tamez Pena AL, Cuz Perez GJ, Proskauer Pena SL. Glucose disturbances in non-diabetic patients receiving acute treatment with methylprednisolone pulses. *Revista da Associacao Medica Brasileira* 2012;58:125–128
16. Brutsaert E, Carey M, Zonszein J. The clinical impact of inpatient hypoglycemia. *J Diabetes Complicat* 2014;28:565–572
17. Vu K, Busaidy N, Cabanillas ME, Konopleva M, Faderl S, Thomas DA, O'Brien S, Broglio K, Ensor J, Escalante C, Andreeff M, Kantarjian H, Lavis V, Yeung SC. A randomized controlled trial of an intensive insulin regimen in patients with hyperglycemic acute lymphoblastic leukemia. *Clin Lymph Myeloma Leukemia* 2012;12:355–362
18. Brunello A, Kapoor R, Extermann M. Hyperglycemia during chemotherapy for hematologic and solid tumors is correlated with increased toxicity. *Am J Clin Oncol* 2011;34:292–296

19. Mathioudakis N, Golden SH. A comparison of inpatient glucose management guidelines: implications for patient safety and quality. *Curr Diab Rep* 2015;15:13
20. Seggelke SA, Gibbs J, Draznin B. Pilot study of using neutral protamine Hagedorn insulin to counteract the effect of methylprednisolone in hospitalized patients with diabetes. *J Hosp Med* 2011;6:175–176
21. Dhital SM, Shenker Y, Meredith M, Davis DB. A retrospective study comparing neutral protamine Hagedorn insulin with glargine as basal therapy in prednisone-associated diabetes mellitus in hospitalized patients. *Endocr Pract* 2012;18:712–719
22. Gosmanov AR, Goorha S, Stelts S, Peng L, Umpierrez GE. Management of hyperglycemia in diabetic patients with hematologic malignancies during dexamethasone therapy. *Endocr Pract* 2013;19:231–235
23. van Raalte DH, van Genugten RE, Linssen MM, Ouwens DM, Diamant M. Glucagon-like peptide-1 receptor agonist treatment prevents glucocorticoid-induced glucose intolerance and islet-cell dysfunction in humans. *Diabetes Care* 2011;34:412–417
24. Matsuo K, Nambu T, Matsuda Y, Kanai Y, Yonemitsu S, Muro S, Oki S. Evaluation of the effects of exenatide administration in patients with T2DM with worsened glycemic control caused by glucocorticoid therapy. *Intern Med* 2013;52:89–95
25. Bevier WC, Zisser HC, Jovanovic L, Finan DA, Palerm CC, Seborg DE, Doyle FJ, 3rd. Use of continuous glucose monitoring to estimate insulin requirements in patients with T1D mellitus during a short course of prednisone. *J Diabetes Sci Technol* 2008;2:578–583
26. Mathiesen ER, Christensen AB, Hellmuth E, Hornnes P, Stage E, Damm P. Insulin dose during glucocorticoid treatment for fetal lung maturation in diabetic pregnancy: test of an algorithm. *Acta Obstetricia et Gynecologica Scandinavica* 2002;81:835–839
27. Umpierrez GE, Hellman R, Korytkowski MT, Kosiborod M, Maynard GA, Montori VM, Seley JJ, Van den Berghe G, Endocrine Society. Management of hyperglycemia in hospitalized patients in non-critical care setting: an endocrine society clinical practice guideline. *J Clin Endocrinol Metab* 2012;97:16–38
28. Baldwin D, Apel J. Management of hyperglycemia in hospitalized patients with renal insufficiency or steroid-induced diabetes. *Curr Diab Rep* 2013;13:114–120
29. Spanakis EK, Shah N, Malhotra K, Kemmerer T, Yeh HC, Golden SH. Insulin requirements in non-critically ill hospitalized patients with diabetes and steroid-induced hyperglycemia. *Hosp Pract* 2014;42:23–30
30. Perez A, Jansen-Chaparro S, Saigi I, Bernal-Lopez MR, Minambres I, Gomez-Huelgas R. Glucocorticoid-induced hyperglycemia. *J Diabetes* 2014;6:9–20

Chapter 8

Transitioning from Intravenous to Subcutaneous Insulin

Lillian F. Lien, MD,[1] Cecilia C. Low Wang, MD,[2] Kathryn Evans Kreider, DNP, APRN, FNP-BC,[3] and David Baldwin, Jr., MD[4]

WHEN IS INTRAVENOUS INSULIN NEEDED?

Regular insulin delivered via the intravenous (IV) route was first studied for use in diabetic ketoacidosis >40 years ago.[1] Since then, the use of IV regular insulin infusion has become the standard of care for hospitalized patients presenting with hyperglycemic emergency (diabetic ketoacidosis [DKA] or hyperglycemic hyperosmolar syndrome [HHS]), for hyperglycemia in critical illness, and for any patient whose clinical situation requires optimal glucose control amid rapidly changing clinical circumstances. Frequent testing of point-of-care (POC) glucose levels allows providers to achieve glycemic control within a fairly narrow target range. Although the use of IV insulin infusion is now commonplace, the success of its use depends on factors such as adequate training of nursing staff, the frequency of POC glucose checks, protocol-driven adjustment of infusion rates along with safe clinical judgment, the alertness of providers and staff to changing clinical situations, and nutrition. Continuing staff education is a key element in the safe and effective use of insulin infusions, because the learning curve required to develop, implement, troubleshoot, and improve insulin infusion protocols is significant.

APPROPRIATE TIME TO TRANSITION FROM INTRAVENOUS TO SUBCUTANEOUS INSULIN

INDICATIONS THAT IT IS SAFE TO TRANSITION

Once a patient's clinical status has improved and stabilized, and she or he is able to begin ingesting food orally, the clinician can consider transitioning patients

[1]Division Chief of Endocrinology, Metabolism, and Diabetes, Professor of Medicine, University of Mississippi Medical Center, Jackson, MS. [2]Associate Professor of Medicine, Division of Endocrinology, Metabolism, and Diabetes, University of Colorado School of Medicine; Director, Glucose Management Team, University of Colorado Hospital, Aurora, CO. [3]Assistant Professor, Duke University School of Nursing; Nurse Practitioner, Endocrinology, Metabolism and Nutrition, Duke University Medical Center, Durham, NC. [4]Professor of Medicine, Division of Endocrinology and Metabolism, Rush University Medical Center, Chicago. IL.

DOI: 10.2337/9781580406086.08

from the IV insulin infusion to a regimen of subcutaneous (SQ)-administered insulin. Factors indicating that a safe transition may be attempted include a blood glucose (BG) within the target range (generally 140–180 mg/dL) and low variability in insulin infusion rates. Some authors suggest that the transition is more likely to be successful if the infusion rate is less than 2 units/h and recent BG are all <130 mg/dL.[2]

INDICATIONS THAT IT IS *NOT* SAFE TO TRANSITION

During important clinical situations, it simply is not safe to attempt an IV to SQ insulin transition. These include hemodynamic instability manifested by hypotension or the need for pressors, significant soft tissue edema preventing effective absorption of injected insulin, high insulin infusion rates (>3 units/h), and markedly variable insulin infusion rates or BG. Clinically unstable patients are not likely to be good candidates for transitioning to SQ insulin. Patients who have undergone tracheostomy and require mechanical ventilation but otherwise are clinically stable likely can tolerate transitioning to an SQ regimen as long as other factors such as soft tissue edema are absent. Other factors that predict difficulty with transition to SQ insulin include advanced age of the patient,[3] high hemoglobin A_{1c} (HbA_{1c}) upon admission,[4] intensive care status, or corticosteroid administration.[5] Generally, if the patient is still on a high insulin infusion rate (>6 units/h), it may be more difficult to transition the patient to SQ-administered insulin without significant rebound hyperglycemia. Patients who are requiring large doses of insulin per hour typically have a clear contributory reason, such as vasopressors, high dose steroids, immediate postoperative status, or sepsis. Patients requiring high insulin doses should be reevaluated in 24 h.

CARE OF THE PATIENT WHO REQUIRES IV INSULIN BUT IS EATING (IV PLUS SQ WITH THE INFUSION)

Occasionally, patients receiving IV insulin infusion therapy are clinically stable enough to eat. Examples of clinical situations in which this might occur include the following: *1*) patients who have undergone solid organ transplant and are requiring an IV infusion because of high doses of glucocorticoids, or *2*) patients who have undergone a nonabdominal surgery and are having their diet advanced while still receiving insulin infusion therapy for severe hyperglycemia. Because insulin infusion rates are adjusted retroactively in response to changes in BG and the half-life of IV insulin is only minutes, food intake while on an IV insulin infusion can result in marked fluctuations in the infusion rate with repeated BG levels outside of the target range.

SQ rapid-acting insulin administered with food while using an insulin infusion for basal insulin coverage is an effective solution to this problem. Some institutions use a conservative dosing regimen such as 2–4 units per meal, with the insulin infusion rate guiding administration of small doses of rapid-acting insulin with food intake. Another practical method is to administer rapid-acting insulin using a carbohydrate-to-insulin ratio to calculate the required dose. A ratio of 1 unit of insulin for every 15 g of carbohydrates would be a reasonable starting point for patients with diabetes or patients with severe insulin resistance on high insulin infusion rates, whereas a ratio of 1 unit insulin for every 25 g of carbohydrates could be used in patients without a prior diagnosis of diabetes. Any additional SQ insulin administration should prompt the care team to discuss transition off the insulin infusion.

PLANNING FOR TRANSITION

FACTORS TO CONSIDER BEFORE CALCULATING AN SQ DOSE

Determining the appropriate amount of insulin to administer is a complex process that involves an assessment of the insulin infusion requirements in addition to individual patient factors such as clinical stability, renal function, postoperative pain, food intake, active clinical issues, and comorbid conditions. The number of units of insulin delivered in a 24-h period via insulin infusion (units/h) does not translate directly to SQ insulin requirements without considering a few scenarios:

Was the infusion rate stable? In many situations, patients who are first placed on an IV infusion have variable rates that indicate the instability of the clinical situation. For example, patients who are admitted with DKA or HHS have high initial infusion rates, but these rates decrease dramatically once circulating insulin levels are restored. Data from the initial hours on the infusion should not be used to calculate total daily requirements.

Was the patient eating while on the insulin infusion? Many patients are NPO while on insulin infusions, allowing a calculation of basal requirements, but certain situations allow for the consumption of food or beverages containing carbohydrates. If the patient is not given prandial coverage with a rapid-acting insulin analog for carbohydrate intake, the BG will rise after food, followed by a significant increase in infusion rate. The provider should understand the patient's clinical scenario, including possible food or drink intake and should realize that the insulin rate is often affected by factors other than baseline metabolic requirements.

How much data are available? Obtaining 24 h of consistent data may be difficult in a hospitalized patient. At least 6 h of data (ideally, overnight while the patient is not eating) is recommended to extrapolate basal insulin requirements from the insulin infusion rates.[5–7]

What is the patient's glycemic control? Even if a patient has had stable insulin infusion rates, it is pertinent to evaluate the degree of glycemic control. If the BG levels have not been at goal (140–180 mg/dL), consider other reasons for this, as listed in the following sections. If the BG levels have not been at target, consider the need to increase the insulin administered to meet target levels.

What other factors are influencing the insulin infusion data? In addition to clinical stability, rate stability, and BG levels, consider other dynamics that may be influencing the data. These factors include the administration of corticosteroids or other medications known to increase BG, insulin resistance, surreptitious intake of food, technical failure of insulin delivery, or poor staff adherence to the insulin infusion protocol.

MECHANICS OF ACTUAL SQ DOSE CALCULATION

Once all the previously noted factors have been considered, one can move on to the mechanics of actual SQ insulin dose calculation, using the following steps:

1. Determine the **24-h *basal* insulin requirement.** Use a 6-h period of overnight (i.e., NPO) insulin infusion rates to determine the 24-h basal insulin requirement. Table 8.1 illustrates an example of the use of insulin infusion rates and BG data for the calculation.
2. Determine **what percentage of the basal insulin requirement** should be given as SQ insulin. Most experts suggest that <100% of the basal insulin requirement should be used as the SQ insulin basal dose to prevent hypoglycemia. Different percentages have been suggested, such as 60% or 80% and other values.[3,7] Still others suggest using weight-based dosing rather percentages.[8] This authorship group agrees with the majority of the literature that suggests **using 80% of the calculated requirement** for initial SQ basal dosing, to provide optimal glycemic control while avoiding hypoglycemia.[5,9–13] See Table 8.2 for an illustration of this percentage calculation.

Table 8.1—Example of Calculating 24-h Basal Insulin Requirement in the NPO Patient

	0000	0100	0200	0300	0400	0500	0600	0700	0800
IV insulin infusion rate	1.2	1.3	1.2	1.3	1.3	1.3	1.3	1.3	1.2
Blood glucose (mg/dL)	155	132	145	125	121	130	132	122	136

Overnight requirements; patient not eating.

- The patient has both good glycemic control as well as stable rates.
- The average rate during this time is 1.3 units/h.
- To complete the calculation, multiply 1.3 units/h × 24 h = 31 units.
- Therefore, the 24-h basal insulin requirement is 31 units.

Table 8.2—Calculating the Percentage of the Basal Insulin Requirement Is Given as SQ Insulin

What is the calculated 24-h basal requirement?	From Table 8.1, the basal requirement is 31 units.
What is 80% of the 24-h basal requirement?	80% × 31 units = (rounded) 25 units.
How would you write the final order for SQ basal insulin?	Give 25 units of detemir or glargine insulin SQ once daily.*

*Long-acting insulin may be given at any time of day, provided that the time is kept consistent from day to day (e.g., 6 P.M. daily).

Table 8.3—Writing the Final Orders for Prandial and Basal SQ Insulin Once the Patient Is Eating

How would you write the final order for SQ basal insulin?	Give 25 units of detemir or glargine insulin SQ once daily.
How would you write the final order for SQ prandial insulin?	Give 5 units* of lispro, aspart, or glulisine insulin SQ TID cc (with meals).**

*As in the text, dosing of prandial insulin can be calculated either via weight-based dosing (Mooradian et al.[14]) or via a small fixed dose of insulin, such as 5 units of rapid-acting insulin with each meal, that is given to cover carbohydrate intake, and then titrated based on patient response.[5,15]
**Rapid-acting insulin should be given immediately before meals or may be given immediately after the patient has finished eating, if the amount of oral intake is uncertain.

3. **SQ prandial insulin can then be added to the SQ basal insulin orders.** Dosing of prandial insulin can be calculated either via weight-based dosing[14] or via a small fixed dose of insulin, such as 5 units of rapid-acting insulin with each meal, that is given to cover carbohydrate intake and then is titrated based on the patient's BG response.[5,15] Another approach is to divide the basal insulin dose by three and use half of this value as the initial fixed dose because of the often poor PO intake of patients in the inpatient setting. Other individual patient factors that influence insulin requirements must be considered, such as renal insufficiency, heart failure, or extreme insulin resistance. See Table 8.3 for an illustration of final SQ orders.

DECIDING WHICH TYPE OF INSULIN TO USE

The type of insulin chosen for individual patients depends on the clinical scenario, patient preferences regarding frequency and timing of injections, financial considerations, and discharge planning. The type of insulin regimen chosen for discharge can have significant implications for the patient and should be chosen carefully. Newer, more physiologic insulin analogs are preferred in the hospital environment because of their more reliable pharmacokinetic and pharmacodynamic profile. A limited number of studies have compared regular-NPH regimens to basal-bolus therapy in the hospital setting. One available study suggested that there was no difference in BG control or rates of hypoglycemia when patients were given detemir or aspart or a regular-NPH regimen.[16] Another randomized controlled trial suggested that transitioning to a regular-NPH regimen from insulin infusion had improvement in glycemic control (compared with glargine), although patients given regular NPH had an increased incidence of hypoglycemia.[17] More evidence is available in the outpatient setting to suggest that basal-bolus regimens result in improved HbA_{1c} values and less glucose variability,[18–20] and decreased incidence of hypoglycemia[18–22] compared with NPH insulin. Furthermore, the use of analogs has been shown to improve adherence and allow for flexibility with dosing in addition to offering an easier delivery method in the pen form.[23,24] Patients may benefit from NPH insulin in certain scenarios, including corticosteroid therapy.[25]

For discharge planning, the patient's financial situation and insurance coverage must be considered. Analog insulins have a higher copay for most patients; a box of aspart pens can cost up to $391.[23] Adherence should be considered before selecting a discharge regimen. Patients who need a higher number of injections are more likely to be nonadherent with medications.[26] Therefore, providers should discuss various options with each patient before discharge and should take into account patient-specific factors, including motivation and ability to self-monitor and administer injections, daily schedule for meals and activity, support system, financial resources, and potentially limiting comorbidities.

HOW TO TRANSITION PATIENTS IN VARIOUS SITUATIONS

THE PATIENT WHO IS NPO

Many patients who require an IV infusion are still not eating by mouth (NPO) when the time for transition occurs. Using only basal insulin to transition off the insulin infusion simplifies the process and allows a stepwise plan of care.

Long-Acting Analogs (Detemir or Glargine)

The administration of either glargine or detemir can facilitate a smooth transition off an insulin infusion. Because of the longer onset of action, these insulins should be administered at least 2 h before discontinuation of the infusion and ideally 2–4 h prior.[5,27] A recent study demonstrated that starting glargine within 12 h of insulin infusion *initiation* (using 0.25 units/kg) resulted in less rebound hyperglycemia than initiating glargine closer to the time of transition.[28] Early administration of the basal analog did not increase rates of hypoglycemia. Another study revealed similar efficacy using insulin detemir 0.25 units/kg/day in medical patients on IV insulin infusion, with a lower incidence of rebound hyperglycemia (18.8% in the detemir group vs. 100% in the control group) and lower average BG in the first 12 h after discontinuation of IV insulin (137.0 ±39.9 mg/dL in the detemir group vs. 219.6 ±57.8 mg/dL in the control group, $P < 0.0001$ between groups) but with more hypoglycemia.[29] These data suggest that early administration of basal insulin in conjunction with the insulin infusion may be an effective approach for transitioning from IV to SQ insulin, but further studies are needed to confirm these findings and determine optimal dosing of simultaneously administered SQ basal insulin in different patient populations.

NPH Insulin Every 12 h

Some authors have suggested that NPH insulin given twice daily can cover basal requirements appropriately when patients are not eating.[30,31] If used for basal coverage, the total daily dose (TDD) should be split into two doses with 50% administered in the morning and 50% given 12 h later. The use of NPH has been linked to higher rates of hypoglycemia,[17,21,32] so this regimen should be used with caution and only if necessary for financial reasons.

Avoiding Sliding-Scale Insulin

The term “sliding-scale” insulin is used when rapid-acting insulin is given in response to a high BG level, rather than administering a scheduled dose to prevent hyperglycemia. Sliding-scale insulin is considered a retroactive rather than a proactive form of glucose control. It is now considered an antiquated and ill-preferred approach to treatment of inpatient hyperglycemia or diabetes.

Multiple studies published in the past several years have demonstrated a lack of efficacy and higher hypoglycemia rates with sliding-scale insulin, and the authors recommend discontinuing sliding-scale insulin as the only form of glucose control in hospitalized patients in favor of scheduled dosing of insulin, which promotes better glucose control.[33–35]

THE PATIENT WHO IS EATING

Basal-Bolus Analogs

Ideally, patients will have a long-acting insulin analog administered SQ several hours before discontinuation of the insulin infusion. If the dose was chosen correctly, IV infusion requirements will decrease gradually and can be discontinued safely. Prandial insulin can be added before infusion discontinuation if the patient is already eating or afterward. Prandial insulins typically are administered before each meal. If the patient is not eating well, the insulin can be administered after the patient has finished eating to ensure that the prandial insulin is matched appropriately to the amount of food consumed.

Regular and NPH Insulin

Regular and NPH insulins often are required for patients who cannot afford the newer agents. As described in the NPO section, patients who are eating and who are transitioned to these insulins should receive a dose of regular insulin 1 h before discontinuation of the infusion, preferably at a meal time. Regular insulin typically covers the usual meals during the day, whereas NPH is administered at night to cover basal requirements. When given in this manner, the dosing is typically as follows: 25% of TDD for each meal (breakfast, lunch, and dinner) plus 25% of TDD for NPH dose to equal 100% of TDD.[4,36]

Early Administration of the SQ Dose

To facilitate a safe transition to SQ insulin, planning for this step should take place proactively once the type of insulin is decided. The half-life of IV insulin is less than 10 min, so SQ insulin must be administered before the discontinuation of the infusion to avoid rebound hyperglycemia.[15] The timing of the SQ insulin depends on the type of insulin given. If regular insulin is given, this should occur 1 h before discontinuing the infusion.[4] If long-acting insulin is administered, this should occur at least 2 h prior, with preference given to earlier administration.[37] As mentioned previously, administering basal insulin as early as possible (close to IV initiation) may facilitate a smooth transition off the insulin infusion and decrease rebound hyperglycemia.[28]

Failure to adhere to these recommendations for early SQ administration can lead to rebound hyperglycemia in patients who lack endogenous insulin production.[38]

TRANSITION TO INSULIN PUMP THERAPY

As continuous SQ insulin pumps (CSII) grow in popularity, the number of hospitalized patients using CSII also will increase. More hospitals are developing plans to safely triage patients admitted with CSII to ensure safe pump handling and optimal glucose control. A critically ill patient in the intensive care unit (ICU) setting receiving an insulin infusion likely will be unable to manage his or her own pump therapy; therefore, the decision to continue CSII during this time should be made with caution.

A key component of pump transition is to ensure that the patient is able to manage his or her own pump without assistance from the staff. Hospital staff are not trained to manage insulin pumps, so it is the primary responsibility of the patient to ensure correct handling and dose administration. Before allowing the patient to resume pump therapy, the provider should assess whether the patient is able to perform basic pump-handling techniques, including manual manipulation of the pump and settings, correct counting of carbohydrates, maintenance of responsibility for all pump supplies, and willingness to adjust pump settings according to provider recommendations.[39,40] The patient should have all of the supplies needed to operate the pump, because hospitals traditionally do not stock CSII supplies. If the patient lacks the ability to carry out these basic tasks or does not have the proper equipment, resumption of pump therapy is not recommended in the hospital setting. Furthermore, mental status should be completely intact and not impaired by pain, medication, or distress. Other factors that suggest the patient is not safe to transition back to CSII therapy include suicide risk, pending operating room procedure, certain radiology procedures, or active DKA or HHS.[41–43]

The provider should establish the 24-h insulin requirement from the insulin infusion rates and compare them with the patient's home basal regimen programmed into the pump. If the rates are similar, it may be appropriate to restart the pump with the same rates. If the rates are dissimilar, the pump settings should be adjusted to match the current requirements (80–100% of current insulin requirements). A temporary basal rate can be utilized, or pump settings can be adjusted manually. For optimal care, an endocrinologist or diabetes specialist should be available to help the patient modify the pump settings, if needed.[10] If the inpatient team is concerned about the safety of restarting the insulin pump, or if the patient's clinical situation remains unstable, the patient may be transitioned to (and discharged on) SQ injections. A follow-up appointment with the outpatient diabetes care team should be arranged shortly after discharge to ensure continuity of care.

INSTITUTION- OR POPULATION-SPECIFIC PROTOCOLS FOR TRANSITIONS

Protocols are designed to standardize the transition process across many different services in the same hospital, as well as to encourage the use of best practices. Although no single protocol will work for every patient, standardized protocols can assist with safety and efficacy in a process as complex as transitioning from IV to SQ insulin for the majority of hospitalized patients. This can be particularly valuable in large teaching institutions that have nonspecialist house staff in training with varying degrees of experience and expertise with insulin therapies. Protocols can be useful in smaller institutions where staff may not have access to on-site endocrinology or diabetes care consultants.

A review of several published institution-specific protocols shows several common themes. These include a tendency to focus particularly on optimizing control in postcardiothoracic surgery patients, the importance of frequent BG monitoring, the need to administer the first dose of SQ insulin at least 1–2 h before stopping the IV infusion, and the utility in giving rapid-acting SQ analogue insulin to cover meals—even while continuing the IV insulin infusion—in patients still on infusion but who also are eating.[3,5,44]

COMPUTERIZED PROTOCOLS

Over the past decade, as the debate over optimal glycemic targets has intensified, there has been growing interest in technological tools that permit the provider to choose a target glucose range and then rely on computerized protocols directing adjustments in IV insulin to achieve that target. Such protocols include those produced by Glucommander©[45] and EndoTool©.[46,47] Some authors have shown that these computerized protocols can achieve a high percentage of BG values within a target range without increasing the risk of hypoglycemia.[45–49] In addition, most recently, Glytec© has developed a computerized module (eGlycemic Management System or eGMS©[50]) to be used with Glucommander©[45] that includes directions for transitioning patients from IV to SQ insulin. Results of a pilot study of patients transitioned from IV to SQ insulin with the eGlycemic Management System suggested that 92% of patients transitioned using the e-management system had BG between 70–180 mg/dL, compared with 79% of patients transitioned using a preestablished paper protocol. The patients transitioned using the e-management system had a low incidence of moderate hypoglycemia (BG <60 mg/dL) and did not demonstrate any severe hypoglycemia (BG <40 mg/dL).[50]

GAPS IN KNOWLEDGE AND RESEARCH NEEDED

Further research is needed to guide and accomplish safe transitions from IV to SQ insulin in hospitalized patients. The particular gaps in knowledge can be placed into the following categories:

- *How to achieve safe transitions in unique patient populations:* Postoperative patients have received much focus to prevent wound infections. Numerous other populations, however, require further study, including patients with type 1 diabetes, patients receiving enteral or parenteral nutrition, patients with end-stage renal disease, and the postpartum patient.
- *The role of standardized protocols in education:* One of the challenges with routine use of protocols is the question of provider autonomy and individual decision making. This issue has been raised as a particular concern in academic training centers. A balance between protocols that promote patient safety and educational independence is necessary. This debate will continue for some time.
- *Cost effectiveness of computerized protocols:* Another major issue is the cost effectiveness of elaborate computerized monitoring systems and complex

titration algorithms. As most hospitals have adopted electronic medical record systems, computerized insulin titration, especially if combined with automated hypoglycemia warnings, could be a reasonable next step in the evolution of inpatient diabetes management.

REFERENCES

1. Genuth SM. Constant intravenous insulin infusion in diabetic ketoacidosis. *JAMA* 1973;223:1348–1351
2. Braithwaite SS. The transition from insulin infusions to long-term diabetes therapy: the argument for insulin analogs. *Semin Thorac Cardiovasc Surg* 2006;18:366–378
3. Avanzini F, Marelli G, Donzelli W, Busi G, Carbone S, Bellato L, Colombo EL, Foschi R, Riva E, Roncaglioni MC, De MM. Transition from intravenous to subcutaneous insulin: effectiveness and safety of a standardized protocol and predictors of outcome in patients with acute coronary syndrome. *Diabetes Care* 2011;34:1445–1450
4. Lien LF, Angelyn BM, Feinglos MN. In-hospital management of type 2 diabetes mellitus. *Med Clin North Am* 2004;88:1085–1105, xii
5. Furnary AP, Braithwaite SS. Effects of outcome on in-hospital transition from intravenous insulin infusion to subcutaneous therapy. *Am J Cardiol* 2006;98:557–564
6. Low Wang CC, Draznin B. Practical approach to management of inpatient hyperglycemia in select patient populations. *Hosp Pract (1995)* 2013;41:45–53
7. Pichardo-Lowden A, Gabbay RA. Management of hyperglycemia during the perioperative period. *Curr Diab Rep* 2012;12:108–118
8. Silinskie KM, Kirshner R, Hite MS. Converting continuous insulin infusion to subcutaneous insulin glargine after cardiac surgery using percentage-based versus weight-based dosing: a pilot trial. *Ann Pharmacother* 2013;47:20–28
9. Bode BW, Braithwaite SS, Steed RD, Davidson PC. Intravenous insulin infusion therapy: indications, methods, and transition to subcutaneous insulin therapy. *Endocr Pract* 2004;10(Suppl. 2):71–80
10. Moghissi ES, Korytkowski MT, DiNardo M, Einhorn D, Hellman R, Hirsch IB, Inzucchi SE, Ismail-Beigi F, Kirkman MS, Umpierrez GE. American Association of Clinical Endocrinologists and American Diabetes Association consensus statement on inpatient glycemic control. *Endocr Pract* 2009;15:353–369
11. Dungan K, Hall C, Schuster D, Osei K. Comparison of 3 algorithms for basal insulin in transitioning from intravenous to subcutaneous insulin in stable patients after cardiothoracic surgery. *Endocr Pract* 2011;17:753–758
12. Schmeltz LR, DeSantis AJ, Schmidt K, O'Shea-Mahler E, Rhee C, Brandt S, Peterson S, Molitch ME. Conversion of intravenous insulin infusions to

subcutaneously administered insulin glargine in patients with hyperglycemia. *Endocr Pract* 2006;12:641–650

13. Ahmann AJ. Inpatient management of hospitalized patients with type 2 diabetes. *Curr Diab Rep* 2004;4:346–351
14. Mooradian AD, Bernbaum M, Albert SG. Narrative review: a rational approach to starting insulin therapy. *Ann Intern Med* 2006;145:125–134
15. Mabrey ME, Lien LF. IV insulin infusions: how to use an "insulin drip." In *Glycemic control in the hospitalized patient: A comprehensive clinical guide*. 1st ed. Lien LF, Cox ME, Feinglos MN, Corsino L, Eds. New York, Springer, 2010, p. 17–27
16. Umpierrez GE, Hor T, Smiley D, Temponi A, Umpierrez D, Ceron M, Munoz C, Newton C, Peng L, Baldwin D. Comparison of inpatient insulin regimens with detemir plus aspart versus neutral protamine hagedorn plus regular in medical patients with type 2 diabetes. *J Clin Endocrinol Metab* 2009;94:564–569
17. Yeldandi RR, Lurie A, Baldwin D. Comparison of once-daily glargine insulin with twice-daily NPH/regular insulin for control of hyperglycemia in inpatients after cardiovascular surgery. *Diabetes Technol Ther* 2006;8:609–616
18. Hermansen K, Fontaine P, Kukolja KK, Peterkova V, Leth G, Gall MA. Insulin analogues (insulin detemir and insulin aspart) versus traditional human insulins (NPH insulin and regular human insulin) in basal-bolus therapy for patients with type 1 diabetes mellitus. *Diabetologia* 2004;47:622–629
19. Bartley PC, Bogoev M, Larsen J, Philotheou A. Long-term efficacy and safety of insulin detemir compared to neutral protamine Hagedorn insulin in patients with type 1 diabetes using a treat-to-target basal-bolus regimen with insulin aspart at meals: a 2-year, randomized, controlled trial. *Diabet Med* 2008;25:442–449
20. Hermansen K, Madsbad S, Perrild H, Kristensen A, Axelsen M. Comparison of the soluble basal insulin analog insulin detemir with NPH insulin: a randomized open crossover trial in type 1 diabetic subjects on basal-bolus therapy. *Diabetes Care* 2001;24:296–301
21. Riddle MC, Rosenstock J, Gerich J. The treat-to-target trial: randomized addition of glargine or human NPH insulin to oral therapy of type 2 diabetic patients. *Diabetes Care* 2003;26:3080–3086
22. Rosenstock J, Ahmann AJ, Colon G, Scism-Bacon J, Jiang H, Martin S. Advancing insulin therapy in type 2 diabetes previously treated with glargine plus oral agents: prandial premixed (insulin lispro protamine suspension/lispro) versus basal/bolus (glargine/lispro) therapy. *Diabetes Care* 2008;31:20–25
23. Grunberger G. Insulin analogs—are they worth it? Yes! *Diabetes Care* 2014;37:1767–1770
24. Seggelke SA, Hawkins RM, Gibbs J, Rasouli N, Wang CC, Draznin B. Effect of glargine insulin delivery method (pen device versus vial/syringe) on glycemic

control and patient preferences in patients with type 1 and type 2 diabetes. *Endocr Pract* 2014;20:536–539

25. Seggelke SA, Gibbs J, Draznin B: Pilot study of using neutral protamine Hagedorn insulin to counteract the effect of methylprednisolone in hospitalized patients with diabetes. *J Hosp Med* 2011;6:175–176
26. Davies MJ, Gagliardino JJ, Gray LJ, Khunti K, Mohan V, Hughes R. Real-world factors affecting adherence to insulin therapy in patients with type 1 or type 2 diabetes mellitus: a systematic review. *Diabet Med* 2013;30:512–524
27. Donaldson S, Villanuueva G, Rondinelli L, Baldwin D. Rush University guidelines and protocols for the management of hyperglycemia in hospitalized patients: elimination of the sliding scale and improvement of glycemic control throughout the hospital. *Diabetes Educ* 2006;32:954–962
28. Hsia E, Seggelke S, Gibbs J, Hawkins RM, Cohlmia E, Rasouli N, Wang C, Kam I, Draznin B. Subcutaneous administration of glargine to diabetic patients receiving insulin infusion prevents rebound hyperglycemia. *J Clin Endocrinol Metab* 2012;97:3132–3137
29. Low Wang CC, Sanagorski R, Hawkins RM, Gibbs J, Tompkins K, Bridenstine M, Seggelke S, Draznin B. Impact of subcutaneous detemir insulin on rebound hyperglycemia in hospitalized patients with diabetes transitioning from a continuous intravenous insulin infusion (Abstract). *Endocrine Reviews* 2015;36
30. Dickerson RN, Wilson VC, Maish GO, III, Croce MA, Minard G, Brown RO. Transitional NPH insulin therapy for critically ill patients receiving continuous enteral nutrition and intravenous regular human insulin. *JPEN J Parenter Enteral Nutr* 2013;37:506–516
31. Weant KA, Ladha A. Conversion from continuous insulin infusions to subcutaneous insulin in critically ill patients. *Ann Pharmacother* 2009;43:629–634
32. Rosenstock J, Schwartz SL, Clark CM, Jr., Park GD, Donley DW, Edwards MB. Basal insulin therapy in type 2 diabetes: 28-week comparison of insulin glargine (HOE 901) and NPH insulin. *Diabetes Care* 2001;24:631–636
33. Braithwaite SS, Edkins R, Macgregor KL, Sredzienski ES, Houston M, Zarzaur B, Rich PB, Benedetto B, Rutherford EJ. Performance of a dose-defining insulin infusion protocol among trauma service intensive care unit admissions. *Diabetes Technol Ther* 2006;8:476–488
34. Umpierrez GE, Smiley D, Zisman A, Prieto LM, Palacio A, Ceron M, Puig A, Mejia R. Randomized study of basal-bolus insulin therapy in the inpatient management of patients with type 2 diabetes (RABBIT 2 trial). *Diabetes Care* 2007;30:2181–2186
35. Datta S, Qaadir A, Villanueva G, Baldwin D. Once-daily insulin glargine versus 6-hour sliding scale regular insulin for control of hyperglycemia after a bariatric surgical procedure: a randomized clinical trial. *Endocr Pract* 2007;13:225–231

36. Barnard K, Batch BC, Lien LF. Subcutaneous insulin: a guide for dosing regimens in the hospital. In *Glycemic control in the hospitalized patient: A comprehensive clinical guide*. 1st ed. Lien LF, Cox ME, Feinglos MN, Corsino L, Eds. New York, Springer, 2010, p. 7–16
37. O'Malley CW, Emanuele M, Halasyamani L, Amin AN. Bridge over troubled waters: safe and effective transitions of the inpatient with hyperglycemia. *J Hosp Med* 2008;3:55–65
38. Hemerson P, Banarova A, Izakovic M, Clancy GM, Richenbacher WE, Beireis L. Transitioning postoperative cardiovascular surgery patients from intravenous to subcutaneous insulin: an improvement project. *J Clin Outcomes Manage* 2011;18:563–567
39. Yogi-Morren D, Lansang MC. Management of patients with T1DM in the hospital. *Curr Diab Rep* 2014;14:458
40. McCrea D. Management of the hospitalized diabetes patient with an insulin pump. *Crit Care Nurs Clin North Am* 2013;25:111–121
41. Evans KJ, Thompson J, Spratt SE, Lien LF, Vorderstrasse A. The implementation and evaluation of an evidence-based protocol to treat diabetic ketoacidosis: a quality improvement study. *Adv Emerg Nurs J* 2014;36:189–198
42. Cook CB, Boyle ME, Cisar NS, Miller-Cage V, Bourgeois P, Roust LR, Smith SA, Zimmerman RS. Use of continuous subcutaneous insulin infusion (insulin pump) therapy in the hospital setting: proposed guidelines and outcome measures. *Diabetes Educ* 2005;31:849–857
43. Morviducci L, Di FA, Lauria A, Pitocco D, Pozzilli P, Suraci C, Frontoni S. Continuous subcutaneous insulin infusion (CSII) in inpatient setting: unmet needs and the proposal of a CSII unit. *Diabetes Technol Ther* 2011;13:1071–1074
44. Stahnke A, Struemph K, Behnen E, Schimmelpfennig J. Pharmacy management of postoperative blood glucose in open heart surgery patients: evaluation of an intravenous to subcutaneous insulin protocol. *Hosp Pharm* 2014;49:164–169
45. Davidson PC, Steed RD, Bode BW. Glucommander: a computer-directed intravenous insulin system shown to be safe, simple, and effective in 120,618 h of operation. *Diabetes Care* 2005;28:2418–2423
46. Cochran S, Miller E, Dunn K, Burgess WP, Miles W, Lobdell K. EndoTool software for tight glucose control for critically ill patients (Abstract). *Crit Care Med* 2006;34:A68
47. Messenger C, Hockley D. Housewide use of EndoTool® computer-based IV insulin management improves glycemic control. Presented at ANA 6th Annual Nursing Quality Conference: Improving the Odds on Quality, 25 January 2012, Las Vegas, NV
48. Newton CA, Smiley D, Bode BW, Kitabchi AE, Davidson PC, Jacobs S, Steed RD, Stentz F, Peng L, Mulligan P, Freire AX, Temponi A, Umpierrez GE. A comparison study of continuous insulin infusion protocols in the

medical intensive care unit: computer-guided vs. standard column-based algorithms. *J Hosp Med* 2010;5:432–437

49. Halpin L, Henry L, Dunning E, Hunt S, Barnett S, White J, Ad N. Comparison of blood glucose management strategies to achieve control following cardiac surgery (computerized versus paper). *AACN Adv Crit Care* 2010;21:146–151
50. Palazzo A, Smith B, Shoun F, et al. Use of the eGlycemic management system by Glytec provides safe and effective transition from IV to subq insulin therapy. Presented at Diabetes Technology Meeting, 6 November 2014, Bethesda, MD

Chapter 9

Preoperative, Intraoperative, and Postoperative Glucose Management

Roma Gianchandani, MD,[1] Elizabeth Dubois, PA-C,[2] Sara Alexanian, MD,[3] and Rob Rushakoff, MD[4]

INTRODUCTION

More than 50 million inpatient surgical procedures are performed in the U.S. every year[1] and at least 20% involve diabetes mellitus as a comorbid condition.[2] Patients with diabetes have increased rates of cardiovascular and microvascular disease, are hospitalized more frequently for surgical procedures, and have longer lengths of stay than the general population. Hyperglycemia portends a higher risk of perioperative morbidity and mortality, namely, via poor wound healing, higher infection rates, and myocardial infarction not only in patients with diabetes but also in those without known diabetes who develop stress hyperglycemia perioperatively. In addition to surgical stress, the type of anesthesia and surgery, hypothermia, steroids, vasopressors, enteral or parenteral feeding, and immunosuppressants all contribute to glucose elevations.[3]

Hyperglycemia in the hospital setting is defined as any glucose level >140 mg/dL. Although numerous studies have associated hyperglycemia with adverse outcomes in hospitalized patients, the impact of glucose control in the perioperative period has not been evaluated extensively. Currently, the goal of pre- and intraoperative diabetes management largely consists of safely getting a patient through surgery while avoiding the hyperglycemia and hypoglycemia that can adversely affect outcomes. Because of the lack of pre- and intraoperative data, most institutions use extrapolated target glucose ranges from inpatient intensive care studies. Targets may further be relaxed because of concerns about hypoglycemia, which is difficult to recognize in sedated patients. Current inpatient guidelines from different professional societies and institutions advocate a moderate glycemic range between 120 and 180 mg/dL.

Hypoglycemia is defined as a glucose level <70 mg/dl, and when severe (<40 mg/dL) can have deleterious effects on the heart and central nervous system,

[1]Associate Professor, Department of Internal medicine/Metabolism, Endocrinology and Diabetes; Director, Hospital Hyperglycemia Program, University of Michigan Medical Center, Ann Arbor, MI. [2]Department of Internal Medicine/Metabolism, Endocrinology and Diabetes, University of Michigan Medical Center, Ann Arbor, MI. [3]Assistant Professor, Department of Endocrinology, Diabetes, Nutrition and Weight Management; Director, Inpatient Diabetes Program, Boston Medical Center, Boston, MA. [4]Professor of Medicine, Director, Inpatient Diabetes, Division of Endocrinology and Metabolism, University of California, San Francisco, CA.

DOI: 10.2337/9781580406086.09

including arrhythmias, seizures, and brain damage. Whether or not iatrogenic hypoglycemia increases mortality is unclear. Patients who are ill, are septic, or have multiorgan dysfunction also may develop hypoglycemia in the absence of exogenous insulin.[4] Although spontaneous hypoglycemia appears to correlate with worse prognosis, several studies evaluating the impact of iatrogenic hypoglycemia have not reached similar conclusions. Regardless, agreement is unanimous that one of the major goals of glucose management in the perioperative period is avoidance of hypoglycemia as much as possible.[4]

PREOPERATIVE GLUCOSE CONTROL

EVIDENCE AND RATIONALE

There are no data on the importance of glucose control within the 12- to 24-h period or weeks leading up to a procedure nor are there prospective trials evaluating the relationship of longstanding preoperative glucose control with outcomes. Several retrospective studies in cardiac and noncardiac surgery patients, using HbA_{1c} as a surrogate of longstanding glucose control, have shown an increase in morbidity and mortality. In patients with high preoperative HbA_{1c} or elevated baseline glucose levels, HbA_{1c} values ≥7 are associated with double the risk of postoperative wound infections.[5] However, other large trials have failed to show this association, especially in noncardiac surgery populations.[6] Conflicting data arising from variations in study size, patient populations, and primary outcomes and difficulty separating the significance of pre- and postoperative effects of glucose management may contribute to the reason that preoperative control has not received much attention.

Of clinical importance is the fact that preoperative hypo- and hyperglycemia may delay a procedure[7] and poor diabetes management decisions, such as holding all insulin before surgery, may compromise specific populations. In patients with type 1 diabetes (T1D), inadequate insulin use can lead to diabetic ketoacidosis (DKA), whereas in those with severe insulin resistance, it can result in hyperosmolar hyperglycemic state (HHS).

PREOPERATIVE CONSIDERATIONS

Well-modified preoperative diabetes regimens can reduce intra- and postoperative hyperglycemia, especially for ambulatory procedures. In the preoperative evaluation of a patient with diabetes, it is important to ascertain the following:

- Type and duration of diabetes mellitus
- Level of glucose control and usual treatment regimen
- History of hypoglycemia, hypoglycemic events requiring assistance, and hypoglycemia unawareness
- Diabetes-related complications, specifically renal, macrovascular, and autonomic neuropathy
- Type, start time, and length of surgery

Patients with T1D are insulinopenic and need basal insulin at all times to prevent DKA and suppress gluconeogenesis and glycogenolysis. They also have significant glucose fluctuations and are more prone to hypoglycemia. T2D patients present along the spectrum of the natural history of T2D, from minimal pharmacologic requirements (control via diet, oral medications only, or combination therapy that may include noninsulin injectables) to multiple daily injections of insulin. Those on diet control or low doses of oral medications tend to normalize their glucose levels when nil by mouth (NPO) and may need no further interventions perioperatively.

The minimum preoperative evaluation of a patient with diabetes undergoing a procedure includes a renal panel, HbA_{1c}, and an electrocardiogram. An HbA_{1c} obtained before a procedure facilitates decision making on diabetes management, points to possible risk of infections, and helps formulate a discharge plan.[8–10] In the setting of recent blood transfusions, hemolysis, or marked anemia, an HbA_{1c} may be inaccurate. Additionally, home glucose monitoring records or meter downloads provide insight into overall glycemic control and help evaluate glycemic patterns.[11] Patients with diabetes have a high incidence of ischemic events, especially silent ischemia. The degree of preoperative workup will depend on the anticipated procedure and patient risk profile. Diabetic nephropathy must be documented as hydration is essential and medications, especially nephrotoxic agents, will need dose adjustments. Patients with autonomic dysfunction can develop several problems: hypotension may occur with anesthesia, gastroparesis can result in vomiting and aspiration, and bladder and bowel dysautonomia can cause urinary retention and constipation, respectively.[8] Lastly, diabetes patients should be placed on the morning list for procedures if possible, as this is the least disruptive to a typical diabetes routine.

PREOPERATIVE TARGETS

There are no published targets for preoperative glucose control. Broad goals of preoperative glucose management include the following:

- Prevention of severe hyperglycemia and hypoglycemia
- Prevention of medical emergencies, specifically DKA and HHS
- Minimization of perioperative morbidity and mortality.

Safe preoperative glucose targets recommended at most institutions range from 120–200 mg/dL. Elderly patients with longstanding diabetes and cardiac comorbidities should have higher glucose targets.[12] A severely hyperglycemic patient presenting for surgery usually has longstanding uncontrolled diabetes and may feel "low" when glucose levels are brought down acutely for the procedural setting.

PREOPERATIVE REGIMENS

GENERAL GUIDELINES

Patients should be instructed to check their BG frequently when NPO in preparation for a procedure and have a glucose monitoring device and treatment for hypoglycemia close at hand, especially when traveling to the hospital. Appropriate hypoglycemia management in the preoperative period must be discussed in advance and usually consists of drinking 15 g of glucose-containing clear liquids and repeating dosing every 15 min until resolution of hypoglycemia or BG is >70 mg/dL. Gels and glucose tablets for treatment should be avoided, as they may contain particulates.

Several institutions use standardized preoperative guidelines for the management of diabetes regimens before surgery. The University of Michigan guidelines are summarized in Table 9.1. University of California, San Francisco has a computerized program available online (ucsf.logicnets.com). Modifications of antidiabetes therapies before surgery are discussed in the following sections for both oral and injectable agents.

Table 9.1—Reoperative/Procedure Diabetes Management

NIGHT BEFORE PROCEDURE	
1. Patient takes oral diabetes medications	Take usual dose
2. Patient takes evening or bedtime insulin	
- **NPH**	Take usual dose
- **Mixed usual dose**	Take usual dose
- **Glargine/Detemir** (insulin monotherapy)	Take 50% of usual dose
- **Glargine /Detemir** (part of basal bolus regimen)	Take 70% of usual dose
- **Regular or aspart or lispro or glulisine**	Take usual dinner dose
3. Patient takes non-insulin injectables	Take usual dose
4. Patient uses insulin pump* **See Perioperative Insulin Pump Guidelines.**	Continue basal rate- unless frequent hypoglycemia Then reduce to temporary basal rate of 70%
MORNING OF PROCEDURE	
1. Patient takes oral diabetes medications	HOLD dose
2. Patient takes evening or bedtime insulin	
- **NPH**	Take 50% of usual dose
- **Mixed insulin**	Take 50% of usual dose
- **Glargine/Detemir** (insulin monotherapy)	Take 50% of usual dose
- **Glargine/Detemir** (part of basal bolus regimen)	Take 70% of usual dose
- **Regular or aspart or lispro or HOLD doses**	HOLD doses
3. Patient takes non-insulin injectables	HOLD doses
4. Patient uses insulin pump* **See Perioperative Insulin Pump Guidelines.**	Reduce to temporary basal rate of 70%

Intraoperative and postoperative use of pump should be addressed on an individual basis in consultation with patient's endocrinologist.
U-500 insulin doses should be changed in conjunction with the patient's endocrinologist.

ORAL ANTIDIABETES DRUGS

Metformin is the most widely used oral antidiabetes agent (OAD). Lactic acidosis is a rare but dreaded complication of metformin and is reported usually in the presence of acute renal failure. Metformin is withheld on the day of the procedure and does not need to be stopped earlier. In procedures requiring radiological contrast or surgeries compromising renal function, metformin is not restarted until 48 h after the procedure or after renal function is rechecked, if required.[13]

Sulfonylureas (e.g., glipizide, glyburide, glimepiride) and nonsulfonylurea secretagogues (e.g., repaginate, meglitinide) increase insulin production and can cause hypoglycemia especially in the fasting state. These drugs are withheld the day of the procedure and typically are restarted when appetite and diet have returned to normal.

Thiazolidinediones (e.g., pioglitazone and rosiglitazone) improve insulin utilization by reducing insulin resistance by their action on the peroxisome proliferator–activated receptors (mostly receptor γ), which are nuclear receptors found predominantly in adipose tissue. Their effects are on gene transcription, and although steady state may be reached in a week, it takes several weeks for the full benefit of their effect on glucose metabolism to occur. Fluid retention, a side effect of these agents, may be a concern in the perioperative setting. No clinical trials have evaluated the duration of withholding thiazolidinediones in advance of surgery; however, in our clinical experience, glucose starts rising within 5 to 7 days following discontinuation.

Dipeptidyl peptidase-4 inhibitors (e.g., sitagliptin, saxagliptin, linagliptin, alogliptin, and vildagliptin) have a glucose-dependent mechanism of action, stimulating insulin release only during hyperglycemia. Therefore, when used as a monotherapy, they have a low risk of hypoglycemia. This risk increases if combined with a sulfonylurea or insulin.[9–11,14] Theoretically, these agents can be continued on the day of surgery if used alone for glucose management. Some experts suggest continuing to use them for inpatient hospitalizations and procedures.[15]

α-Glucosidase inhibitors (acarbose and miglitol) inhibit intestinal saccharidases and reduce glucose excursions caused by absorbed carbohydrates. These drugs are withheld when oral intake is discontinued. Furthermore, the gastrointestinal side effects associated with these agents make them less desirable in the immediate perioperative period.

Sodium-glucose linked transporter-2 inhibitors (e.g., canagliflozin, dapagliflozin, empagliflozin), the newest class of OADs, reduce urinary glucose reabsorption and cause glycosuria. They are not contraindicated with intravenous (IV) contrast agents, but because of the diuresis caused by glycosuria, it is recommended that they be held on the day of surgery to prevent dehydration, hypotension, and hypoglycemia.[11] Combination OADs should be managed following the recommendations of their individual components.

The group of *noninsulin injectable drugs* largely consists of the glucagon-like peptide-1 receptor agonists (GLP-1RA; e.g., exenatide, liraglutide, lixisenatide, and albiglutide and dulaglutide). These can be used at normal doses the day before but should be withheld the day of the surgical procedure given their significant impact on postprandial glucose levels as well as gastrointestinal motility. In patients needing a preprocedure bowel preparation, it may be advisable to hold these drugs beginning the day of the bowel prep. One recent group has published their experience of starting GLP-1RAs before a procedure to reduce hyperglycemia during hospitalization but currently there are no studies to support this. Other noninsulin injectable drugs (e.g., pramlintide) should be managed similarly to the GLP-1 receptor agonists.[9,11,14] Long-acting GLP-1RA when dosed before a procedure, require no change. If the typical redosing day coincides with the day of the procedure, these agents should be held.

INSULIN

Basal insulin is produced by the body in the fasting state and suppresses gluconeogenesis and glycogenolysis and prevents DKA and hyperketotic states. Replacement basal insulin is often injected at bedtime and the preoperative dose is based on the patient's weight, level of insulin resistance, level of diabetes control, and whether used alone or in concert with mealtime boluses of fast-acting insulin.

Glargine (U-100 and U-300) detemir and degludec are currently available long-acting insulins. Glargine and levemir are dosed via a standardized guideline, which recommends a 20–30% reduction, if given the night before the operation or the morning of the operation. A small study suggests that degludec, if dosed in the mornings, should be held the morning of surgery.[16] It then could be given after the procedure is completed or the morning after because of its long half-life. If given at night, the dose of degludec may need to be reduced for 2 days before the procedure. This reduction is generally adequate to prevent fasting hypoglycemia while avoiding marked hyperglycemia. It is most appropriate for patients on multidose insulin therapy with long-acting basal and short-acting meal insulin.[7,17] Variations are appropriate in a patient with significantly uncontrolled diabetes who, despite the current dosing, is severely hyperglycemic. In this situation, a reduction in basal insulin dosing may not be necessary. On the other hand, a patient using basal insulin only without mealtime insulin with a tendency toward fasting hypoglycemia may require up to a 50% reduction in their basal insulin.[7]

Neutral protamine Hagedorn (NPH) is an intermediate-acting insulin with a shorter duration of action and higher peak than long-acting insulin. The bedtime dose can be kept unchanged (or reduced by 30% if the preoperative fasting period starts before the dose); on the morning of procedure, this dose should be reduced by 50% to prevent hypoglycemia. Although other complex calculations have been proposed, this dose decrease works well.[14]

Fast-acting *bolus insulins* include regular and the rapid insulin analogues aspart, glulisine, and lispro. These are given with meals to cover the prandial glucose excursions and for correction of hyperglycemia.[2] Mealtime doses can be used until the fasting period begins, after which they are withheld. Correction doses may be used carefully in a fasting state to correct marked hyperglycemia (e.g., glucoses >200 mg/dL) and to avoid resultant hypoglycemia on the day of procedure.

Mixed insulin preparations available in the U.S. include NPH/regular insulin 70/30 and 50/50 and two insulin analogue mixed insulins—Humalog 75/25 and NovoLog 70/30. Some 70–75% of these insulins consist of an intermediate-acting component and 25–30% consist of a fast-acting component. Because of the peak effect of the intermediate insulin and the fast-acting component, patients can experience significant hypoglycemia when these insulins are used in the absence of oral intake. Mixed insulin doses can be given unchanged with dinner the night before the procedure and should be reduced to half of the usual dose on the morning of procedure. In a hospitalized patient, it is safest to convert the mixed insulin to a long-acting basal and short-acting bolus regimen before a procedure. The basal dose is calculated by using half of the total daily dose (TDD) as basal insulin and reducing this dose appropriately the night before procedure.[11]

U-500 insulin should be managed by reducing the usual bedtime dose by 30% the night before the procedure and reducing the morning dose by 50%.

INSULIN PUMPS

Continuous subcutaneous insulin infusion (CSII) via an insulin pump is increasingly used for management of T1D and much less often for management of T2D. Insulin pumps provide a continuous subcutaneous delivery of a basal dose, with boluses given via the pump before meals, typically based on current glycemia and carbohydrate intake (carbohydrate counting). The decision to continue an insulin pump during surgery depends on the length and type of surgery and the familiarity and comfort of the surgical and anesthesia teams with insulin pumps. For a short outpatient procedure (≤2 h), continuing basal insulin via an insulin pump is advisable.[11,14,18] If the patient has a history of several recent hypoglycemic episodes and must be fasting for the procedure, a temporary reduction in the basal rate by 30% may be necessary. The patient is asked to change the insulin infusion and site the day before the procedure and check at least two glucose values to ensure that the infusion set and site are working. The infusion site also needs to be at a distance from the surgical area—for example, if the procedure involves the abdomen, the pump site should be placed in the arm or leg. The patient must bring extra infusion sets and syringes to the procedure in case of infusion site or set malfunction. When the patient arrives to preoperative holding area, glucose is checked and if values are between 80 and 200 mg/dL, basal delivery from the insulin pump is continued. If the glucose is <70 mg/dL, the patient is treated by institutional hypoglycemia protocol with oral or IV glucose as appropriate for that surgery and BG rechecked within 15 min. The insulin pump rate is then reduced to 50%, or the insulin pump is discontinued and replaced with an IV infusion of insulin. For a procedure >2–3 h or for major surgeries, an IV insulin infusion generally is used to control glucose levels.[10,11,14,18] If the patient will be admitted to the hospital after surgery, the pump can be continued during and after the operative procedure only if the patient is expected to be alert and able to manage the pump and also to be able to eat soon after surgery (see Chapter 24 for more detail).

INTRAOPERATIVE GLUCOSE CONTROL

EVIDENCE AND RATIONALE

In observational studies, intraoperative hyperglycemia was determined to be an independent risk factor for morbidity and mortality when adjusted for postoperative

Table 9.2–Insulin Pump Guidelines for Perioperative Management

T1DM patients must have basal insulin at all times

The decision to continue an insulin pump during procedure depends on the length and type of procedure and on the surgical and anesthesia teams' familiarity with this technology.

PREOPERATIVE MANAGEMENT

Night before the procedure

Instruct patients to:

- Continue pump basal rate unless they experience frequent hypoglycemic episodes. Then reduce to a temporary basal rate of 70%.
- Change insulin infusion and site the day before the procedure and have at least 2 BG values checked after site change, to make sure that the infusion and site are working.
- Move site away from the surgical area, e.g., if an abdomen surgery, move site to arm or leg.
- Bring extra infusion sets, tubing, and syringes to the procedure.

Day of the procedure

Instruct patients to:

- Use a temporary basal rate of 70%. Hold meal insulin.
- Check BG every 2 hours
- If BG > 250 mg/dl at home, patient should take half of a correction insulin dose.
- If BG < 70 mg/dl at home, patient should treat by using clear liquids which have no particulate matter. Recheck in 15 minutes. Reduce basal pump rate further by 30%.
- In case of severe hypoglycemia (BG < 40 mg/dl) or loss of consciousness, family should use glucagon, and call ________for further instructions

HOLDING AND INTRAOPERATIVE MANAGEMENT

Outpatient procedures or those < 2 hours

- Staff should check BG in Holding Room
- BG is between 80-200 mg/dl, continue pump for procedure.
- Monitor BG at least every 1 hour
- If BG > 250 mg/dl
  - Correct with moderate scale using rapid acting insulin (Humalog).
  - If BG continues to rise, discontinue pump and start intravenous insulin drip protocol.
- If BG < 70 mg/dl,
  - Treat patient via hypoglycemia protocol using appropriate route (oral or IV), and recheck in 15 minutes.
  - Discontinue pump and start intravenous insulin drip protocol.

Major procedures, or those > 2 hours or inpatients who will be unable to manage pump or eat after procedure

- Staff should check BG in Holding Room.
- Initiate intravenous insulin drip protocol.
- Stop and disconnect insulin pump, and return it safely back to family.
- Pump infusion set insertion in the body can remain intact if away from surgical site.
- For inpatients, the pump should be removed, stored safely with patient belongings or with family and intravenous insulin initiated in am of surgery.
- Glucose checks should be performed hourly and drip rate titrated per protocol in holding and during surgery.
- More frequent checks may be necessary if clinical condition requires.

POSTOPERATIVE PACU MANAGEMENT

Procedures of < 2 hours, outpatient procedures

- If insulin pump has remained intact during procedure
  - Glucose is checked and pump continued in PACU
  - Patient is discharged when awake and able to manage insulin pump.
- If insulin pump was discontinued before or during surgery and replaced by an insulin infusion,
  - Pump is restarted in PACU when patient is alert and able to manage it.
  - **OVERLAP insulin drip and pump for at least an hour before discontinuing insulin drip.**
  - Glucose is checked prior to discharge to confirm that the pump is delivering insulin.
- Patient is instructed to resume normal basal and bolus pump rates when they start to eat.

glucose control.[19] In a single small prospective trial of cardiac surgery patients, intensive intraoperative glucose targets of 80–110 mg/dL did not improve outcomes or length of stay, but in fact increased the incidence of hypoglycemia and stroke.[20] Insulin resistance during surgery is associated with poor outcomes, but prospective treatment trials are not available.[21]

INTRAOPERATIVE CONSIDERATIONS

The stress of surgery and anesthesia releases a large number of neurohumoral and inflammatory factors into the circulation. These include catecholamines, cortisol, growth hormone, cytokines (interleukin-6 and tumor necrosis factor-α), and metabolic by-products (of lipolysis and protein catabolism), all of which increase insulin resistance, decrease peripheral utilization of glucose, and impair insulin secretion, thus causing hyperglycemia.[2] The degree of intraoperative hyperglycemia is based on a number of factors, including the length and nature of the procedure, the induction and anesthetic agent used, drugs and nutrients administered (steroids, parenteral nutrition, β-blockers), and patient factors (infection or trauma).[8] General anesthesia—especially with volatile agents (halothane, enflurane, isoflurane)—releases counterregulatory hormones and raises glucose levels. In contrast, epidural anesthesia has a minimal effect on glucose metabolism, and induction agents such as etomidate, benzodiazepines, and opioids block the effects of stress on cortisol and sympathetic hormones and thus do not adversely affect glucose levels.[22]

Hypothermia is a strong stimulus for insulin resistance and can increase insulin requirements during induction of hypothermic circulatory arrest. With rewarming, insulin resistance starts to improve and the drip rates of IV insulin need to reduced. This is an important management issue immediately after cardiac surgery when the patient is transferred to the intensive care unit (ICU). In addition, IV steroids used intraoperatively to prevent nausea and vomiting can raise glucose levels significantly. The hyperglycemic effect of a single large dose of solumedrol or dexamethasone can cause prolonged perioperative hyperglycemia, especially in patients with poorly controlled diabetes.

INTRAOPERATIVE TARGETS

Because of a lack of evidence-based guidelines and the inability of a sedated patient to recognize or respond to hypoglycemia, most institutions use a safe intraoperative glucose target range of 120–200 mg/dL.[14,23]

Preoperative glucose >250 mg/dL, especially in patients with T1D, may trigger an evaluation for DKA, hyperglycemic states, or other metabolic abnormalities. Procedures generally are canceled when glucose levels are >400 mg/dL and are not based on evidence-based guidelines (e.g., >500 mg/dL; Boston University).[23] Because metabolic stability and the risk of postoperative infection are of concern at these high glucose levels, the clinical judgment of the anesthesiology and surgical provider should guide this decision. Surgery in a severely hyperglycemic case associated with a septic focus should not be postponed, as surgical removal of the infected tissue will improve glucose values, as in an amputation or cholecystectomy.

INTRAOPERATIVE REGIMENS

For procedures of <2 h, monitoring glucose levels every hour and using a short-acting insulin analog correction scale may be adequate to maintain glucose goals in moderately sensitive hyperglycemic patients. For major procedures and those requiring long periods of NPO status, IV insulin infusions are required to control glucose. Trigger glucose levels for insulin drip initiation vary among institutions and again have no evidence-based data to support them: University of Michigan proposes 160 mg/dL, Boston University uses 180 mg/dL, and Yale uses 200 mg/dL.[23] Standardized insulin infusion protocols and computer-guided algorithms can help improve glucose control and may reduce hypoglycemia and glucose variability.[2,3] An institution's insulin drip protocol should specify the frequency of glucose monitoring (i.e., hourly) and outline the conditions for increasing or decreasing the monitoring frequency based on the glucose response. Dosing should be based on the glucose value obtained and also the change in value in the last time period. The safety and efficacy of the protocol also should have been validated.

POSTOPERATIVE GLUCOSE CONTROL

RATIONALE AND EVIDENCE

In the ambulatory setting, no data on the impact of postoperative control on outcomes is available. In patients hospitalized after a procedure, hyperglycemia is associated with an increased risk of adverse outcomes, irrespective of whether the patient has diabetes or stress hyperglycemia.[24–26] In cardiac and noncardiac surgery patients, hyperglycemia is associated with a high risk of nosocomial infections and renal dysfunction. Poor wound healing results from the formation of advanced glycation end products and cytokines, which interfere with collagen formation and fibroblast proliferation.[27] In situations of reduced chemotaxis and phagocytosis, bacteria proliferate, leading to surgical site infections, the most common health-associated infections.

Cardiac surgery populations were the initial group in which glucose levels controlled to <200 mg/dL were found to reduce the incidence of deep sternal wound infection and mortality.[28,29] In a randomized controlled study of surgical critically ill patients, morbidity and mortality were reduced significantly with intensive glucose control to 80–110 mg/dL.[30] Several trials that followed failed to show the same risk reduction with intensive control, whereas others were stopped because of a very high incidence of hypoglycemia. The Normoglycemia in Intensive Care Evaluation-Survival Using Glucose Algorithm Regulation (NICE-SUGAR) study was the largest trial evaluating intensive glucose control in large surgical and medical populations. It reported increased mortality at 90 days from cardiovascular causes in the intensive control group. On the basis of these results, current guidelines recommend a glucose target of 140–180 mg/dL, which can be achieved by most institutions with minimal hypoglycemia.[31] In a meta-analysis of ICU trials, the risk of hypoglycemia was increased with intensive glucose control, but when separated by type of ICU setting, the surgical ICUs continued to show benefit from intensive glucose control.[32]

In the inpatient general unit setting, several retrospective studies have linked hyperglycemia with poor outcomes in varied patient populations, but few prospective trials are available.[3,33] In one randomized controlled trial of postsurgical patients, basal-bolus insulin therapy with a goal of maintaining premeal and fasting glucose values to <140 mg/dL improved outcomes when compared with sliding-scale insulin but had higher rates of hypoglycemia. This morbidity reduction was attributed to lower postsurgical infection rates and renal failure, whereas mortality was not different among the groups.[34]

POSTOPERATIVE CONSIDERATIONS

Important issues that affect glucose control and management strategies in postoperative patients include the following: *1)* whether a patient has stress-induced hyperglycemia or diabetes, and the type of diabetes; *2)* the patient's nutrition plan (NPO, enteral or total parenteral nutrition); and *3)* the patient's use of medications that contribute to hyper- or hypoglycemia (including vasopressors, steroids, octreotide, and pentoxyphiline).

POSTOPERATIVE TARGETS

No targets for ambulatory surgery are available. For hospitalized patients, moderate postoperative glucose control is used in the ICU setting with an emphasis on safe and effective glucose management with the prevention of hypoglycemia.[35] The American Diabetes Association and the Society of Thoracic Surgeons currently recommend starting insulin infusions in ICU patients at a threshold no greater than 180 mg/dL and then maintaining the glucose range between 140 and 180 mg/dL. The Critical Care Society recommends that insulin drips should be started when glucose values are >150 mg/dL and that glucose be maintained <180 mg/dL with drip titration.[36] Data exist that targeting the lower end of this range may be beneficial in certain patient populations, such as postsurgical, posttrauma, or those on steroids,[3,37] and a goal of 120–140 mg/dL was shown to offer the metabolic advantage of reduced negative nitrogen balance.[38] Agreement is unanimous that a glucose goal of <110 mg/dL is not routinely recommended.

Outside the intensive care setting, there are no data for BG goals in postsurgical patients. General guidelines from the American Diabetes Association suggest a premeal or fasting goal of <140 mg/dL and a postprandial and bedtime target of <180 mg/dL. Therapy should be reassessed when glucose levels are <100 mg/dL and should be modified when glucose values go <70 mg/dL to reduce the risk of future hypoglycemia. For patients who are clinically stable and have excellent outpatient glucose levels, more stringent goals may be used, whereas those with hypoglycemia unawareness or other comorbidities (coronary artery disease, terminal illness) need higher targets.[33]

POSTOPERATIVE REGIMENS

Ambulatory Procedure

In the postanesthesia care unit (PACU), glucose should be monitored postoperatively and before discharge to screen for hypoglycemia. If an insulin drip was used during the ambulatory procedure, glucose should be checked an hour after drip discontinuation. The patient should be instructed to resume oral agents or subcutaneous insulin when they start eating. This is particularly important for patients with T1D to ensure that they do not go into DKA. For patients on metformin who received a contrast agent or underwent a procedure that could compromise renal function, the metformin should be started 48 h after the procedure, and in some circumstances, a follow-up creatinine level may be required before restarting the metformin.[10,11,13]

Insulin Pump Therapy

For an ambulatory procedure in patients whose insulin pump was continued through the procedure, the patient is discharged when awake, with a stable glucose level, and the patient is able to manage the pump safely. If the pump was discontinued before or during surgery and replaced by an insulin infusion, the patient must be alert and able to manage the insulin pump before restarting it.[18] The insulin drip should overlap with the pump for at least an hour before the drip is discontinued. A glucose check before discharge should confirm that the pump is delivering insulin. If the pump basal rates were reduced before surgery, patients can resume their normal basal and bolus rates once they begin eating.

Hospitalization after a Procedure

A continuous IV insulin infusion is the best method of controlling hyperglycemia in postsurgical patients being admitted to the ICU. In addition, subcutaneous basal insulin (insulin glargine or detemir) can be given along with an insulin drip and can be helpful in several circumstances. Starting basal insulin 12–24 h before discontinuing the IV insulin drip may help to smooth the transition to subcutaneous insulin regimens.[9] Experiences at the University of Michigan have demonstrated reduced glucose variability and smoother transitions to subcutaneous insulin with the addition of a small dose of subcutaneous basal insulin to support an insulin infusion that has a high and erratic drip rate. For a subcutaneous basal dose, 10–20% of patient's TDD of insulin, based on their weight in kilograms, is a reasonable starting point.

In patients with T1D, adding a small dose of subcutaneous basal insulin (10% of TDD) under the drip will ensure that the patient always has insulin on board and helps prevent DKA in case the drip is discontinued for prolonged periods of time. In addition, a study evaluating the effect of basal insulin given to cardiac surgery patients with stress hyperglycemia on admission to the ICU found that the length of the insulin infusion was reduced significantly. This may have implications for nursing workload reduction.[39]

To cover postprandial excursions when a patient starts to eat while on an insulin drip, use of rapid-acting subcutaneous and carbohydrate counting or IV insulin doses adjusted based on the drip rate can moderate these elevations.

Transitioning an insulin drip to subcutaneous insulin is done once the patient is stable, off vasopressors, extubated, and eating or being maintained on a stable regimen of enteral or parental nutrition. Specific guidelines and doses for drip transition are outlined in Chapter 8. To transition a patient to subcutaneous insulin, the insulin drip needs to be continued for a few hours after giving the subcutaneous insulin. To prevent rebound hyperglycemia in situations in which there is concern that the insulin drip will be prematurely discontinued, a "bridging dose" of short-acting insulin may be given. This bridging dose can be based on the drip rate or calculated as 10% of the basal dose and the drip should be stopped immediately after it is administered.[40]

For patients with stress hyperglycemia and a normal HbA_{1c} who are on a low insulin drip rate (<2 units/h), basal insulin may not be required and they can be transitioned to an insulin correction scale and glucose levels followed.[33] The University of Michigan guideline to transition patients with stress hyperglycemia uses tapering doses of NPH. The TDD is calculated based on the last 8 h of the drip rate and is divided equally into two injections of NPH. One dose is given at transition time and the next dose is 20% less and is given at bedtime. Each subsequent dose of NPH is again reduced by at least 20%, until reaching 0.

Inpatient Management

Patients transferred to the inpatient floor after a procedure can be placed back on their preoperative insulin regimen if HbA_{1c} was <7.5% preoperatively. Otherwise, a new insulin regimen should be considered (see Chapter 5).

CONCLUSION

Perioperative glucose management can reduce surgical morbidity especially by reducing infectious complications. This process starts with well-planned modification of the preoperative diabetes regimen to prevent hyperglycemia, hypoglycemia, and acute metabolic derangements. This brings the patient into surgery with a reasonable glucose value that then can be monitored and treated more effectively. A correction scale is usually adequate for short procedures, whereas an IV insulin infusion is used for major procedures and those with a duration of >2 h. Intraoperative glucose treatment targets are liberal, suggested to range from 120 to 200 mg/dL, and hypoglycemia must be avoided. Postoperative management in ambulatory patients consists of insulin drips with or without basal insulin and restarting oral hypoglycemic agent and mealtime insulin when the patient begins eating.

REFERENCES

1. Cullen KA, Hall MJ, Golosinskiy A. Ambulatory surgery in the United States, 2006. *Natl Health Stat Report* 2009;11:1–25

2. Clement S, et al. Management of diabetes and hyperglycemia in hospitals. *Diabetes Care* 2004;27(2):553–591

3. Moghissi ES, et al. American Association of Clinical Endocrinologists and American Diabetes Association consensus statement on inpatient glycemic control. *Endocr Pract* 2009;15(4):353–369

4. Kosiborod M, et al. Relationship between spontaneous and iatrogenic hypoglycemia and mortality in patients hospitalized with acute myocardial infarction. *JAMA* 2009;301(15):1556–1564

5. Dronge AS, et al. Long-term glycemic control and postoperative infectious complications. *Arch Surg* 2006;141(4):375–380; discussion 380
6. King JT, Jr, et al. Glycemic control and infections in patients with diabetes undergoing noncardiac surgery. *Ann Surg* 2011;253(1):158–165
7. Rosenblatt SI, et al. Insulin glargine dosing before next-day surgery: comparing three strategies. *J Clin Anesth* 2012;24(8):610–617
8. McAnulty GR, Robertshaw HJ, Hall GM. Anaesthetic management of patients with diabetes mellitus. *Br J Anaesth* 2000;85(1):80–90
9. Meneghini LF, Perioperative management of diabetes: translating evidence into practice. *Cleve Clin J Med* 2009;76(Suppl. 4):S53–S59
10. Joshi GP, et al. Society for Ambulatory Anesthesia consensus statement on perioperative blood glucose management in diabetic patients undergoing ambulatory surgery. *Anesth Analg* 2010;111(6):1378–1387
11. Bodnar TW, Gianchandani R. Preprocedure and preoperative management of diabetes mellitus. *Postgrad Med* 2014;126(6):73–80
12. Gerstein HC, et al. Glycemia treatment strategies in the Action to Control Cardiovascular Risk in Diabetes (ACCORD) trial. *Am J Cardiol* 2007;99(12A):34i–43i
13. Duncan AI, et al. Recent metformin ingestion does not increase in-hospital morbidity or mortality after cardiac surgery. *Anesth Analg* 2007;104(1):42–50
14. Vann MA. Perioperative management of ambulatory surgical patients with diabetes mellitus. *Curr Opin Anaesthesiol* 2009;22(6):718–724
15. Schwartz SS, DeFronzo RA, Umpierrez GE. Practical implementation of incretin-based therapy in hospitalized patients with type 2 diabetes. *Postgrad Med* 2014:1–7
16. Takeshi S, et al. Evaluation of safety of insulin degludec on undergoing total colonoscopy using continuous glucose monitoring. *J Diabetes Investig* 2014;63(Suppl. 1A). Available online at http://onlinelibrary.wiley.com/doi/10.1111/jdi.12409/abstract
17. Professional Practice Committee for the standards of medical care in diabetes—2015. *Diabetes Care* 2015;38(Suppl. 1):S88–S89
18. Boyle ME, et al.. Insulin pump therapy in the perioperative period: a review of care after implementation of institutional guidelines. *J Diabetes Sci Technol* 2012;6(5):1016–1021
19. Gandhi GY, et al. Intraoperative hyperglycemia and perioperative outcomes in cardiac surgery patients. *Mayo Clin Proc* 2005;80(7):862–866
20. Gandhi GY, et al. Intensive intraoperative insulin therapy versus conventional glucose management during cardiac surgery: a randomized trial. *Ann Intern Med* 2007;146(4):233–243

21. Sato H, et al. The association of preoperative glycemic control, intraoperative insulin sensitivity, and outcomes after cardiac surgery. *J Clin Endocrinol Metab* 2010;95(9):4338–4344
22. Wolf AR, et al. Effect of extradural analgesia on stress responses to abdominal surgery in infants. *Br J Anaesth* 1993;70(6):654–660
23. Alexanian SM, McDonnell ME, Akhtar S. Creating a perioperative glycemic control program. *Anesthesiol Res Pract* 2011;2011:465974
24. Capes SE, et al. Stress hyperglycaemia and increased risk of death after myocardial infarction in patients with and without diabetes: a systematic overview. *Lancet* 2000;355(9206):773–778
25. Umpierrez GE, et al. Hyperglycemia: an independent marker of in-hospital mortality in patients with undiagnosed diabetes. *J Clin Endocrinol Metab* 2002;87(3):978–982
26. Falciglia M. Causes and consequences of hyperglycemia in critical illness. *Curr Opin Clin Nutr Metab Care* 2007;10(4):498–503
27. Tsourdi E, et al. Current aspects in the pathophysiology and treatment of chronic wounds in diabetes mellitus. *Biomed Res Int* 2013;2013:385641
28. Zerr KJ, et al. Glucose control lowers the risk of wound infection in diabetics after open heart operations. *Ann Thorac Surg* 1997;63(2):356–361
29. Furnary AP, et al. Continuous insulin infusion reduces mortality in patients with diabetes undergoing coronary artery bypass grafting. *J Thorac Cardiovasc Surg* 2003;125(5):1007–1021
30. Van den Berghe G, et al. Intensive insulin therapy in the critically ill patients. *N Engl J Med* 2001;345(19):1359–1367
31. Finfer S, Heritier S. The NICE-SUGAR (Normoglycaemia in Intensive Care Evaluation and Survival Using Glucose Algorithm Regulation) Study: statistical analysis plan. *Crit Care Resusc* 2009;11(1):46–57
32. Griesdale DE, et al. Intensive insulin therapy and mortality among critically ill patients: a meta-analysis including NICE-SUGAR study data. *CMAJ* 2009;180(8):821–827
33. Umpierrez GE, et al. Management of hyperglycemia in hospitalized patients in non-critical care setting: an Endocrine Society clinical practice guideline. *J Clin Endocrinol Metab* 2012;97(1):16–38
34. Umpierrez GE, et al. Randomized study of basal-bolus insulin therapy in the inpatient management of patients with type 2 diabetes undergoing general surgery (RABBIT 2 surgery). *Diabetes Care* 2011;34(2):256–261
35. Finfer S, et al. Intensive versus conventional glucose control in critically ill patients. *N Engl J Med* 2009;360(13):1283–1297
36. Jacobi J, et al. Guidelines for the use of an insulin infusion for the management of hyperglycemia in critically ill patients. *Crit Care Med* 2012;40(12):3251–3276

37. Lazar HL, et al. The Society of Thoracic Surgeons practice guideline series: blood glucose management during adult cardiac surgery. *Ann Thorac Surg* 2009;87(2):663–669
38. Hsu CW, et al. Moderate glucose control results in less negative nitrogen balances in medical intensive care unit patients: a randomized, controlled study. *Crit Care* 2012;16(2):R56
39. Aggarwal A, et al. Long-acting subcutaneously administered insulin for glycemic control immediately after cardiac surgery. *Endocr Pract* 2011;17(4):558–562
40. Schmeltz LR, et al. Conversion of intravenous insulin infusions to subcutaneously administered insulin glargine in patients with hyperglycemia. *Endocr Pract* 2006;12(6):641–650

Chapter 10

Treatment of Hyperglycemia on Medical and Surgical Units

Robert J. Rushakoff, MD,[1] Heidemarie Windham MacMaster, PharmD, CDE, FCSHP,[2] Mercedes Falciglia, MD, FACP,[3] and Kristen Kulasa, MD[4]

INTRODUCTION

Effective inpatient glycemic management limits the risks of severe hypo- and hyperglycemia and has the potential to reduce rates of morbidity and mortality. Even in patients who have had excellent outpatient glucose control, achieving this goal can be challenging as the inpatient environment and the patient's metabolic status is fundamentally different from the patient's outpatient daily life. Nutritional intake may be ever changing, delayed, and unpredictable because of the underlying medical or surgical reason for admission. Patients who use exercise as a cornerstone of their treatment may be at bed rest. Elevated counterregulatory hormones resulting from stress, relative physical inactivity, medications such as pressors or glucocorticoids, and agents administered with intravenous (IV) dextrose all represent scenarios and factors that increase blood glucose values. A patient who may have sepsis, renal failure, or hepatic failure or who may receive insulin before a meal that ultimately is not consumed, is placed at risk for hypoglycemia. Insulin directions from preadmission medication lists for patients often reflect the prescription order, not the current dosing regimen and thus may not be appropriate to resume on admission. Finally, some patients who have had considerable self-control of their diabetes management, given these constraints, will not have the knowledge to translate their outpatient regimens to safe inpatient care adjustments. Additionally, there may be conflict with patients who wish to maintain control of their inpatient diabetes management. It is in this environment that appropriate orders need to be written to safely manage diabetes during hospitalization.

As of this time, treatment goals for blood glucose remain controversial. Although organizations have published goals that premeal glucoses should be <140 mg/dL and <180 mg/dL at other times, evidence is insufficient to support

[1]Professor of Medicine, Director, Inpatient Diabetes, Division of Endocrinology and Metabolism, University of California, San Francisco, CA. [2]Diabetes Management Specialist, Institute of Nursing Excellence, Assistant Clinical Professor, Department of Clinical Pharmacy, School of Pharmacy, University of California, San Francisco Medical Center, San Francisco, CA. [3]Associate Professor of Medicine, Endocrinology, Diabetes & Metabolism, University of Cincinnati College of Medicine, Acting Chief, Endocrinology, Diabetes & Metabolism, Cincinnati VA Medical Center, Cincinnati, OH. [4]Assistant Clinical Professor of Medicine, Director, Inpatient Glycemic Control, Division of Endocrinology, Diabetes, and Metabolism, University of California, San Diego, CA.

DOI: 10.2337/9781580406086.10

the lower limit for blood glucose in which benefit outweighs the potential risk of hypoglycemia. In addition, despite a variety research studies with dedicated diabetes teams using protocols to aggressively lower glucose levels, these suggested goals have not been met[1–3] and therapy was modified if the HbA_{1c} targets for blood glucose (BG) in the inpatient setting are based largely on extrapolation of research conducted in the critical care setting as no clinical studies directly compare different glycemic targets in this patient population.[4] In general, a goal for glucoses between 110 and 180 mg/dL remains reasonable as long as these targets can be safely achieved, but glucoses will be outside this range at times despite the best management skills. It is important to note that the recommendations from professional organizations emphasize the need to individualize BG targets, based on the clinical circumstances of each patient.

To successfully manage inpatient diabetes, institutional infrastructure must be in place with institution-specific guidelines and protocols for educating all nursing staff, pharmacists, physicians, and other health-care team members. Without this comprehensive underlying structure in place, it will be difficult to safely manage patients with hyperglycemia. The general guidelines and following methods are appropriate for most institutions.

PHYSIOLOGIC INSULIN REGIMEN

All patients have "basal, nutritional, and correctional" insulin requirements that must be met with endogenous or exogenous insulin. All of these are utilized for writing inpatient insulin orders.

- **Basal:** Insulin needed even when patient is not eating (to control gluconeogenesis).
  Use glargine (usually once daily in the morning or at bedtime), NPH (once daily at bedtime, or in the morning and bedtime), detemir (once daily or q 12 h), or a continuous subcutaneous (SQ) insulin infusion with rapid-acting insulin (insulin pump).
- **Nutritional:** Insulin needed to cover carbohydrate intake from food, dextrose in intravenous fluid (IVF), tube feeds, and total parental nutrition (TPN).
  Use rapid-acting insulin (aspart, lispro, or glulisine) or short-acting insulin (regular).
- **Correctional:** Insulin given to bring a high blood glucose level down to target range. For example, for a patient who is eating, the target range would be usually < 150 mg/dL premeal and <200 mg/dL at bedtime or 2 A.M.
  Use rapid-acting insulin (aspart, lispro, or glulisine) or short-acting insulin (regular); this insulin type should be the same as the nutritional insulin.

GENERAL GUIDELINES

Patients with type 1 diabetes (T1D) always need exogenous basal insulin or an IV infusion to cover basal needs even when they receive no nutrients. Failure to provide insulin will invariably lead to diabetic ketoacidosis (DKA).

AVOID EXCLUSIVE USE OF SLIDING-SCALE INSULIN

With the few exceptions, arbitrary sliding-scale insulin should be avoided as it is not only ineffective but also potentially dangerous. Originally proposed sliding-scale methodology dates to diabetes monitoring by urine glucose levels. Urine monitoring methods would change colors depending on how much glucose was in the urine, and insulin was then given based on the change in color. This method was called "rainbow coverage" and inevitably resulted in "roller coaster glucose control." Under this protocol, the patient would not receive insulin when their glucose level was normal and a few hours later their glucose level would predictably increase (Figure 10.1).

Of great concern, patients with T1D were at risk for periods of insulin deficiency and subsequent DKA with use of this sliding scale. Furthermore, patients who are thought to have type 2 diabetes (T2D), but who actually have T1D or latent autoimmune diabetes of adults (LADA) or who may be relatively insulinopenic, are also at increased risk of DKA with use of sliding scale. The Institute of Safe Medication Practices (ISMP) recommends that hospitals implement safe practices to prevent these avoidable DKA events.

Historically, sliding-scale insulin was given on a "nurse-centric" fixed-time schedule to standardize dosing and documentation, with no relation to if or when a patient may be eating and not making any physiologic sense. Now, these types of correctional orders generally are written for use at meals intended for patients who are eating; in some cases, the doses of insulin may be much more aggressive, approaching what actually would be considered a nutritional dose. As will be discussed, however, nutritional premeal insulin is most often required and is more physiologically sound. In the movement to provide patient-centric meals and patient satisfaction scores, many hospitals are moving to feeding patients at the time they want to eat (see the next section). Hospitals must put safety nets in place to prevent insulin stacking from back-to-back meals and overcorrection of a postprandial blood glucose reading. In addition, patients who skip or miss meals with mealtime insulin orders should still have their glucose monitored to assess for correctional insulin and to optimize glycemic control.

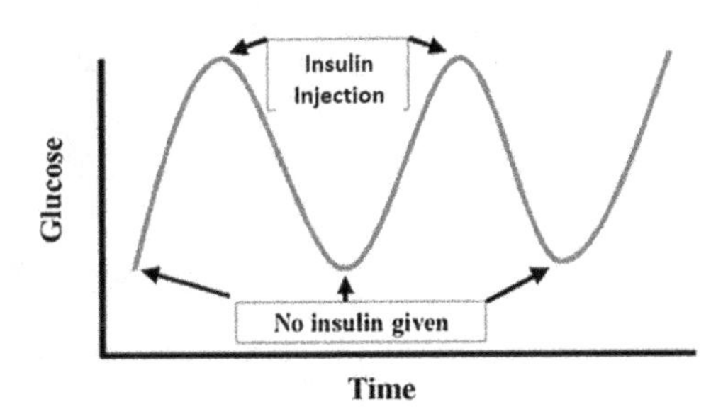

Figure 10.1—Sliding-scale insulin.

ORAL HYPOGLYCEMIA AGENTS AND OTHER NONINSULIN AGENTS

In general, oral diabetes medications and noninsulin injectables (e.g., glucagon-like peptide agonists) are discontinued during an acute hospitalization of a patient with diabetes and are inappropriate for initial management of the nondiabetic hyperglycemic patient in the inpatient setting. Table 10.1 describes various risks associated with use of these agents in the hospital setting.

In the rare hospitalized patient who is clinically stable and who has normal nutritional intake, normal blood glucose levels, and stable renal and cardiac

Table 10.1—Potential Disadvantages Associated with Specific Oral Antihyperglycemic Agents in the Hospital Setting

Agent	Potential disadvantages
Insulin secretagogues (sulfonylureas, including glyburide, glipizide, and glimepiride; and nonsulfonylureas, including repaglinide and nateglinide)	Hypoglycemia if caloric intake is reduced Increased risk of prolonged hypoglycemia in those that are long-acting, especially in the setting of acute renal failure
Metformin	Increased risk of lactic acidosis when used in the setting of renal dysfunction, circulatory compromise, or hypoxemia Relatively slow onset of action Possible GI upset, nausea, diarrhea
Thiazoladinediones (e.g., rosiglitazone and pioglitazone)	Very slow onset of action (2–3 weeks) Possible fluid retention (particularly when used with insulin) and increased risk for CHF Contraindication in presence of liver disease or transaminitis
α-Glucosidase inhibitors (e.g., acarbose, miglitol)	No clinical benefits in the fasting patient Possible abdominal bloating and flatus Requirement for treatment with pure dextrose should hypoglycemia occur in the setting of the agent
GLP-1 mimetics (e.g., exenatide)	Limited inpatient data Possible abdominal bloating and nausea secondary to delayed gastric emptying
DPP-4 inhibitors (e.g., sitagliptin)	Limited inpatient data
SGLT-2 inhibitor	Limited inpatient data Low risk of hypoglycemia
Other: colesevelam; dopamine agonists	Limited data Gastrointestinal side effects Colesevelam binds medications

CHF, congestive heart failure; GLP, glucagon-like peptide; DPP-4, dipeptidyl peptidase 4; SGLT, sodium-glucose linked transporter.

function, it is possible that the medications may be continued safely. Oral agents may be started or resumed in the hospital if they are to be included in the discharge medication regimen, once the patient is clinically stable and once it has been ensured that contraindications to their use no longer exist.

INSULIN ORDERS

Whether paper-based or computer order entry, standardized comprehensive insulin orders are recommended. The orders should include orders for glucose monitoring, insulin dosing, and hypoglycemia treatment that are familiar to the providers, pharmacy, and nursing staff.

As shown in Figure 10.2, an example of an insulin order set for a patient eating is shown. The components previously discussed and nutritional, correctional, and basal insulin are all easily ordered.

BASICS ON INSULIN REGIMENS FOR HOSPITALIZED PATIENTS

This section discusses the methods we have found useful to determine both the initial insulin doses and ongoing adjustments of insulin doses. The general components of insulin regimens are the basal, nutritional, and correctional dosing. For all of the following, it is imperative that insulin doses must be reevaluated at least

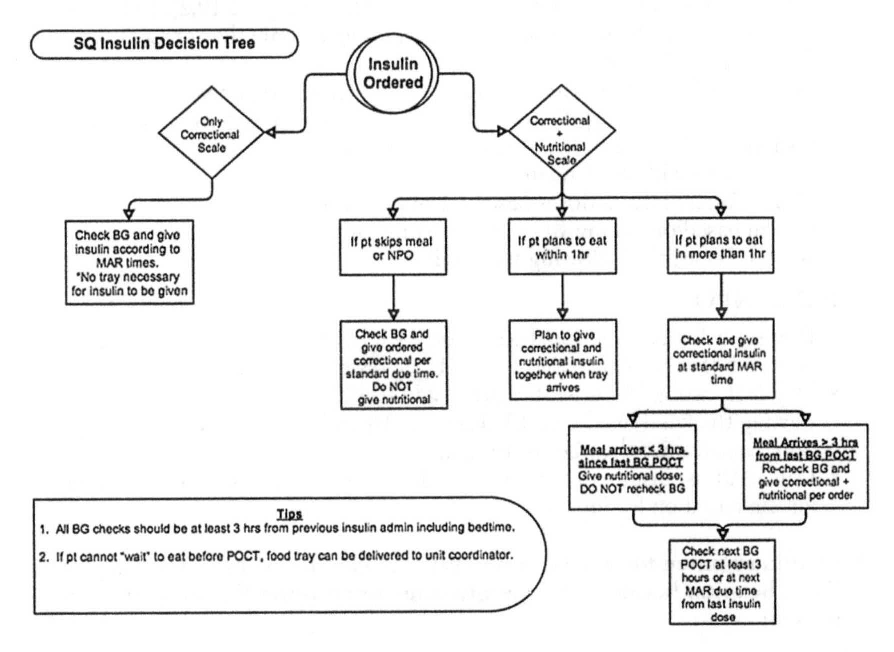

Figure 10.2—The decision tree for insulin administration for patients with meals on demand. BG, blood glucose; MAR, medication administration record; SQ, subcutaneous.

daily and adjusted to adapt to the patients' changing clinical situation and to achieve glycemic goals.

- Nutritional coverage: Short-acting regular insulin is given 30 min before each meal. The rapid-acting insulins, lispro, aspart, or apidra, are given with each meal or immediately after eating (the dose then may be based on amount eaten).
- Total daily dose of insulin needed for patients with T1D require approximately 0.2 to 0.4 units/kg/day; patients with T2D vary in their insulin resistance and may require from 0.5 to 2 units/kg/day.

1. **Insulin regimen for a patient controlled only with diet at home but needing insulin in hospital:**
The patient with diabetes but not requiring oral medications or insulin at baseline may be the one circumstance in which correctional insulin alone may be a sufficient initial order. Although some advocate for automatically starting insulin in these patients, we believe that this places some patients at risk for initial hypoglycemia. These patients may need significant insulin as their hospitalization progresses.

Patient eating

- Day 1: Order a correctional scale for meals and bedtime (with lispro, aspart, apidra, or regular) based on BMI (see order form; Figure 10.2). In this instance, no nutritional dose is written for a meal, only the correction dose for an elevated glucose is delivered.
- Day 2: If BG pre-meals are >150 mg/dL, add nutritional insulin. *Also*, if fasting BG is >150 mg/dL, add basal insulin. For most patients, starting the insulin at 0.2–0.3 units/kg/day, with half given as basal and half divided for meal dosing will be adequate.
- Day 3: Adjust insulin doses based on BG pattern; increase or decrease basal insulin based on fasting BG, and adjust nutritional insulin based on premeal BG levels (see the following for details).

Patient NPO

- Day 1: Order a correctional scale every 4 h (with lispro, aspart, apidra) or every 6 h (for regular) based on BMI (see order form; Figure 10.2).
- Day 2: If fasting BG is >150 mg/dL, add basal insulin. For most patients, starting the basal insulin at 0.1–1.5 units/kg will be adequate. The correctional insulin can then be continued.
- Day 3: Adjust insulin doses based on BG pattern. Increase or decrease basal insulin based on fasting BG.

2. **Insulin regimen for a patient on oral agents at home but requiring insulin in hospital because of hyperglycemia or contraindications to the oral agents:**

Patient eating

- Day 1: Generally start with basal/nutritional dosing. Starting dose is 0.3–0.5 units/kg/day, with half given as basal and half divided for premeal dosing. Some caution must be used. The effect of the patient's home oral agents still may have a significant glucose-lowering effect based on the agent used. If glucose on admission is low or low normal, correctional insulin alone may be appropriate for the first day or so. Glucoses generally will begin to increase thereafter and insulin should be initiated as described previously.

- Day 2: Adjust insulin doses based on BG pattern. Increase or decrease basal insulin based on fasting BG and adjust nutritional insulin based on pre-meal BG levels (see the following for details).

Patient NPO

- Day 1: Generally start with basal and correctional insulin. Starting basal dose is 0.15–0.25 units/kg/day. Order a correctional scale every 4 h (with lispro, aspart, apidra) or every 6 h (for regular) based on BMI (see order form; Figure 10.2). Some caution must be used. The effect of the patient's home oral agents still may have a significant glucose-lower effect based on the agent used. If glucose on admission is low or low normal, correctional insulin alone may be appropriate for the first day or so. Glucoses generally will begin to increase thereafter and insulin should be initiated as described previously.
- Day 2: Adjust insulin doses based on BG pattern. Increase or decrease basal insulin based on fasting BG.

3. **Insulin regimen for a patient on insulin at home:**
For patients previously on insulin, there needs to be consideration of type of diabetes, home BG control, appetite, renal function, and risk for hypoglycemia. All three components of insulin replacement must be addressed: basal, nutritional, and correctional.

Patient eating

- Day 1
  - Basal requirements: Continue home regimen, and consider decreasing the total dose by 20–30% to reduce the risk of in-hospital hypoglycemia if the patient has been well controlled at home. Often the larger the basal dose used at home, the greater the need to decrease this on admission. For some patients on large doses of basal insulin, the basal insulin may be covering a portion of their nutritional needs. With decreased nutritional intake, they are at significant risk for hypoglycemia.
  - If the patient is on premixed insulin at home, convert to basal and mealtime insulin, starting with about half of this as basal insulin and half divided for meals. Inpatient use of premixed insulin has been associated with an increased risk for hypoglycemia.[5]
  - If the patient is on mealtime insulin at home, then this dose, or 80% of the home dose, can be continued.
  - If no mealtime insulin is used at home, then starting at 0.1–0.2 units/kg/day, divided for meals, is a reasonable starting approach.
  - Correctional need: Order a correctional scale based on total insulin dose or BMI (see Table 10.1).

- Day 2: Adjust insulin doses based on BG pattern. Increase or decrease basal insulin based on fasting BG, and adjust nutritional insulin based on premeal BG levels (see the following for details).

Patient NPO

- Day 1
  - Basal requirements: Continue home basal regimen and consider decreasing the total dose by 20–30% to reduce the risk of in-hospital hypoglycemia if the patient has been well controlled at home. Often, the larger the basal dose used at home, the greater the need to decrease this on admission. For some patients on large doses of basal insulin, the basal dose may cover their nutritional intake. With decrease nutritional intake, they are at significant risk for hypoglycemia.
  - If the patient is on premixed insulin at home, convert to basal and mealtime insulin, starting with about half of this as basal insulin and half divided for meals.
  - Correctional need: Order a correctional scale based on total insulin dose or BMI (see Table 10.1).
  - If patient has T1D, then consider starting IV insulin infusion.
- Day 2: Adjust insulin doses based on BG pattern. Increase or decrease basal insulin based on morning fasting BG and adjust correction insulin based on glucose levels during the day.

4. **Insulin regimen when a patient is made NPO for a procedure:** A patient always will require his or her basal insulin, even while NPO, and should not become hypoglycemic if that basal insulin is dosed appropriately. For safety purposes, however, adhere to the following:
   - The night before the procedure, give the usual dose of bedtime NPH, if applicable, or decrease the usual dose of bedtime glargine by up to 25%.
   - The morning of the procedure, if applicable, decrease the usual dose of morning NPH by 50%, or decrease the usual dose of morning glargine by up to 25%.
   - Do not give nutritional insulin (as the patient is not eating) but continue the usual correctional insulin.

5. **Special circumstances:**

   Insulin based on carbohydrate counting: Some outpatients will calculate their nutritional insulin dose based on the amount of carbohydrate they ingest. For example, a person may use a ratio of 1:10 (1 unit of insulin for every 10 g of carbohydrate). For a typical meal with 40 g of carbohydrate, a patient would take 4 units of nutritional insulin, in addition to what is required for correction. This same type of order can be used for inpatients with the nutritional insulin dose based on the carbohydrate in their meals. Depending on the patient preferences and needs, the amount of carbohydrate eaten at meals may be a set amount, or may vary, with nutritional insulin determined accordingly. Registered dietitian nutritionists (RDs or RDNs) are integral to determining the best method to be used, along with the patient. Nursing staff needs to be trained to understand the basic principles of counting if this method is to be utilized. The standardized practice of insulin dosing through carbohydrate counting should be considered carefully prior to implementation based on the resources and familiarity of staff with carbohydrate counting.

Patient with irregular or unpredictable nutritional intake: Administering the full nutritional dose to patients experiencing nausea or advancing from a limited diet may place the patient at risk for hypoglycemia, and correction insulin dosing also may not be adequate. We provide two potential scenarios that are best operationalized with standard order sets and nursing staff trained on use.

- Write orders so that the nutritional insulin dose of rapid-acting insulin is given after the meal. Rapid-acting insulin has an onset of action within minutes as opposed to regular insulin, which has a delayed onset of action that could predispose the patient to hypoglycemia if given after the meal. If the patient does not eat, only correction insulin is given. If 50% of the meal is eaten, 50% of the nutritional insulin would be given.
- Use postmeal insulin dosing based on carbohydrate counting as noted.
- Once the patient resumes regular eating, then the dose of insulin is given premeal and is based on the carbohydrate to be consumed.

Meals on demand: At many institutions, patients now have the option to order their meals at the time they wish, not based on any specific or predetermined institutional schedule. Although this has been shown to improve caloric intake and patient satisfaction, matching insulin use with these irregular meal times may be problematic. Some institutions implement an algorithm to minimize incorrect timing of insulin, but ensure that the patient receives insulin (Figure 10.2).

6. **Daily insulin adjustments:**

There are no validated formulas to make these daily insulin adjustments (see Table 10.2). Some clinicians will take the amount of extra (correctional) insulin used in the previous day and then add that evenly into the next day's dosing. Although this is appealing for its simplicity, it may lead to significant mismatched dosing as the patients' actual glucose pattern may call for a significantly different insulin order. For example, if only the fasting glucose is elevated, and extra insulin is given later in the day, the patient will be risk for hypoglycemia and the fasting elevation will not be addressed. Thus, adjusting the insulin based on glucose patterns with the following guidelines works well:

- **Basal Insulin:** Generally, the basal insulin dose is adjusted based on fasting glucose levels. For example, if fasting blood glucose (FBG) <140 mg/dL, no change. If FBG 141–160 mg/dL, increase the basal dose by 2–3 units. If FBG 160–180 mg/dL, increase basal dose by 4–5 units. If FBG 180–200 mg/dL, increase basal dose by 6–7 units. If FBG >200 mg/dL, increase basal dose by 8 units. Following this approach, the basal insulin can be titrated up to the patient's actual requirement relatively quickly. For patients on significantly large doses of basal insulin (e.g., >50 units), larger incremental changes may be appropriate. For patients with T1D, smaller

Table 10.2—Daily Insulin Adjustments

Prebreak-fast glu-cose (mg/dl)	Insulin given for breakfast (nutritional + correctional)	Prelunch glucose (mg/dl)	Intervention for next day	Nutritional prebreak-fast dose next day
220	5 + 2 = 7 units	210	If there is no significant change in the glucose level from before breakfast to before lunch, then the dose of insulin the patient received at breakfast (nutritional plus correction) would be an appropriate nutritional dose for breakfast the next day	7 units
220	5 + 2 = 7 units	260	If there is a significant increase in the glucose level from before breakfast to before lunch, then the dose of insulin the patient received at breakfast (nutritional plus correction) would need to be increased and become the nutritional dose for breakfast the next day	8 units
220	5 + 2 = 7 units	138	If the glucose level before break-fast had been high, and the glu-cose level at lunch is at goal, then no change in the nutritional dose will be required for the next day	5 units
220	5 + 2 = 7 units	60	If a meal was consumed, then no matter what the glucose level was at breakfast, if the glucose level after breakfast or before lunch is low, then the breakfast nutritional dose needs to be decreased for the next day	3 units

incremental changes may be appropriate based on the usual amount of basal insulin.

- **Nutritional Insulin:** The adequacy of the nutritional insulin dose is based on the glucose level before the next meal or bedtime. For example, the glucose level just before lunch will indicate whether the insulin given at breakfast was appropriate. The glucose level at bedtime will indicate whether the insulin given at dinner was appropriate. A simple approach is as follows: If there was no significant change in the glucose level from before breakfast to before lunch, then the total dose of insulin the patient received at breakfast (nutritional plus correctional) should be used as the nutritional dose for breakfast the next day. If there was a significant increase in the glucose level from before breakfast to before lunch, then the total dose of insulin the patient received at breakfast (nutritional plus correctional) should be increased and should become the nutritional dose for breakfast the next day. If the glucose level before breakfast was high, and the glucose level at lunch was at goal, then no change in the nutritional dose will be required for the next day. Finally, no matter what the glucose level was at breakfast, if the glucose level after breakfast or before lunch was low, then the breakfast nutritional dose should be decreased for the next day.

For this example, the patient has 5 units aspart ordered for breakfast. He or she is on a sensitive correction dose (see the previous order set).

SPECIFIC USE OF ORAL AGENTS FOR INPATIENTS

Data on use of noninsulin medications in the hospital setting remains limited. Although we suggest caution, medications such as sulfonylureas and metformin often can be safely restarted before discharge in a patient previously on these medications. The patient needs to be stable and reliably eating. In some patients, a meglinitide may be used in the inpatient setting until nutritional intake is stabilized. These are short-acting secretagogues and specific orders can be written so they are not given unless the patient eats, thus limiting the risk for hypoglycemia.

More recently there has been interest is using the dipeptidyl peptidase-4 (DPP-4) inhibitors as part of inpatient diabetes management.[6] As a class, these agents pose minimal risk for hypoglycemia when used without insulin or insulin secretagogues. These agents may be useful for patients with minimally elevated glucoses. Because of the expense, the addition of these agents to insulin regimens to reduce the amount of insulin needed may not be a justifiable addition to the inpatient diabetes regimen.

INHALED INSULIN

As of this time, the use of inhaled insulin for patients in the hospital setting in not recommended. Patients who have any pulmonary issues cannot use this form of insulin. Pulmonary function tests are required before initiating use and after 6 and then every 12 months. Dosing units are currently limited to 4 and 8 units, limiting titration. Manufacturer package inserts can help guide conversion to SQ insulin for patients using inhaled insulin during hospitalization. If the decision is made to continue inhaled dosing during hospitalization, nursing and pharmacy staff need to be educated on how the inhaled insulin devices are used; with the small numbers of patients using inhaled insulin, maintaining competency may prove challenging.

HYPOGLYCEMIA PROTOCOL

Adhere to the following hypoglycemia protocol:

- D50%, glucose tabs, and carbohydrates such as juice should be quickly available on all units. Consider adding D50% and glucose tablets to the override list for the automatic dispensing machines on each unit.

- BG <70 mg/dL: If patient taking po, give 20 g of oral fast-acting carbohydrate either as glucose tablets or 6 ounces fruit juice. If patient cannot take po, give 25 mL D50% IV push.
- Check BG every 15 min and repeat previous treatment until BG is ≥100 mg/dL.

Create a culture of safety and encourage staff to investigate hypoglycemic events (severe, glucose levels <40 mg/dL) to evaluate for potential system errors. Seize the opportunity to teach the patient about signs and symptom awareness and treatment plans.

REFERENCES

1. Baldwin D, Villanueva G, McNutt R, Bhatnagar S. Eliminating inpatient sliding-scale insulin: a reeducation project with medical house staff. *Diabetes Care* 2005;28(5):1008–1011
2. Umpierrez GE, Smiley D, Zisman A, et al. Randomized Study of Basal Bolus Insulin Therapy in the inpatient management of patients with type 2 diabetes (RABBIT 2 Trial). *Diabetes Care* 2007;30(9):2181–2186
3. Vellanki P, Bean R, Oyedokun FA, et al. Randomized controlled trial of insulin supplementation for correction of bedtime hyperglycemia in hospitalized patients with type 2 diabetes. *Diabetes Care* 2015;38(4):568–574
4. American Diabetes Association. Diabetes care in the hospital, nursing home, and skilled nursing facility. *Diabetes Care* 2015;38(Suppl. 1):S80–S85
5. Bellido V, Suarez L, Rodriguez MG, Sanchez C, Dieguez M, Riestra M, Casal F, Delgado E, Menendez E, Umpierrez GE. Comparison of basal-bolus and premixed insulin regimens in hospitalized patients with type 2 diabetes. *Diabetes Care* 2015;38:2211–2216
6. Umpierrez GE, Gianchandani R, Smiley D, et al. Safety and efficacy of sitagliptin therapy for the inpatient management of general medicine and surgery patients with type 2 diabetes: a pilot, randomized, controlled study. *Diabetes Care* 2013;36(11):3430–3435

Chapter 11

Hospital Glucose Management of Post-Transplant Patients

Archana Sadhu, MD, FACE,[1] Abhishek Kansara, MD,[2]
Umesh Masharani, MD,[3] David Baldwin, MD,[4] Robert Rushakoff, MD,[5]
and Amisha Wallia, MD, MS[6]

Organ transplantation is a rapidly growing field with a significant increase in cases in centers performing various types of transplants including kidney, liver, heart, lung, bone marrow, and multiple organs. As of January 2015, the Organ Procurement and Transplantation Network (OPTN) reported that more than 624,000 organ transplants have been performed since 1998.[1] Glycemic management in this setting can be complex with an interplay of multiple factors, including initiation of potent diabetogenic drugs, rapidly changing organ function, insulin resistance postoperatively, numerous drug–drug interactions and unstable nutritional status. To compound this clinical dilemma, there are limited data and no evidence-based guidelines for the optimal management of post-transplant patients. Therefore, glucose management in the hospital setting for these patients is a growing challenge at many institutions. This chapter proposes an evaluation and management strategy to address the current challenges of post-transplant patients using available research and our institutional clinical experience until definitive guidelines are established.

PRETRANSPLANT RISK ASSESSMENT

It is important to understand the mechanisms that result in hyperglycemia after solid organ transplantation. With the exception of pancreas transplant, which will not be discussed here, the post-transplant treatment plan begins with an assessment of pretransplant glycemic control as well as risk factors for post-transplant hyperglycemia and for new onset diabetes after transplant (NODAT). Many patients have preexisting diabetes, either contributing to the organ failure or as a

[1]Director, Transplant Endocrinology Program, Director, System Diabetes Management Program Assistant Professor, Division of Endocrinology, Diabetes and Metabolism, Weill Cornell Medical College, Houston Methodist, Houston, TX. [2]Assistant Professor, Division of Endocrinology, Diabetes and Metabolism, Weill Cornell Medical College, Houston Methodist, Houston, TX. [3]Professor, University of California, San Francisco, San Francisco, CA. [4]Professor of Medicine, Division of Endocrinology and Metabolism, Rush University Medical Center, Chicago, IL. [5]Professor of Medicine, Medical Director for Inpatient Diabetes, Division of Endocrinology and Metabolism, University of California, San Francisco, CA. [6]Assistant Professor, Division of Endocrinology, Metabolism and Molecular Medicine, Center for Health Care Services, Northwestern University Feinberg School of Medicine, Chicago, IL.

DOI: 10.2337/9781580406086.11

result of insulin resistance related to chronic organ failure. Furthermore, end-stage kidney, liver, and heart failure can confer changes to insulin resistance and glucose metabolism and mask the diagnosis of diabetes until after transplantation. The traditional risk factors of age, gender, BMI, non-Caucasian ethnicity, hepatitis C infection and a family history of diabetes are still relevant to the development of post-transplant hyperglycemia and NODAT. However, unique to the transplant setting are additional factors such as human leukocyte antigen (HLA) subtype mismatches, deceased donor organs, male donors, cytomegalovirus, and of course, the diabetogenic effects of immunosuppressive medications.[2,3] Therefore, it is imperative to assess pretransplant risk factors by obtaining an extended personal and family history of diabetes or prediabetes and screen patients with a fasting plasma glucose and hemoglobin A_{1c} (HbA_{1c}) before transplant, should their underlying condition allow. Note that HbA_{1c} levels in the postoperative period may not be accurate because of anemia or transfusions and therefore give incorrect estimations of pretransplant glycemic control.

IMMEDIATE POSTOPERATIVE PERIOD

All patients respond to the stress of surgery with an acute increase in counter-regulatory hormones that increases gluconeogenesis, inflammation, and insulin resistance, while decreasing glucose uptake into peripheral tissues.[4–8] Additionally in the transplant patient, the rapid introduction of high doses of immunosuppressive induction therapy such as corticosteroids and calcineurin inhibitors immediately post-transplant exacerbate this physiologic condition. It is well established that corticosteroids induce hyperglycemia by increasing hepatic gluconeogenesis, insulin resistance in the peripheral tissues, and inhibition of insulin secretion from the β-cell.[9–12] The most commonly used immunosuppressive drugs are calcineurin inhibitors (CNI) such as tacrolimus and cyclosporine, and mammalian target of rapamycin (mTOR) inhibitors, such as sirolimus and everolimus. The CNIs decrease insulin secretion by inhibiting the calcium-dependent release of insulin from the β-cell and increase β-cell apoptosis over time.[13–16] mTOR inhibitors decrease insulin secretion as well as β-cell mass, specifically in the hyperglycemic state, by disrupting the usual protein synthesis pathways related to the mTOR pathway in the β-cell.[17]

Glycemic management is further challenged by unpredictable post-transplant organ function. For instance, following kidney transplantation, normalization of renal function within hours to days alters the response to glucose-lowering therapies. In liver transplant recipients, immediate function of the graft results in gluconeogenesis and glycogenolysis that is enhanced by the diabetogenic effects of the immunosuppressive drugs. Additionally, initial delays or sudden changes in allograft function may cause dramatic and erratic changes in metabolic control. Therefore, close monitoring of the allograft function and the immunosuppressive regimen are critical to management of hyperglycemia.

Nutritional status is another important factor and can be significantly altered immediately post-transplant. Patients often have chronic malnutrition during the pretransplant period. Post-transplantation, nutritional regimens can vary widely from oral intake within 24 h of surgery to prolonged NPO status, or supplementation with enteral or parenteral nutrition for patients with complications or significant malnutrition. To further complicate the nutritional intake, commonly encountered gastrointestinal side effects of the new immunosuppressive drugs can result in inconsistent absorption of calories and require frequent changes to the nutritional treatment. Therefore, when assessing glycemic control for post-transplant patients, all of these issues must be evaluated and considered carefully in the decision making of the treatment regimen.

Evidence-based guidelines on organ-specific transplant inpatient glycemic goals have not been outlined in depth. In the nontransplant arena, glucose targets have been studied and established for the critically ill patients. In a surgical intensive care unit (ICU), the Van den Berghe study showed reduced morbidity and mortality in the intensive treatment group with the glucose goal of 80–110 mg/dL as compared to those with a goal of 180–200 mg/dL.[18] In contrast, the NICE-SUGAR (Normoglycemia in Intensive Care Evaluation-Survival Using Glucose Algorithm Regulation) trial showed increased mortality with a goal of 80–110 mg/dL and thus proposed a glycemic target of 140–180 mg/dL.[19] A glucose goal of 110–140 mg/dL in the ICU for transplant patients can be considered in those institutions that can safely achieve such goals without an increased risk of hypoglycemia. If an experienced team is not available, 140–180 mg/dL may be a safer target, as outlined by the 2009 American Academy of Clinical Endocrinologists/American Diabetes Association (AACE/ADA) consensus guidelines for inpatient glycemic control.[20]

Studies of glycemic control following transplant have shown mixed results. In kidney transplant recipients, a randomized controlled trial of 93 subjects that compared a tight glycemic target of 70–110 mg/dL using IV insulin to a target of 70–180 mg/dL with using SQ insulin for the first 3 postoperative days after kidney transplantation showed improved glycemic control with IV insulin but no difference in the primary outcome of delayed graft function or an increase in graft rejection in the long term.[21] In another retrospective study of 202 kidney transplant patients, no association was found between the mean in-hospital glucose (157 ± 34 mg/dL) and the occurrence of rejection, infection, or readmission. Intensive control between 80 and 110 mg/dL also did not show a significant relationship in any of the transplant outcomes.[22] Poor glycemic control (>200 mg/dL), however, has been associated with an increased rate of rejection in liver and liver–kidney transplant recipients.[23] Given the absence of larger, randomized controlled trials, we suggest using the usual glycemic targets for hospitalized nontransplant patients for transplant patients with additional consideration for both hyperglycemia and hypoglycemia, both of which occur more frequently in the post-transplant patient. At this time, it is reasonable to maintain blood glucose <180 mg/dL while avoiding blood glucose <70 mg/dL after transplantation.

In the hospital setting, many of the oral hypoglycemic agents are not effective or safe to use in the rapidly changing clinical environment of the post-transplant patient. They often cause significant side-effects or drug–drug interactions with other immunosuppressive therapies initiated during this time. Limited data are available for the non-insulin-based therapies in the acute post-transplant setting. Therefore, insulin is generally the mainstay of therapy. Both IV and SQ insulin regimens have been demonstrated to be effective.[24] The decision regarding route of administration should be guided by institutional practices typically used for nontransplant hospitalized patients. Critically ill patients with glucose >180 mg/dL should be managed with IV insulin per current guidelines for nontransplant patients.[20] This is most often necessary for heart, lung, and liver transplant recipients who are always admitted to the ICU. In contrast, kidney transplant patients are clinically more stable and usually are admitted to non-ICU units in many centers. Even in these patients, however, a rapid improvement in renal function along with concurrent administration of high-dose immunosuppressive therapy may result in a rapid and severe hyperglycemia that is most effectively managed with IV insulin. Some institutions have implemented insulin infusion protocols for the non-ICU setting to manage these patients who otherwise do not require ICU care.

For any glycemic management team (pharmacists, endocrinologists, internists, hospitalists) developing a treatment protocol for transplant patients, it is imperative that the insulin protocol(s) established take into account post-transplant immunosuppression, steroid protocols, and the available in-hospital insulin formulary. In our experience, patients often require IV insulin infusion, often for 48–96 h after heart, lung, and liver transplantation. Transition to SQ insulin is then considered depending on other factors that include nutritional status, need for vasopressor support, medication changes, and renal function.

Patients on intravenous insulin are usually ready for transition to SQ insulin when postoperative progress is stable, generally after steroids are decreased and nutrition is stable. We recommend a basal and bolus SQ insulin regimen using ~50–70% of the total IV insulin dose for the prior 24-h period with consideration of any upcoming changes in steroid dosing, nutrition, or organ function. When starting an SQ insulin regimen de novo, a reasonable starting total dose can be 0.4–0.6 units/kg/day with accommodation for other risk factors for hyperglycemia and hypoglycemia. Daily monitoring with further titration is critical to maintain glucose in the desired target range.

Basal insulin options include intermediate-acting insulin, NPH, and the long-acting insulin analogs, glargine and detemir. NPH insulin has the advantage that its pharmacodynamics closely mimic the hyperglycemic effect of prednisone/methylprednisolone on glucose, having a peak effect 4–8 h after administration and a duration of action of 12–16 h after administration.[25] NPH usually is dosed twice daily, but some patients without preexisting diabetes who have steroid-induced postprandial hyperglycemia may not require any overnight basal insulin when the steroids have their least effect. In these cases, using an intermediate-acting insulin dosed once daily in the morning will avoid fasting hypoglycemia that can occur with long-acting basal insulin analogs. NPH also can be dosed more frequently, as often as every 6–8 h, when needed to match a similar dosing schedule of IV corticosteroids. The basal insulin always should be combined with a bolus dose of rapid-acting insulin, especially for patients with oral intake. This rapid-acting dose usually consists of a scheduled prandial dose with an additional scale-based correction dose for hyperglycemia, if needed. Often times, incrementally increasing doses of rapid-acting insulin are needed for the lunch and dinner meals to match the glucose excursions caused by a steroid dosed every morning. For regimens with NPH and a rapid-acting insulin, we generally provide 60% of the total daily insulin requirements as NPH with 40% as rapid-acting insulin dosed three times daily before meals. If a long-acting basal insulin analog is used, there is often a need for an increased ratio of bolus to basal dosing of up to 70% bolus and 30% basal insulin. Nurses also need to have parameters to modify or need to hold the insulin in the event of sudden changes in the nutritional regimen, along with orders for supplementation with dextrose-containing fluids to avoid hypoglycemia.

For patients on continuous parenteral or enteral nutrition, a regimen of NPH insulin dosed every 6–12 h is effective at providing the continuous insulin coverage for the basal needs, carbohydrate exposure, and steroid therapy. The more frequent dosing intervals along with a correction scale using rapid-acting insulin minimizes hypoglycemia in the event of sudden changes to nutrition or unexpected glucose trends. To prevent hypoglycemia, a nursing protocol is necessary to initiate 10% dextrose at a similar rate to that of tube feeds or TPN when NPH insulin already has been given and the nutrition suddenly has been discontinued. Adding regular insulin to the bags of hyperalimentation best treats patients experiencing hyperglycmemia who are receiving parenteral feedings.

Of note, kidney transplant recipients provide an additional challenge as they generally are discharged home in 72–96 h of surgery if there is adequate allograft function. Several factors act simultaneously and can result in unstable glucose control in this setting. Rapid tapering of steroids results in lower insulin requirements, while concurrent improvement in allograft function and an increasing appetite and oral intake will increase insulin requirements. During this time, close monitoring and frequent adjustments to insulin dosing may be needed. As renal function improves and steroids are tapered, insulin doses may increase or decrease.

The use of noninsulin antidiabetic agents after transplantation can be challenging because of possible side effects and drug–drug interactions. Although insulin is the most frequently used drug for glycemic control immediately post-transplant, clinicians should be familiar with the risks and benefits of noninsulin therapies, particularly in the setting of a readmission or when choosing a discharge regimen. Caution should be used with glucose-lowering drugs that are metabolized by CYP3A4 as they will alter the serum levels of calcineurin inhibitors and mTOR inhibitors. This can result in increased side effects, changes in graft function, and potentially graft rejection. Sulfonylureas are constituently active insulin secretagogues and have an increased risk of hypoglycemia whenever significant renal dysfunction is present. Additionally, the limited titration of these drugs, interactions with other medications (e.g., sulfamethoxazole-trimethaprim), and unstable nutrition make this class difficult to use immediately after transplant. Shorter acting sulfonylureas that are predominately metabolized by the liver, such as glipizide, may be used safely once the patient is stable after transplant. Meglitinides, such as nateglinide and repaglinide, have not been well studied in this setting but can be useful in patients with mild postprandial hyperglycemia related to carbohydrate intake. These agents are dosed more frequently than other oral therapies but have less risk of hypoglycemia and fewer contraindications to renal or hepatic impairment than sulfonylureas.

Metformin may seem a useful candidate but is limited by the potential risk of lactic acidosis in settings of renal and hepatic dysfunction, the presence of hypoxia, or use of IV contrast, all of which are common in the immediate post-transplant setting. Thiazolidinediones (TZDs) have been studied in the long-term post-transplant setting, but their therapeutic effects are not seen until weeks after initiation.[26,27] They also have the well-known side effect of volume expansion that is already common after kidney, liver, and heart transplantation. The gastrointestinal (GI) side effects of α-glucosidase inhibitors make this class difficult to use because of the similar common side effect with other immunosuppressive drugs, particularly mycophenalate mofetil. Medications that induce GI intolerance have the potential to decrease the absorption of the immunosuppressive regimen, which can contribute to rejection in the immediate post-transplant period. Bromocriptine has not been described in transplant-related diabetes or the hospital setting and has significant drug interactions with calcineurin inhibitors and mTOR inhibitors. Sodium-glucose linked transporter (SGLT-2) inhibitors are the newest class in diabetes pharmacotherapy and also have not yet been studied in the transplant setting. Although the mechanism of action is novel and synergistic to other glucose-lowering therapies, the increased risk of genitourinary infections in the immunocompromised patient is a concern, particularly after renal transplant in which urinary tract infections causing graft dysfunction are a common cause for readmission.

The incretin class of agents may target the pathogenesis of β-cell dysfunction caused by immunosuppressive drugs. Their mechanism of action improves glucose-dependent insulin secretion by directly counteracting the effects of the immunosuppressive drugs on glucose sensitivity and calcium-dependent insulin release, thereby restoring β-cell function.[28] Again, like many of the other non-insulin therapies, they have not been studied during the immediate post-transplant period. Data, however, are demonstrating their safety and efficacy in nontransplant hospitalized patients, including postoperative patients.[29,30] Dipeptidyl peptidase-4 (DPP-4) inhibitors have been demonstrated to be safe and efficacious in kidney and heart transplant patients for the treatment of transplant-related diabetes in the chronic outpatient setting.[31,32] Nevertheless, caution should be used, especially in post–liver transplant patients who may have biliary complications that predispose to the potential for pancreatitis. The initial concerns of DPP-4 inhibitors and a possible association with heart failure has now been disproven by more recent studies. Glucagon-like peptide 1 (GLP-1) receptor agonists have been less well studied in transplant patients. In a small retrospective review of heart, liver, kidney, and lung transplant recipients who were treated with GLP-1 receptor agonists, there was no difference in immunosuppressive drug levels or renal function.[33] GLP-1 receptor agonists do cause GI intolerance that could affect absorption of other immunosuppressive medications, if these symptoms are severe. The delayed gastric emptying caused by GLP-1 receptor agonists should be a special consideration in lung transplant patients, as these patients are already at increased risk of aspiration and resultant allograft lung injury. More data are needed on the optimal time and setting to use these therapies.

Many institutions have recognized the importance of a dedicated team to assist with the successful management of inpatient hyperglycemia and diabetes. In a study at Dartmouth-Hitchcock Medical Center in New Hampshire, the glucose profiles of patients that were managed by a dedicated team were compared with patients managed in the usual way. The mean glucoses were slightly lower in the patients cared for by the dedicated team, and they also had a lower incidence of hypoglycemia.[34] Wallia et al. were the first to publish the benefits of a glucose management service specifically in liver transplant recipients.[35] They demonstrated lower length of ICU stays, lower mean glucoses, and lower rates of infection in the cohort of patients managed by a glucose management service (an advanced practice nurse overseen by endocrinologists) as compared with those managed by the primary team.[35] Given the complexity of the post-transplant patient, a team of clinicians who are expert in diabetes management can have a positive impact in their hospital outcomes.

Endocrinologists, hospitalists, physician assistants or advanced practice nurses, and pharmacists can serve as an effective inpatient management team; however, it is advisable that they have experience in dosing insulin in the setting of steroids and organ dysfunction. Regardless, the team should utilize insulin infusions when necessary or basal-bolus SQ insulin, regardless of diabetes status. The teams should follow these patients closely, throughout the hospital stay, as it is imperative to adjust the insulin regimen with changes in patient status.

It is important to focus attention on diabetes management at the time of hospital discharge.[36] Most often, patients require insulin upon discharge. In some cases, based on the drug–drug interactions, side effect profiles, hypoglycemia risk, and patient factors, a noninsulin therapy can be selected. In our anecdotal experience, this is generally the case when the patient's in-hospital total daily insulin dose is <20 units/day or <0.3 units/kg/day on the day of discharge. In these cases, an appropriate oral agent can be selected based on the risk profile discussed in the previous section on noninsulin therapies. When insulin dosing is >0.4 units/kg per day, insulin is generally recommended. All transplant patients should receive education regarding their potential risk for NODAT in the future if diabetes is not already present. For those requiring glucose-lowering therapy, additional education on glucose monitoring, medication administration, and dietary management is critical. Insulin doses upon discharge are determined based on their total daily dose for the previous 24–48 h. Regimens are further defined if patients are going home on a steroid taper with a reduction by 30–50% during the steroid taper. For de novo insulin dosing, Clore and Thurby-Hay have proposed a weight-based insulin regimen starting at 0.4 units/kg for prednisone doses >40 mg/day with subsequent reduction in insulin dose by 0.1 units/kg for each 10 mg/day decrease in prednisone.[37] Insulin requirements may be much higher depending on other risk factors for insulin resistance. Regardless of the discharge dosing plan, close outpatient follow-up is required as further adjustments often are needed to maintain euglycemia.

Glucose management of a post-transplant patient requires a collaborative effort of multiple disciplines, including physicians, nurses, and pharmacists as well as the patient. The interventions may begin in the pretransplant setting and need ongoing intensive management perioperatively as well upon discharge from the hospital. Optimal glucose control can be achieved with well-defined therapeutic protocols and access to a dedicated transplant team of clinicians with experience in the glucose management challenges of the transplant setting. More investigation is needed in this population to define the optimal glucose targets and therapeutic regimens that will result in improved outcomes for these patients.

REFERENCES

1. Organ Procurement and Transplantation Network. U.S. Department of Health and Human Services. http://optn.transplant.hrsa.gov

2. Salifu M, Tedla F, Murty PV, Aytug S, McFarlane SI. Challenges in the diagnosis and management of new-onset diabetes after transplantation. *Curr Diabetes Rep* 2005;5:194–199

3. Hjelmesaeth J, Sagedal S, Hartmann A, et al. Asymptomatic cytomegalovirus infection is associated with increased risk of new-onset diabetes mellitus and impaired insulin release after renal transplantation. *Diabetologia* 2004; 47:1550–1556

4. Gerich J, Cryer P, Rizza R. Hormonal mechanisms in acute glucose counter-regulation: the relative roles of glucagon, epinephrine, norepinephrine, growth hormone, and cortisol. *Metabolism* 1980;29:1164–1175

5. Shamoon H, Hendler R, Sherwin RS. Synergistic interactions among anti-insulin hormones in the pathogenesis of stress hyperglycemia in humans. *J Clin Endocrinol Metab* 1981;52:1235–1241

6. Sacca L, Vigorito C, Cicala M, Ungaro B, Sherwin RS. Mechanisms of epinephrine-induced glucose intolerance in normal humans. *J Clin Invest* 1982;69:284–293

7. Bratusch-Marrain PR. Insulin-counteracting hormones: their impact on glucose metabolism. *Diabetologia* 1983;24:74–79

8. Gelfand RA, Matthews DE, Bier DM, Sherwin RS. Role of counterregulatory hormones in the catabolic response to stress. *J Clin Invest* 1984;74: 2238–2248

9. Yuen KC, Chong LE, Riddle MC. Influence of glucocorticoids and growth hormone on insulin sensitivity in humans. *Diab Med* 2013;30(6):651–663

10. Hjelmesaeth J, Hartmann A, Kofstad J, et al. Glucose intolerance after renal transplantation depends upon prednisolone dose and recipient age. *Transplantation* 1997;64:979–983

11. Rizza RA, Mandarino LJ, Gerich JE. Cortisol-induced insulin resistance in man: impaired suppression of glucose production and stimulation of glucose utilization due to a postrreceptor defect of insulin action. *J Clin Ednocrinol Metab* 1982;54:131–138

12. Ekstrand A, Schalin Jantii C, Lofman M, et al. The effect of (steroid) immunosuppression on skeletal muscle glycogen metabolism in patients after kidney transplantation. *Transplantation* 1996;61:889–893

13. Soleimanpour SA, Crutchlow MF, Ferrari AM, et al. Calcineurin signaling regulates human islet β-cell survival. *J Biol Chem* 2010;285(51):40050–40059

14. Penfornis A, Kury-Paulin S. Immunosuppressive drug-induced diabetes. *Diabetes Metab* 2006;32(5 Pt 2):539–546 [Review]

15. Mora PF. Post-transplantation diabetes mellitus. *Am J Med Sci* 2005; 329(2):86–94

16. Crutchlow MF, Bloom RD. Transplant-associated hyperglycemia: a new look at an old problem. *Clin J Am Soc Nephrol* 2007;2(2):343–355

17. Fraenkel, M, Ketzinel-Gilad M, Ariav, Y, et al. mTOR inhibition by rapamycin prevents β-cell adaptation to hyperglycemia and exacerbates the metabolic state in type 2 diabetes. *Diabetes* 2008;57:945–957

18. Van den Berghe G, Wouters P, Weekers F, et al. Intensive insulin therapy in critically ill patients. *N Engl J Med* 2001:345(19):1359–1367
19. NICE-SUGAR Study Investigators. Intensive versus conventional glucose control in critically ill patients. *N Engl J Med* 2009;360:1283–1297
20. Moghissi E, Korytowski M, DiNardo M, et al. American Association of Clinical Endocrinologists and American Diabetes Association consensus statement on inpatient glycemic control. *Diabetes Care* 2009;32(6):1119–1131
21. Hermayer KL, Egidi M, Finch N, et al. A randomized controlled trial to evaluate the effect of glycemic control on renal transplantation outcomes. *J Clin Endocrinol Metab* 2012;97(12):1–8
22. Ramirez SC, Maaske J, Kim Y, et al. The association between glycemic control and clinical outcomes after kidney transplantation. *Endocr Pract* 2014;20(9):894–900
23. Wallia A, Parikh ND, Moltich ME, et al. Post-transplant hyperglycemia is associated with increased risk of liver allograft rejection. *Transplantation* 2010;89(2):222–226
24. Wallia A, Gupta S, Garcia C, et al. Examination of implementation of intravenous and SQ insulin protocols and glycemic control in heart transplant patients. *Endocr Pract* 2014;20(6):527–535
25. Magee MH, Blum RA, Lates CD, et al. Prednisolone pharmacokinetics and pharmacodynamics in relation to sex and race. *J Clin Pharmacol* 2001;41: 1180–1194
26. Baldwin D Jr., Duffin KE. Rosiglitazone treatment of diabetes mellitus after solid organ transplantation. *Transplantation* 2004;77(7):1009–1014
27. Luther P, Baldwin D Jr. Pioglitazone in the management of diabetes mellitus after transplantation. *Am J Transplant* 2004;4(12):2135–2138
28. Sadhu A, Schwartz SS, Herman ME. The rationale for use of incretins in the management of new onset diabetes after transplantation (NODAT). *Endocr Pract* 2015;21(7):814–822
29. Umpierrez GE, Gianchandani R, Smiley D, et al. Safety and efficacy of sitagliptin therapy for the inpatient management of general medicine and surgery patients with type 2 diabetes: a pilot, randomized controlled study. *Diabetes Care* 2013;36(11):3430–3435
30. Umpierrez, GE, Schwartz SS. Use of incretin-based therapy in hospitalized patients with hyperglycemia. *Endocr Pract* 2014;20(9):933–944
31. Haidinger M, Werzowa J, Hecking M, Antlanger M, Stemer G, Pleiner J, Kopecky C, Kovarik JJ, Döller D, Pacini G, Säemann MD. Efficacy and safety of vildagliptin in new-onset diabetes after kidney transplantation—a randomized, double-blind, placebo-controlled trial. *Am J Transplant* 2014;14(1):115–123
32. Werzowa J, Hecking M, Haidinger M, Lechner F, Döller D, Pacini G, Stemer G, Pleiner J, Frantal S, Säemann MD. Vildagliptin and pioglitazone in

patients with impaired glucose tolerance after kidney transplantation: a randomized, placebo-controlled clinical trial. *Transplantation* 2013;95(3): 456–462

33. Krisl J, Gaber AO, Sadhu AR. Long acting glucagon like peptide-1 (GLP-1) agonist therapy in post solid organ transplant patients. *Am J Transplant* 2014;15(S3):523
34. Comi R, Jacoby J, Basta D, et al. Improving glucose management by redesigning the care of diabetic inpatients using a nurse practitioner service. *Clinical Diabetes* 2009;27(2):78–81
35. Wallia A, Parikh N, O'Shea-Mahler E, et al. Glycemic control by a glucose management service and infection rates following liver transplantation. *Endocr Pract* 2011;17(4):546–551
36. Kimmel B, Sullivan MM, Rushakoff RJ. Survey on transition from inpatient to outpatient for patients on insulin: What really goes on at home? *Endoc Pract* 2010;16(5):785–791
37. Clore J, Thurby-Hay L. Glucocorticoid-induced hyperglycemia. *Endocr Pract* 2009;15:469–474

Chapter 12

Hyperglycemia in Patients Undergoing Hematopoietic Stem Cell Transplantation

Sara J. Healy, MD,[1] Boris Draznin, MD, PhD,[2] and Kathleen M. Dungan, MD, MPH[1]

INTRODUCTION

Worldwide, more than 30,000 autologous hematopoietic stem cell transplantations (HSCT) are performed annually, most for multiple myeloma or non-Hodgkin's lymphoma, and more than 15,000 allogenic transplantations are performed, nearly half for acute leukemias.[1,2] The prevalence of diabetes mellitus is reported to be as high as 30% within 2 years of HSCT.[2] In long-term follow-up studies, metabolic syndrome has been observed at higher frequencies in survivors of HSCT compared with age-matched controls.[2] Furthermore, hyperglycemia is common in patients undergoing HSCT because of frequent use of glucocorticoids and antirejection medications, as well as illness-related factors including total parenteral nutrition, stress hyperglycemia, and graft-versus-host disease (GVHD).

Glucocorticoid and antirejection medications, as well as illness-related factors such as total parenteral nutrition (TPN) and stress hyperglycemia may contribute to the development of hyperglycemia following HSCT.[3,4] GVHD and its treatment are associated with hyperglycemia and post-transplant diabetes, at least in part via inflammatory mechanisms.[5] Treatment factors also may play a role, including administration of glucocorticoids, which are first-line therapy for severe acute GVHD and may be continued for up to 2 years.[1,2] Tacrolimus is prescribed frequently for GVHD prophylaxis in patients with unrelated or human leukocyte antigen–mismatched HSCT and may improve overall survival.[6,7] Tacrolimus may lead to hyperglycemia through reduced insulin secretion, and toxic levels have been shown to induce islet cell apoptosis.[8] Finally, total body irradiation in the setting of HSCT is associated long-term with insulin resistance and features of the metabolic syndrome; one proposed mechanism is long-standing growth hormone deficiency.[9]

ADVERSE OUTCOMES

Hyperglycemia occurring throughout the HSCT period has been associated with poor outcomes. Before the neutropenic period, hyperglycemia is reported to be

[1]Division of Endocrinology, Diabetes and Metabolism, Ohio State University Wexner Medical Center, Columbus, OH. [2]Division of Endocrinology, Diabetes and Metabolism, University of Colorado Anschutz Medical Campus, Aurora, CO.

DOI: 10.2337/9781580406086.12

associated with later risk of infection, particularly in the presence of corticosteroids,[10] and during the neutropenic period, it is a significant predictor of organ dysfunction, acute GVHD, and nonrelapse mortality (NRM).[11] Following HSCT, severe hyperglycemia is associated with higher risk of GVHD.[5] In one study, hyperglycemia did not have a significant effect on time to engraftment, but it was associated with longer hospital length of stay following HSCT.[12,13] Moreover, hyperglycemia, as well as hypoglycemia and glycemic variability, were important predictors of NRM in patients with HSCT.[14] In patients treated with steroids for acute GVHD, dysglycemia is associated with worse overall survival and higher NRM.[15]

Hyperglycemia during TPN therapy is associated with higher risk of cardiovascular events, infection, renal failure, and mortality.[3] Following HSCT, hyperglycemia in TPN recipients is associated with higher frequency of infection, red cell and platelet transfusions, and delayed engraftment times.[3,4]

The mechanism for poor outcomes among HSCT patients is unknown, although it is likely multifactorial. One possibility may be that hyperglycemia leads to immune dysfunction, increasing infection risk in this vulnerable population. Further research is needed to establish glucose targets, identify causal relationships, and optimize treatment strategies.

DIAGNOSIS AND MONITORING

Diagnostic testing should be performed with a few caveats. First, short- to intermediate-acting glucocorticoids such as prednisone and hydrocortisone may result in short-term hyperglycemia that may lead to isolated postprandial hyperglycemia when dosed once daily. This limits the utility of a fasting glucose measurement.[16] Second, HbA_{1c} may be affected by recent blood transfusions or alterations in hematopoiesis and must be interpreted with caution. HbA_{1c} otherwise may be quite useful for differentiating illness or steroid-induced hyperglycemia from established diabetes.

Glucose monitoring should be conducted in most patients following HSCT, particularly those with known diabetes, critical illness, glucocorticoid therapy, or enteral nutrition or TPN. The frequency of point-of-care glucose monitoring is generally four times per day in the hospital, but this should be tailored to the type of glucose-lowering therapy and the needs of the patient.[17] Professional guidelines from the American Association of Clinical Endocrinologists and American Diabetes Association and the Endocrine Society recommend a glucose target of 140–180 mg/dL for most hospitalized patients, and glucose <200 mg/dL may be reasonable for those receiving glucocorticoids.[18,19]

TREATMENT STRATEGIES

Data from well-designed, controlled studies to guide the treatment of hyperglycemia in HSCT patients are limited. Glucose management therefore should follow recommendations for other hospitalized patient populations.[18,19]

GENERAL APPROACH

Most hospitalized noncritically ill patients should receive insulin therapy for management of hyperglycemia, and most noninsulin therapies should be discontinued.[18,19] Increasing attention has centered on the role of oral and noninsulin injectable agents, such as dipeptidyl peptidase inhibitors, although noninsulin therapies may have limited efficacy or tolerability or may present other concerns that limit use. An initial total daily insulin dose of 0.3–0.5 units/kg is recommended for hospitalized patients with type 2 diabetes, and should be individualized based on factors such as age, weight, renal function, prior insulin exposure, severity of hyperglycemia, and risk for hypoglycemia.[18,19] In one study of patients with type 2 diabetes receiving high-dose dexamethasone, a mean daily insulin dose of 1.2 unit/kg was required.[20] Traditionally, half of the total daily dose (TDD) is delivered as basal insulin and the other half is divided evenly over three meals. Daily dose adjustments of 10–20% of the total daily insulin dose are suggested.

Experts recommend an intravenous (IV) insulin infusion for management of hyperglycemia in critically ill patients. IV insulin should be continued ideally until the patient is hemodynamically stable, is on a stable nutritional source, and has glucose measures that are well controlled for a period of time that is sufficient to calculate basal insulin requirements (typically at least 24 h).

GLUCOCORTICOID-INDUCED HYPERGLYCEMIA

A variety of management strategies for steroid-induced hyperglycemia may be employed, depending on the severity of hyperglycemia and type of glucocorticoid (see also Chapters 7 and 13). Depending on the type of glucocorticoid, NPH insulin, basal insulin analog, or prandial insulin alone are reasonable options for mild hyperglycemia, whereas basal-bolus insulin typically is advised for more significant hyperglycemia. IV insulin may be useful for more severe hyperglycemia (Figure 12.1). Among patients already receiving insulin, dose increases of 20–100% may be necessary.[17]

Influence of Type of Glucocorticoid

The insulin regimen should reflect the duration of glucocorticoid effect and dosing interval. For example, prednisone once daily may respond to once-daily NPH or prandial insulin alone. In contrast, hydrocortisone dosed at 6-h intervals or dexamethasone once daily generally requires long-acting basal insulin. In hospitalized patients with hematologic malignancies, basal-bolus insulin was reported to be safe and effective for the management of dexamethasone-induced hyperglycemia.[20]

Although once-daily short- to intermediate-acting glucocorticoids appear to predominantly affect postprandial glucoses, hyperglycemia patterns reflect the steroid exposure period and not prandial requirements per se. Because many patients undergoing HSCT have unreliable oral intake, NPH may be a more effective approach than prandial-heavy insulin regimens. The peak action of NPH is 4–8 h with a duration of 12–16 h, and matches that of prednisone and prednisolone.[8]

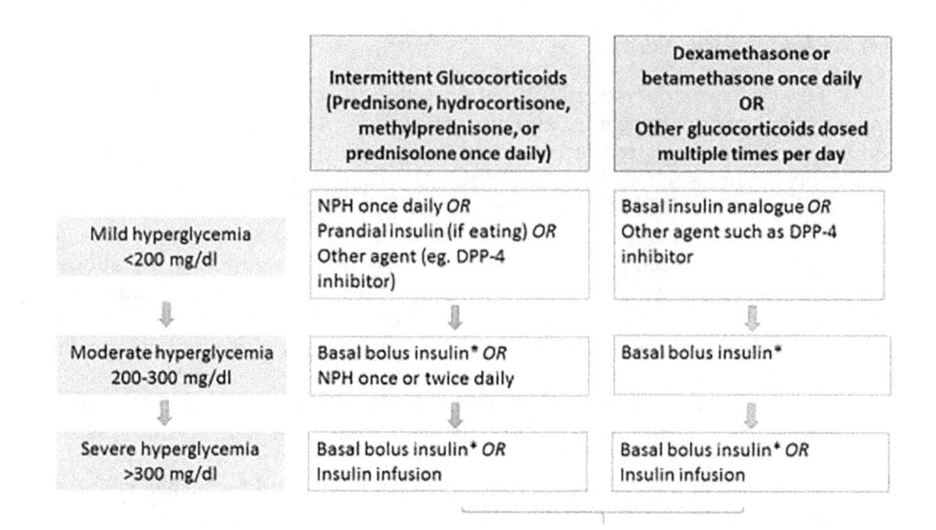

Figure 12.1—Approach to insulin therapy in HSCT patients receiving glucocorticoids. *Typical initial dose is 0.3–0.5 unit/kg, 30% of the total dose provided as basal insulin, 70% provided as prandial/correction insulin divided evenly over three meals, *if the patient is eating normally*. If the patient is not eating normally, the bolus component should be reduced or NPH should be used.

Adjustments in Therapy

Insulin should be titrated daily by at least 10–20% of the TDD, customized for the glucose pattern. During high-dose glucocorticoid therapy, hypoglycemia is uncommon. Hypoglycemia risk increases as the glucocorticoid dose is tapered, however; therefore, proactive insulin dose reduction should accompany any decrease in the glucocorticoid dose in the absence of marked hyperglycemia. When hypoglycemia occurs, a reduction in insulin of 20–50% of the TDD is advised.

ADDITIONAL CONSIDERATIONS

Among solid organ transplant patients receiving tacrolimus, switching to cyclosporine may reduce hyperglycemia[2] and may be a consideration for some HSCT patients. In addition, HSCT patients receiving TPN may benefit from lower dextrose-containing or lower calorie infusions.[4] Inadequate oral nutritional intake is typical for many patients treated on the bone marrow transplant unit. Not infrequently these patients consume only high-sugar containing fluids or supplements requiring reductions in TDD of insulin or recalculations of basal and bolus amounts of insulin. Frequent adjustments are essential to prevent both significant hyperglycemia and dangerous hypoglycemia in these patients.

The hospital inpatient diabetes management team may be consulted for patients with refractory hyperglycemia or hypoglycemia, particularly those with complex insulin regimens (including coverage for enteral or parenteral nutrition or insulin pumps), those with any new diagnosis of diabetes, patients who are new to insulin, and patients with type 1 diabetes. Early consultation ensures more effective management in the hospital and at discharge.

HOSPITAL DISCHARGE

The HbA_{1c} is recommended as a guide for adjusting preadmission glucose-lowering therapies for hospitalized patients with diabetes.[19] Unfortunately, the HbA_{1c} may be less useful in HSCT patients, because the result may not be accurate, and hyperglycemia mediated by other short-term factors, such as short-term glucocorticoid use, may not be reflected. Therefore, other approaches are needed.

Diabetes education should begin as early as possible in the hospital course to provide opportunities for reinforcement of survival skills. Topics should focus on glucose monitoring, injection technique, carbohydrate awareness, and treatment targets, as appropriate. Many such skills can be taught during routine care by nursing staff.

NONINSULIN THERAPIES

Mild hyperglycemia may respond to oral medications, with careful consideration of tolerability and contraindications. GVHD may be associated with hepatic or renal dysfunction, limiting the use of metformin and thiazolidinediones. Metformin is also contraindicated in any condition known to increase the risk of lactic acidosis, such as decompensated heart failure or hypoxia. Sulfonylureas should be avoided in patients with poor or erratic oral intake.[2] Thiazolidinediones may be effective for management of hyperglycemia post-transplant,[8] but have a slow onset, and increase the risk of volume overload, heart failure, and long-term fractures. HSCT patients already may have increased fracture risk as a consequence of glucocorticoid therapy and other factors.

Several newer drug classes may be attractive in that they do not cause hypoglycemia or weight gain. GLP-1 receptor agonists are highly effective agents for type 2 diabetes and steroid-induced hyperglycemia, but their use may be limited by gastrointestinal side effects. Dipeptidyl peptidase-4 inhibitors are well tolerated but have modest efficacy compared with other agents. Sodium-glucose cotransport 2 inhibitors reduce glucose levels through promotion of renal glucose excretion. They increase the risk for lower genital infection, particularly mycotic infections, and although infections are self-limited and respond well to standard treatment, their safety is not established in potentially immune-compromised patients. In addition, these agents may lower blood pressure and have a mild diuretic effect, which may be clinically relevant in HSCT patients. Use of all of these newer agents may be limited by higher costs.

INSULIN REGIMENS

The discharge regimen for patients with moderate hyperglycemia may consist of an oral agent plus basal insulin, NPH only, or a basal-bolus insulin regimen depending on the presence and type of glucocorticoid, glucose control, and patient preference or capacity. NPH once daily may be an effective option for patients receiving short- or intermediate-acting steroids. Long-acting insulin with or without prandial insulin is required for fasting or more marked hyperglycemia, especially with long-acting glucocorticoids or shorter acting steroids dosed multiple times per day. Patients should have close follow-up and receive written and verbal directions for adjusting insulin in concert with the steroid dose.

LONG-TERM FOLLOW-UP

Long-term monitoring of glycemic control should be conducted at least every 3–6 months. As noted, HbA_{1c} levels should be interpreted with caution and factors that may confound measurement or interpretation should be recognized. Additional glycemic measures may be considered, including fasting serum glucose or alternate glucose biomarkers (such as fructosamine, glycated albumin, or 1,5-anhydroglucitol), depending on whether reliable self-monitored blood glucose measures are available.

Patients without hyperglycemia during HSCT are at increased long-term risk of the metabolic syndrome and diabetes, even after discontinuation of immunosuppressant therapy.[2] Screening should be conducted regularly, using fasting glucose, oral glucose tolerance test, or both, as well as HbA_{1c} provided that disorders of hematopoiesis have resolved.[2]

CONCLUSION

Patients undergoing HSCT may develop hyperglycemia during hospitalization and thereafter. Although causal relationships have not been proven, hyperglycemia has been linked to poor outcomes, including mortality, infections, disease relapse, and GVHD. Treatment strategies should be targeted to the glucose patterns and glucocorticoid regimens. Future research should focus on disease outcomes.

REFERENCES

1. Copelan EA. Hematopoietic stem-cell transplantation. *N Engl J Med* 2006;354(17):1813–1826

2. Griffith ML, Jagasia M, Jagasia SM. Diabetes mellitus after hematopoietic stem cell transplantation. *Endocr Pract* 2010;16(4):699–706

3. Sheean PM, Braunschweig C, Rich E. The incidence of hyperglycemia in hematopoietic stem cell transplant recipients receiving total parenteral nutrition: a pilot study. *J Am Diet Assoc* 2004;104(9):1352–1360

4. Sheean PM, et al. Adverse clinical consequences of hyperglycemia from total parenteral nutrition exposure during hematopoietic stem cell transplantation. *Biol Blood Marrow Transplant* 2006;12(6):656–664
5. Gebremedhin E, et al. Severe hyperglycemia immediately after allogeneic hematopoietic stem-cell transplantation is predictive of acute graft-versus-host disease. *Inflammation* 2013;36(1):177–185
6. Hiraoka A, et al. Phase III study comparing tacrolimus (FK506) with cyclosporine for graft-versus-host disease prophylaxis after allogeneic bone marrow transplantation. *Bone Marrow Transplant* 2001;28(2):181–185
7. Paczesny S, Choi SW, Ferrara JL. Acute graft-versus-host disease: new treatment strategies. *Curr Opin Hematol* 2009;16(6):427–436.
8. Clore JN, Thurby-Hay L. Glucocorticoid-induced hyperglycemia. *Endocr Pract* 2009;15(5):469–474
9. Frisk P, et al. Glucose metabolism and body composition in young adults treated with TBI during childhood. *Bone Marrow Transplant* 2011;46(10): 1303–1308
10. Derr RL, Hsiao VC, Saudek CD. Antecedent hyperglycemia is associated with an increased risk of neutropenic infections during bone marrow transplantation. *Diabetes Care* 2008;31(10):1972–1977
11. Fuji S, et al. Hyperglycemia during the neutropenic period is associated with a poor outcome in patients undergoing myeloablative allogeneic hematopoietic stem cell transplantation. *Transplantation* 2007;84(7):814–820
12. Garg R, et al. Hyperglycemia and length of stay in patients hospitalized for bone marrow transplantation. *Diabetes Care* 2007;30(4):993–994
13. Karnchanasorn R, et al. Association of hyperglycemia with prolonged hospital stay but no effect on engraftment after autologous hematopoietic stem cell transplantation. *Endocr Pract* 2012;18(4):508–518
14. Hammer MJ, et al. The contribution of malglycemia to mortality among allogeneic hematopoietic cell transplant recipients. *Biol Blood Marrow Transplant* 2009;15(3):344–351
15. Pidala J, et al. Dysglycemia following glucocorticoid therapy for acute graft-versus-host disease adversely affects transplantation outcomes. *Biol Blood Marrow Transplant* 2011;17(2):239–248
16. Lansang MC, Hustak LK. Glucocorticoid-induced diabetes and adrenal suppression: how to detect and manage them. *Cleve Clin J Med* 2011;78(11):748–756
17. Baldwin D, Apel J. Management of hyperglycemia in hospitalized patients with renal insufficiency or steroid-induced diabetes. *Curr Diab Rep* 2013;13(1):114–1120
18. Moghissi ES, et al. American Association of Clinical Endocrinologists and American Diabetes Association consensus statement on inpatient glycemic control. *Endocr Pract* 2009;15(4):353–369

19. Umpierrez GE, et al. Management of hyperglycemia in hospitalized patients in non-critical care setting: an Endocrine Society clinical practice guideline. *J Clin Endocrinol Metab* 2012;97(1):16–38
20. Gosmanov AR, et al. Management of hyperglycemia in diabetic patients with hematologic malignancies during dexamethasone therapy. *Endocr Pract* 2013;19(2): 231–235

Chapter 13

Management of Hospitalized Adult Patients with Cystic Fibrosis–Related Diabetes

Boris Draznin, MD, PhD,[1] and Roma Gianchandani, MD[2]

INTRODUCTION

Cystic fibrosis (CF) is one of the most common life-threatening autosomal recessive diseases and causes significant morbidity and shortens life expectancy.[1] Approximately 1 in 30 Caucasian Americans is a CF carrier and 1 in 3,500–4,000 children in the U.S. is born with CF.[2] Advances in medical and nutritional treatment of CF have dramatically improved the life expectancy of affected individuals.[3,4] Survival into their fifth and sixth decades of life is no longer a medical miracle but a realistic expectation for many individuals with CF.

With improved longevity, CF-related diabetes (CFRD) has emerged as the most common nonpulmonary complication of CF, adding more complexity to therapy and negatively affecting overall outcome.[5] The prevalence of CFRD is only 5–8% in children between 5 and 10 years of age, but rises sharply after puberty.[5,6] It is estimated that approximately half of CF adult patients develop CFRD.[3,4]

The pathogenesis of CFRD is incompletely understood. Clearly, insulin insufficiency, particularly in the postprandial state, plays a principal role in the pathogenesis of CFRD.[7–9] In many patients, insulin secretory response to oral glucose (and meals) declines progressively over time. Even though the prevalence of fasting hyperglycemia rises with age,[6] most patients with CFRD do not develop complete absence of insulin secretion. Additionally, patients with CFRD demonstrate varying degrees of insulin resistance, especially during episodes of acute infection or steroid therapy.[10,11]

The clinical course of diabetes in CFRD patients is generally mild. In many patients, it may remain undetected for years. Clinical care guidelines for CFRD have been developed by the joint effort of the American Diabetes Association with the Cystic Fibrosis Foundation and endorsed by the Lawson Wilkins Pediatric Endocrine Society.[12] Recent publication of the consensus statement on diagnosis, pathophysiology, and treatment of CFRD is a contemporary milestone in our approach to this dreaded disease.[12] A few simultaneously published reviews on various aspects of CFRD have strengthened the importance of maintaining good glycemic control in patients with CFRD.[3,13]

[1]Division of Endocrinology, Diabetes, and Metabolism, Department of Medicine, University of Colorado School of Medicine, Aurora, CO. [2]Division of Metabolism, Endocrinology and Diabetes, University of Michigan School of Medicine, Ann Arbor, MI.

DOI: 10.2337/9781580406086.13

Even though most CF and CFRD care occurs on an outpatient basis, patients frequently are admitted to the hospital, primarily with infections and deterioration of pulmonary function. In fact, one of the critical components of improved therapy is efficacious inpatient treatment of CF exacerbations. These hospitalizations not only are crucial for the effective treatment of hyperglycemia associated with acute illness, use of steroids, or clinical nutrition, but also provide a unique opportunity for patient education and selection of appropriate therapy for the outpatient setting. Knowing that CFRD has a negative impact on pulmonary function, recovery from infection, and survival,[3,4,14–16] it is imperative to achieve the best possible glycemic control in hospitalized patients with CF.

Analysis of 410 admissions among 121 patients with CFRD during 32 consecutive months[17] revealed that the majority of the CFRD patients were treated with insulin (87.6% of all admissions). Of these, 39% of patients were treated with basal-bolus regimen, 39.6% were treated with rapid-acting prandial insulin only, 1.1% with long-acting insulin alone, 16.4% were on insulin pump, and 3.8% on NPH insulin alone.

During 238 admissions (58% of all admissions), patients with CFRD were treated with steroids, either injectable (methylprednisolone) or oral (prednisone).

Adequate caloric intake is critical for the health and survival of patients with CF with and without diabetes. CF patients frequently require a high-calorie diet to compensate for increased resting energy expenditure and inadequate absorption of calories related to pancreatic insufficiency. The catabolic state in patients with CFRD is frequently more severe than in a CF patient without diabetes. Not infrequently, hospitalized patients with CFRD receive enteral or parenteral nutritional support, which is an important element of therapy for patients with CFRD who display greater nutritional needs. Involvement of the registered dietitian nutritionist on the CF team is critical to ensuring that the nutritional needs of the patient are fully assessed and positive outcomes are achieved.

BASAL AND MEALTIME INSULIN

CFRD patients with fasting hyperglycemia are likely to benefit from basal insulin. At least initially, a small dose of long-acting insulin administered at bedtime is sufficient to control fasting hyperglycemia. Patients without fasting hyperglycemia may do well for many years on prandial insulin only.

One way of dosing rapid-acting insulin for CFRD patients is to use a carbohydrate-to-insulin (C:I) ratio for meals and snacks with an adequate correction factor. Although a C:I ratio is designed to provide adequate doses of insulin based on the amount of carbohydrate (CHO) consumed, a correction factor allows the patient to correct for preprandial hyperglycemia using an estimated ratio of how much 1 unit of rapid-acting insulin will lower the patient's glucose values. In most patients, the C:I ratio and correction factor typically used at home are a good place to start. For those not on insulin therapy at home or who have not previously used a C:I ratio, we suggest a starting ratio of 20:1 with a correction factor of 60:1 (i.e., an estimate that 1 unit of rapid-acting insulin will lower blood glucose level by 60 mg/dL) when the patient's glycemia is >150 mg/dL. These conservative starting doses account for the retained insulin sensitivity of CFRD patients. Adjustments then are made daily as needed based on blood glucose monitoring results.

Erratic meal patterns represent one of the most prevalent difficulties in the management of hospitalized patients with CFRD. Many hospitals encourage patients to order meals at the time of their own choosing, thus creating unpredictable intervals of time between meals. Depending on the level of hunger or gastrointestinal symptoms, patients with CFRD may either skip meals or double up on meals. Many younger adults with CFRD stay awake late into the morning hours and sleep until either late morning or afternoon hours. In addition to scheduled meals, many CFRD patients consume high sugar–containing snacks and beverages throughout the day to increase their caloric intake. Some patients forgo regular meals and continuously graze on snacks and beverages throughout the day and require alternate insulin dosing strategies to safely manage blood glucose levels.

Education of patients and of the nursing staff about the importance of coordinating food intake and insulin delivery is critical for proper management of hospitalized patients with CFRD. Many hospitals require that prandial insulin be given immediately after the meal and not before or at the beginning of the meal as most patients do at home. This policy is designed to increase patient safety and to prevent hypoglycemia if a patient, for whatever reason, does not eat the full meal after receiving insulin intended to cover that meal. This approach works well if the prandial insulin is given immediately following the meal. If, however, the prandial insulin is administered too long after the meal is completed, the delayed injection of rapid-acting insulin will not match the patient's glycemic excursion and may result in either hyper- or hypoglycemia. Furthermore, communication between patients and the nursing staff may not be optimal, with patients neglecting to inform their nurses when the tray arrives or when they finish their meal.

STEROIDS IN PATIENTS WITH CFRD

Most of the CFRD patients receive 40 to 60 mg of intravenous methylprednisolone between one and four times a day followed by a subsequent taper. Acute or short-term administration of methylprednisolone causes predominantly postprandial hyperglycemia that lasts 6 to 12 h. Because NPH insulin has duration of action of ~6 to 12 h, it frequently has been used at the time of methylprednisolone administration to counteract the hyperglycemic effect of this steroid. The doses of NPH insulin in CFRD patients for steroid-induced hyperglycemia are typically lower than in patients with other types of diabetes, because patients with CFRD are generally much more insulin sensitive than patients with type 1 or type 2 diabetes. NPH insulin is administered in addition to the basal-bolus insulin these patients receive. It appears that adding NPH insulin to a standard basal-bolus regimen in patients receiving glucocorticoids results in better glycemic control than increasing long- or rapid-acting insulins.[17] Because the NPH insulin is stopped as soon as methylprednisolone is discontinued, this provides a safer option than having residual effects from high doses of long-acting insulin on board. Use of insulin to counteract steroid-induced hyperglycemia in hospitalized patients is detailed elsewhere in this volume (Chapter 7). Empirical evidence suggests that in CFRD patients receiving methylprednisolone, the starting doses of NPH (given in addition to their standard doses of insulin) are usually in the following range: 0.6 to 1 unit/mg of methylprednisolone for the first 20 mg of steroid; 0.3–0.5 unit/mg for the next 20 mg of steroid; and 0.2–0.25 unit/mg of steroid exceeding 40 mg/dL.

Even though most patients with CFRD are insulin-sensitive, a few display significant insulin resistance. This group includes patients with longer duration of diabetes and those with frequent infections.

TUBE FEEDING

Adequate nutrition is a cornerstone of successful therapy for CF. Provision of appropriate caloric content may be challenging at times and patients are placed on supplemental tube feeds, frequently overnight, to meet nutritional needs. In the hospital, CF and CFRD patients may be placed on either bolus tube feeding or continuous tube feeding. Insulin therapy during the periods of tube feeding not only is helpful in controlling hyperglycemia, but also is essential for better utilization of administered CHO. Appropriate use of insulin in patients on enteral or parenteral nutrition is described in Chapter 6 of this book.

It is important to realize that continuous tube feeding as well as periods of time during or immediately after bolus tube feeding corresponds to a postprandial state. For this reason, glycemic goals while patients are on tube feeding must be in the range of 140 to 180 mg/dL. Lower glycemic goals incorrectly assume a fasting state and increase the risk of hypoglycemia if and when the tube feeding is discontinued. In the event of interruption of enteral nutrition in patients receiving insulin, an infusion of D10% must be initiated to prevent hypoglycemia.

CONTINUOUS SUBCUTANEOUS INSULIN INFUSION

As long as the patient is alert, oriented, and cognitively stable, we recommend allowing continuous subcutaneous insulin infusion (CSII, an insulin pump therapy) in the hospital under the supervision of the Glucose Management Team (GMT) or the clinician managing the patient's diabetes. Patients on CSII must keep a log of their blood glucose values and insulin rates at the bedside for review by those responsible for overseeing glucose management. All adjustments in CSII settings are done only in consultation with the GMT. The GMT rounds on these patients daily and is available by pager or cell phone to patients, nursing staff, and house staff 24 h a day, 7 days per week, every day of the year.

CFRD patients on CSII and treated with steroids will need to adjust basal rates by ~30–40% to control glycemia.[18] Alternatively, presteroid basal rates can be continued and NPH insulin added concomitantly with steroid administration as described earlier. Adjustments to the C:I ratio are also recommended because postprandial hyperglycemia is the hallmark of steroid-induced derangements in glycemic control.

CONCLUSION

Significant improvements in therapy and longevity of patients with CF have occurred. Concurrently, CFRD has emerged as the most common nonpulmonary

Table 13.1—Stepwise Approach to Use of SQ Insulin in CF-Related Diabetes Hospitalized Patients

Step	Target/Instructions
1. Target blood glucose (BG) range	Fasting: 110–180 mg/dL Bedtime: <200 mg/dL (should be checked >2 h after eating)
2. Oral and noninsulin SQ agents for diabetes/hyperglycemia are usually *discontinued on admission*	These agents are inappropriate for rapid titration to treat hyperglycemia in the hospital setting (especially for CFRD).
3. Bolus insulin for postprandial and correction of hyperglycemia (lispro, aspart, glulisine)	CFRD patients can be treated with meal coverage and correction insulin alone for many years.
	For patients who know how to count carbs, instruct them to use an insulin:carb ratio.
	Starting insulin carbohydrate ratio of 1:20 (units:gm).
	Starting insulin correction factor 1:50 (units/mg/dl >150 or 200 mg/dl).
4. Basal insulin for fasting hyperglycemia (glargine daily [ideal], detemir daily or twice daily, or NPH twice daily)	If NPO, patient should get 50% of ordered glargine dose. *Do not hold basal insulin entirely!*
5. Basal/bolus regimen for CFRD patients	Divide the *total daily dose* (TDD) into the appropriate *basal* and *bolus* components.
	For CFRD patients, we recommend starting with *30% basal* and *70% bolus*, divided for meals/snacks and determined by use of I:C ratio.
6. CFRD patients receiving glucocorticoids	Steroid-induced hyperglycemia can be attenuated with higher nutritional insulin doses (more "bolus-heavy") and/or use of additional NPH insulin given with the steroid.
7. Tube feeding	There are several regimens of insulin coverage in patients receiving enteral nutrition (see Chapter 6). ■ For *continuous tube feeding*, we recommend NPH insulin (or pre-mixed 70/30 insulin) administered every 8 hours. Others recommend either regular insulin (not rapid-acting analogues) four times daily or NPH two to four times daily. ■ *For nocturnal tube feeding*, we recommend either NPH or pre-mixed 70/30 insulin at the beginning of the feeding. ■ *For short bolus feedings*, rapid acting analogues may be most efficacious.

complication of this disease. Patients with CFRD have lower lung function and more frequent hospitalizations than CF patients without diabetes.[3,5,14] Increased frequency of hospitalization among CFRD patients most likely reflects the presence of more severe disease.[5] It has been suggested that both insulin deficiency and hyperglycemia negatively affect pulmonary disease in CF.[3,19]

CFRD is unique in pathophysiology and clinical course. Although sensitive to insulin at baseline, patients with CFRD experience significant postprandial hyperglycemia, frequently because of high-dose steroids or acute-on-chronic illness. CHO intake must not be limited because of their high metabolic requirements, but limitation of simple sugars can be recommended,[20] if deemed appropriate for the ongoing circumstances. Although exocrine pancreatic function typically fails early in CF, endocrine function may wax and wane for years.

Inpatient therapy for CFRD requires a customized approach uniquely different from that of type 1 or type 2 diabetes (Table 13.1). We believe that every hospital admission presents an opportunity to educate patients and optimize the treatment of diabetes. As patients with CF continue to have frequent admissions and prolonged hospital stays, it is clear that the inpatient management of CFRD is just as important as outpatient care to the patient's overall health.

REFERENCES

1. The cystic fibrosis genotype—phenotype consortium. Correlation between genotype and phenotype in patients with cystic fibrosis. *New Eng J Med* 1993;329:1308–1313
2. Welsh MJ, Tsui LC, Boat TF, Beaudet AL. Cystic fibrosis. In Scriver CR, Beaudet AL, Sly WS, Vall D, Eds., *Metabolic and Molecular Basis of Inherited Diseases*, 7th ed., New York, McGraw-Hill, 1995, p. 3799–3876
3. Moran A, Becker D, Casella SJ, Gottlieb PA, Kirkman MS, Marshall BC, Slovis B. Epidemiology, pathophysiology, and prognostic implications of cystic fibrosis-related diabetes. *Diabetes Care* 2010;33:2677–2683
4. Stacenko AA, Moran A. Update on cystic fibrosis-related diabetes. *Curr Opin Pulm Med* 2010;16:611–615
5. Moran A, Dunitz J, Nathan B, Saeed A, Holme B, Thomas W. Cystic fibrosis-related diabetes: current trends in prevalence, incidence, and mortality. *Diabetes* 2009;32:1626–1631
6. Marshall BC, Butler SM, Stoddard M, Moran AM, Liou TG, Morgan WJ. Epidemiology of cystic fibrosis-related diabetes. *J Pediatr* 2005;146:681–687
7. Moran A, Diem P, Klein DJ, Levitt MD, Robertson RP. Pancreatic endocrine function in cystic fibrosis. *J Pediatr* 1991;118:715–723
8. Arrigo T, Cucinotta D, Nibali CS, Di Cesare E, Di Benedetto A, Magazzu G, De Luca F. Longitudinal evaluation of glucose tolerance and insulin secretion in non-diabetic children and adolescents with cystic fibrosis: results of a two-year follow-up. *Acta Paediatr* 1993;82:249–253

9. Lombardo F, De Luca F, Rosano M, Sferlazzas C, Lucanto C. Arrigo T, Messina MF, Crisafulli G, Wasniewska M, Valenzise M, Cucinotta D. Natural history of glucose tolerance, beta-cell function and peripheral insulin sensitivity in cystic fibrosis patients with fasting euglycemia. *Eur J Endocrinol* 2003;149:53–59

10. Hardin DS, LeBlanc A, Lukenbough S, Seilheimer DK. Insulin resistance is associated with decreased clinical status in cystic fibrosis. *J Pediatr* 1997;130: 948–956

11. Hardin DS, LeBlanc A, Marshall G, Seilheimer DK. Mechanism of insulin resistance in cystic fibrosis. *Am J Physiol* 2001;281:E1022–E1028

12. Moran A, Brunzell C, Cohen R, Katz M, Marshall BC, Onady G, Robinson K, Sabadosa KA, Stecenko A, Slovis B. Clinical care guidelines for cystic fibrosis-related diabetes. *Diabetes Care* 2010;33:2697–2708

13. Frohnert BI, Ode KL, Moran A, Nathan BM, Laguna T, Holme B, Thomas W. Impaired fasting glucose in cystic fibrosis. *Diabetes Care* 2010;33:2660–2664

14. Koch C, Rainisio M, Madessani U, Harms HK, Hodson ME, Mastella G, McKenzie SG, Navarro J, Strandvik B, Investigators of the European Epidemiology Registry of Cystic Fibrosis. Presence of cystic fibrosis-related diabetes mellitus is tightly linked to poor lung function in patients with cystic fibrosis: data from the European Epidemiology Registry of Cystic Fibrosis. *Pediatr Pulmonol* 2001;32:343–350

15. Adler AI, Shine B, Haworth C, Leelerathna L, Bilton D. Hyperglycemia and death in cystic fibrosis-related diabetes. *Diabetes Care* 2011;34:1577–1578

16. Chamnan P, Shine BS, Haworth CS, Bilton D, Adler AI. Diabetes as a determinant of mortality in cystic fibrosis. *Diabetes Care* 2010;33:311–316

17. Rasouli N., Seggelke S, Gibbs J, Hawkins RM, Casciano M, Cohlmia E, Taylor-Cousar J, Wang C, Pereira R, Hsia E, Draznin B. Cystic fibrosis-related diabetes in adults: inpatient management of 121 patients during 410 admissions. *J Diab Sci Technol* 2012;6:1038–1044

18. Bevier WC, Zisser HC, Jovanovic L, Finan DA, Palerm CC, Seborg DE, Doyle FJ, 3rd. Use of continuous glucose monitoring to estimate insulin requirement in patients with type 1 diabetes mellitus during a short course of prednisone. *J Diabetes Sci Technol* 2008;2:578–583

19. Brennan AL, Gyi KM, Wood DM, Johnson J, Holliman R, Baines DL, Phillips BJ, Geddes DM, Hodson ME, Baker EH. Airway glucose concentration and the effect on growth of respiratory pathogens in cystic fibrosis. *J Cyst Fibros* 2007;6:101–109

20. Nathan BM, Laguna T, Moran A. Recent trends in cystic fibrosis-related diabetes. *Curr Opin Endocrinol Diabetes Obesity* 2010;17:335–341

Chapter 14

Improving the Safety and Effectiveness of Insulin Therapy in Hospitalized Patients with Diabetes and Chronic Renal Failure

Jill Apel, MD,[1] and David Baldwin, MD[1]

INTRODUCTION

Chronic renal failure is frequently encountered in hospitalized patients with diabetes and is an important risk factor for hypoglycemia, especially if these patients are treated with a sulfonylurea or with insulin. A study of a large database from the U.S. Veterans Health Administration revealed that the rate of blood glucose (BG) <70 mg/dL was twice as high in patients with diabetes and estimated glomerular filtration rate (eGFR) <60 mL/min per 1.73 m^2 as compared with patients with diabetes and normal renal function after adjustment for age, race, and other comorbidities. Of 2,040,206 glucose measurements in this database, 57% were from patients during hospitalization.[1] Mortality within 1 day of the hypoglycemic episode was increased in all patients with chronic renal failure, odds ratio (OR) 1.85 for BG 60–69 mg/dL, OR 4.10 for BG 50–59 mg/dL, and OR 6.09 for BG <50 mg/dL (all $P < 0.0001$).

Current guidelines for management of diabetes in the hospital setting recommend avoiding oral antidiabetic agents, especially sulfonylureas in the hospital setting and using either intravenous (IV) insulin infusion in critical care units or subcutaneous (SQ) basal and prandial insulin in general medical-surgical units.[2] Chronic renal failure is a challenging comorbidity for safe and effective dosing of insulin for hospitalized patients, especially for patients with end-stage renal disease (ESRD) who are maintained with either hemodialysis (HD) or peritoneal dialysis (PD). Hypoglycemia, especially in the fasting state, is a common complication of ESRD treated with intermittent HD whether or not background diabetes is present.[3] Explanations include decreased insulin clearance, reduced hepatic and renal gluconeogenesis, gastroparesis, hypoglycemic unawareness, protein malnutrition, and decreased food intake because of poor appetite.[4] Patients with diabetes and renal failure are known to have decreased insulin requirements and a specific approach for insulin dosing in this population of hospitalized patients is needed to reduce the incidence of hypoglycemia, while avoiding uncontrolled hyperglycemia.

[1]Division of Endocrinology, Rush University Medical Center, Chicago, IL.

 DOI: 10.2337/9781580406086.14

INSULIN CLEARANCE IN RENAL FAILURE

Multiple alterations in insulin and glucose metabolism occur in chronic renal failure. Because endogenous insulin is secreted via the portal vein, the liver metabolizes ~50% of insulin in the first pass. The kidney plays a secondary role in the metabolism of endogenous insulin but will clear ~65% of insulin reaching it. In contrast, exogenous insulin is absorbed systemically and thus the kidney plays a primary role in the metabolism of injected therapeutic insulin.[5] Renal clearance of insulin is dramatically reduced when GFR is <20 mL/min.[3] Additionally, hepatic clearance of insulin also may be reduced in ESRD, likely because of the effect of uremic toxins and insulin resistance, both of which are improved by chronic dialysis.

DECREASED GLUCONEOGENESIS IN RENAL FAILURE

In ESRD, both hepatic and renal glucose production is reduced. In the nonfasting state, the liver is the site of all endogenous glucose production through glycogenolysis (75%) and gluconeogenesis (25%).[6] Reduced caloric intake associated with uremia decreases glycogen stores and thus decreases glycogenolysis.[7] Renal gluconeogenesis normally contributes 10–25% of glucose production in the fasting state, but this protective process is lost in ESRD because of acidosis and uremia[7] and predisposes this group to fasting hypoglycemia.[8]

GLYCEMIC CONTROL AND CHRONIC RENAL FAILURE

Ricks et al.[9] analyzed glycemic control and mortality in 54,757 patients with diabetes and ESRD. They included all HbA_{1c} values for a 6-year period of time and adjusted their analysis for multiple comorbidities, including length of time on dialysis, anemia, and malnutrition. They found a statistically significant correlation between HbA_{1c} and survival, with mortality increased with either HbA_{1c} <7% or >8% as compared with 7–7.9%. The finding of an increased mortality associated with HbA_{1c} <7% is particularly important in light of the increased incidence of hypoglycemia in renal failure patients (Figure 14.1).

It is controversial whether HbA_{1c} is a reliable assessment of mean BG in patients with diabetes with renal failure as compared with those who have normal renal function. HbA_{1c} can be falsely decreased because of anemia, blood transfusions, and erythropoietin-stimulating agents.[10] Despite these caveats, the Kidney Disease Quality Outcomes Initiative (KDQOI) and Kidney Disease Improving Global Outcomes (KDIGO) clinical practice guidelines recommend using HbA_{1c}, in combination with home BG monitoring, to guide the management of diabetes in ESRD patients.[11]

INSULIN THERAPY IN PATIENTS WITH CHRONIC RENAL FAILURE AND ESRD

Bisenbach et al.[12] studied 20 patients with type 1 diabetes (T1D) and 20 patients with type 2 diabetes (T2D) from the onset of overt nephropathy (creatinine clearance 80 mL/min) to ESRD. They found that insulin requirements decreased in

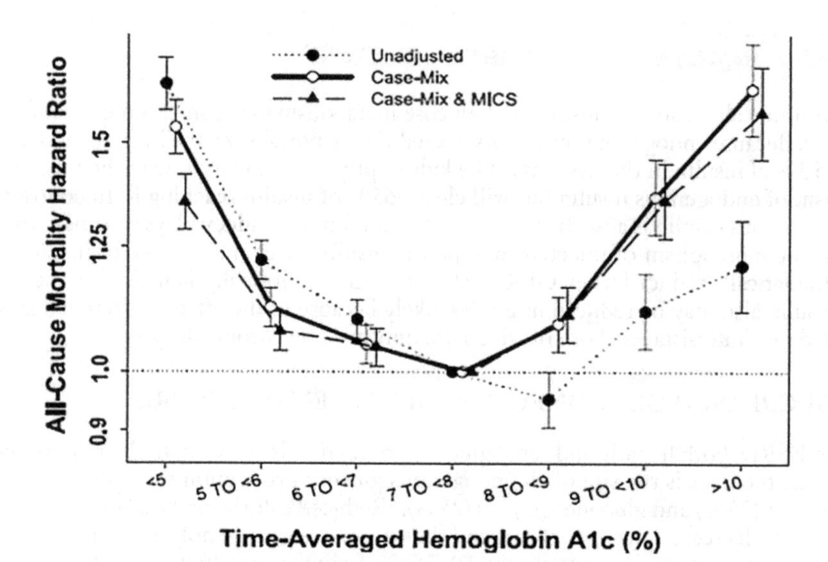

Figure 14.1—The hazard ratios of all-cause mortality of the entire range of HbA_{1c} in 54,757 patients on maintenance hemodialysis in a time-averaged model. The case-mix model is adjusted for age, sex, race, ethnicity, categories of dialysis vintage, primary insurance, martial status, dialysis dose, and residual renal function during the entry quarter. The case-mix and Medicare case-mix index model adds BMI, nPCR, serum albumin, total iron-binding capacity, ferritin, creatinine, phosphorus, calcium, bicarbonate, white blood cell count, lymphocyte percentage, and hemoglobin.

Source: Reprinted with permission from Ricks et al.[9]

patients with T1D from 0.72 units/kg/day to 0.45 units/kg/day, a 38% decline, whereas the decrease in patients with T2D was 51%, from 0.68 units/kg/day to 0.33 units/kg/day. Although patients with T1D would not be expected to have greater reductions in insulin requirements because of their absolute degree of insulin deficiency, many patients with T2D may progress to needing no therapy for hyperglycemia after developing ESRD. This phenomenon has been termed "burnt out" T2D.[13] Support for this concept comes from studies of patients with diabetes on chronic dialysis, in which 95% have T2D. Between 33 and 39% of such patients have HbA_{1c} levels that are <6%, implying that little or no therapy should be needed for hyperglycemia.[11] Indeed, it also implies that those patients who are still receiving therapy, despite HbA_{1c} <6%, may well be receiving unnecessary and, in the case of sulfonylurea or insulin, potentially deleterious treatment.

The role of the newer insulin analogues has not been well studied in patients with chronic renal failure because these patients were excluded from registration trials. A small study of insulin lispro in patients with T1D with mean GFR 54 mL/min showed that the pharmacodynamics were unchanged as compared with patients with diabetes with mean GFR 90 mL/min.[14] No published pharmacodynamic studies exist for insulin aspart, glulisine, glargine, or detemir, and further studies clearly are needed.

Baldwin et al.[15] reported the results of a prospective trial comparing two dosing regimens using insulin glargine and glulisine in noncritically ill hospitalized subjects with T2D and chronic renal failure (eGFR <45 mL/min). The trial included 107 subjects not yet requiring dialysis who were randomized to a total daily insulin dose of 0.5 units/kg versus 0.25 units/kg. Fifty percent of the total dose was given daily as insulin glargine, and subjects who were eating also received one-sixth of the total dose as insulin glulisine with each meal. Insulin glulisine doses were titrated daily based on premeal and bedtime BG measurements. No other antidiabetic agents were continued while hospitalized. Data were analyzed for up to 6 hospital days as long as the subject was hospitalized for >48 h. Mean HbA_{1c} on admission was 8%, and 76% of patients were treated with insulin before admission. Mean eGFR was 30±9 mL/min. Mean BG was the same for both insulin dose groups on day 1 (196±62 mg/dL) and decreased to mean 174±49 in both groups on subsequent days. Although the glucose-lowering effect of the different insulin doses was not different, less hypoglycemia occurred in the total daily dose 0.25 units/kg: 15.8% of subjects as compared with 30% of subjects who received 0.5 units/kg ($P = 0.08$). Although the result did not reach statistical significance, it likely represents a clinically relevant difference.

In a recent study of a computerized IV insulin infusion program used in medical and surgical intensive care units, patients with ESRD requiring HD were significantly more likely to have BG levels <79 mg/dL than patients without ESRD.[16] Patients with ESRD achieved a mean BG of 147±16 mg/dL versus 152±23 mg/dL in patients without ESRD. However, 41% of the ESRD patients had one or more BG <79 mg/dL as compared with 17.8% of the patients without ESRD ($P < 0.01$). The authors suggested that the BG target range for patients with ESRD treated with IV insulin infusion should be set higher than patients without ESRD to offset the increased risk of hypoglycemia with insulin therapy in the ESRD population.

CHANGES IN GLYCEMIA WITH HEMODIALYSIS

Two studies have found significant changes in insulin sensitivity and glycemic control in patients with T2D and ESRD when these parameters were compared before and after HD. Kazempour-Ardebili et al.[17] used continuous glucose monitoring in 19 subjects and found that the mean BG was 12.6±5.6 mmol/L in the 24 h before dialysis but dropped to 9.8±3.8 mmol/L in the 24 h after dialysis. There was no change in dose or frequency of diabetes medications. Four subjects had hypoglycemia (BG <45 mg/dL for ≥30 min), and this occurred within 24 h of dialysis in three subjects.

Sobngwi et al.[18] used the euglycemic clamp to study insulin requirements in 10 subjects for 24 h before HD and 24 h after HD while the subjects were eating standard meals. They found a 25% reduction ($P = 0.01$) in basal insulin requirements on the day after dialysis as compared with the day before dialysis. There was no difference in the bolus insulin needed for meals and no significant difference between recorded dietary caloric intakes for the day on dialysis and the day off dialysis.

PERITONEAL DIALYSIS IN PATIENTS WITH DIABETES

PD creates an osmotic gradient across the peritoneal lining usually using dextrose-containing fluids. The traditional approach of continuous ambulatory peritoneal dialysis is to instill a 2,000 mL bag of dialysate and to drain and replace it every 6 h around the clock. Typically dextrose concentrations of 1.5 or 2.5% are used in the dialysate during the three daytime exchanges and 2.5 or 4.25% dextrose dialysates are used in the overnight exchange. Depending on the amount of peritoneal dextrose, a typical patient may absorb up to 200 g of dextrose per 24 h.[19] Although this is still the dominant approach of peritoneal dialysis in the hospital setting, two new developments in PD technology have added to the complexity of managing hyperglycemia in patients with diabetes. First, many outpatients have their dialysate instilled and drained by an automatic cycling machine during their hours of sleep. During their waking hours, these patients may receive one 2,000 mL bag of dialysate or commonly no dialysate at all. Second, a new peritoneal dialysate has been developed that uses icodextrin instead of dextrose to generate an osmotic gradient across the peritoneal lining. Icodextrin is more slowly absorbed than dextrose and is metabolized to maltose, maltotriose, and maltotetraose. Icodextrin typically is substituted for 4.25% dextrose in automated overnight PD regimens. Maltose and other metabolites of icodectrin subsequently can be metabolized to glucose, but the amount of new glucose appearing in the intravascular compartment is less as compared with 4.25% dextrose, and BG levels with the use of icodextrin generally are unchanged.[20] In a study by Li et al.[20] the use of icodextrin versus dextrose for 6 months resulted in a 0.5% mean decrease in HbA_{1c} without a change in the insulin requirement. One has to be careful when caring for patients with diabetes receiving icodextrin who may be using older BG meters with the glucose dehydrogenase-PQQ (pyrroloquinoline quinone) methodology. This methodology measures maltose as glucose and produces falsely elevated BG levels, which may prompt insulin dosing when unnecessary and increase the risk of hypoglycemia.[21]

DOSING OF INSULIN FOR PATIENTS WITH DIABETES RECEIVING HEMODIALYSIS

The typical outpatient with T1D treated with HD should be treated with low doses of glargine or detemir once daily as well as low doses of rapid-acting analog with each meal, or via continuous SQ insulin infusion (CSII) using a pump. The required total daily doses are typically less than half of the doses of insulin needed before the patient developed significant renal dysfunction. When patients with T1D treated with HD are admitted to the hospital, their usual daily dose of glargine or detemir or their usual CSII basal rates should be continued and titrated daily to achieve a morning BG level of 120–150 mg/dL. This target is set a little higher than for patients with T1D and normal renal function to reduce the increased risk of hypoglycemia in patients with ESRD. These patients may continue outpatient doses of a rapid-acting analog as long as they are eating well;

otherwise, the rapid-acting analog should be held and used only for correction dosing until the patient resumes a normal diet.

The typical outpatient with T2D treated with HD often requires no pharmacological therapy for hyperglycemia. If therapy is required, pioglitazone or dipeptidyl peptidase-4 (DPP-4) inhibitors are reasonable choices for patients who do not require insulin. Sulfonylureas are best avoided because of their prolonged duration (often 2–3 days) and the high risk of hypoglycemia in patients with ESRD. When insulin is required, NPH every morning, or glargine or detemir once daily with or without a rapid-acting analog, usually can be titrated to achieve an HbA_{1c} in the 7–8% range with an acceptably low risk of hypoglycemia. When patients with T2D treated with HD are admitted to the hospital, pioglitazone or a DPP-4 inhibitor can be continued as long as BG control is reasonable. If the patient is taking a sulfonylurea, hospitalization represents an ideal opportunity to transition the patient to a safer therapy for diabetes. Patients previously treated with insulin initially can continue on their usual outpatient doses, but these doses should be titrated daily to achieve a morning BG of 120–150 mg/dL and prelunch, predinner, and bedtime BG levels of 140–180 mg/dL. HbA_{1c} measurement is mandatory and provides crucial data to guide insulin doses for hospital discharge.

DOSING OF INSULIN FOR PATIENTS WITH DIABETES RECEIVING PERITONEAL DIALYSIS

There are two routes for delivery of insulin for patients receiving PD. Regular insulin can be added to each bag of dialysate or a regimen of SQ insulin can be given utilizing rapid-acting insulin, intermediate-lasting NPH insulin, or basal glargine or detemir. Both approaches have been demonstrated to be effective in the outpatient setting with subtle advantages and disadvantages.[22–23]

The typical outpatient with diabetes treated with PD usually will receive dialysis via an automatic cycling machine overnight. If dextrose-based dialysate is used, patients with T1D usually will be best treated with a dose of NPH given in the evening before the start of dialysis, and either a smaller dose of NPH or glargine or detemir should be given every morning. A low dose of rapid-acting analog should accompany meals. The evening dose of NPH is adjusted to achieve a reasonable morning BG level, balancing the absorbed load of peritoneal dextrose overnight. Outpatients with T2D generally are best treated with a dose of NPH given in the evening before the start of dialysis, and they may not require any other insulin during the day or may need low doses of rapid-acting analog with meals similar to people with T1D. Patients with T2D who receive an icodextrin-based dialysate typically will not need any evening NPH but may need a low dose of glargine or detemir once daily to meet overall basal needs.

Less commonly, outpatients with diabetes may receive PD by traditional continuous ambulatory delivery. Because the overnight dwell of dialysate typically has more dextrose (i.e., 2.5 or 4.25%) than the three daytime dwells (1.5 or 2.5%), NPH twice daily will work for most patients with T1D or T2D. The morning dose of NPH with or without a rapid-acting analog will be smaller than the evening dose of NPH with or without a rapid-acting analog, and the four components of insulin can be adjusted individually to move the four daily BG levels into their target ranges. The alternative strategy of adding regular insulin directly to the bags of dialysate can be employed; three-times larger doses of insulin are required as compared with SQ dosing. This approach will not be discussed further because its complexity makes it ill suited for use in the hospital setting.

The BG target range for any individual patient should be as close as possible to the 100–180 mg/dL range, while limiting the frequency of any BG <80 mg/dL (ideally, less than monthly). Even a single episode of severe hypoglycemia should raise any individual patients BG targets by 40 mg/dL. It is difficult to titrate glargine or detemir for patients with T1D receiving continuous ambulatory PD but, potentially, an evening dose of NPH could supplement once-daily glargine or detemir and a rapid-acting analog with meals. For patients using CSII, the overnight basal rate will need to be higher than during the waking hours of the day.

Automatic overnight PD cyclers are rarely used in the hospital. When the typical patient with insulin-treated diabetes dialyzed at home with an automatic PD cycler is admitted to the hospital, the potential for uncontrolled hyperglycemia or hypoglycemia is greatly increased. These patients usually are converted to around-the-clock exchanges of dextrose-based dialysate every 6 h or, uncommonly, to HD if there is technological obstacle to continuing PD. This necessitates a significant adjustment of insulin doses to accommodate around-the-clock dialysis. BG levels should be checked every 6 h at the time of each new dialysate exchange; a 6 A.M. to 12 P.M. to 6 P.M. to 12 A.M. schedule is usually best and comes close to the conventional inpatient BG testing times of 6 A.M. to 12 P.M. to 5 P.M. to 10 P.M. If the daytime exchanges have 1.5% dextrose and the overnight exchange has 2.5 or 4.25%, then start by giving 40% of their usual outpatient evening dose of NPH at 6–8 P.M., 20% of their usual outpatient evening dose of NPH at 7–8 A.M., and 10% of their usual outpatient evening dose of NPH as rapid-acting analog with each meal. If all four exchanges of dialysate are 1.5% or are 1.5% alternating with 2.5% then the morning and evening doses of NPH can be the same, 30% of their usual outpatient evening dose of NPH. On subsequent days, the evening dose of NPH is titrated according to the 6 A.M. BG. The daytime doses of NPH and rapid-acting analog are titrated according to the 12 P.M., 6 P.M., and bedtime BG levels as well as how well a patient may be eating. The most common problem encountered with this approach relates to the clinical necessity for nephrology to change the dextrose concentration of different exchanges on different days to achieve adequate fluid removal. Matching the optimal amount of insulin with a given dialysate at different times of the day can be a challenge, and dynamic study of BG levels with frequent insulin dose changes are necessary. Standing orders for insulin doses are not recommended for patients receiving PD. Real-time dosing that incorporates rapid-acting insulin corrections is a safer and more effective approach.

CONCLUSION

The management of hospitalized patients with hyperglycemia complicated by chronic renal failure presents clinicians with multiple challenges. Table 14.1 summarizes several recommendations to meet these challenges. The use of consistent algorithms for this commonly encountered patient population has led to significant improvements in their quality of care both in the hospital and after discharge.

Table 14.1—Recommendations for the Treatment of Diabetes in Hospitalized Patients with Renal Failure

1. Elderly patients may have a substantial decrease in eGFR despite having a mild elevation in serum creatinine. Always incorporate eGFR into dosing decisions of noninsulin therapies and into weight-based initiation of insulin dosing.
2. When beginning insulin in patients with eGFR <45 mL/min, reduce the total daily insulin dose to 0.25 units/kg/day, 50% basal insulin and 50% rapid acting, to reduce the frequency of hypoglycemia.
3. For patients with T2D receiving hemodialysis, once-daily morning dosing with NPH will often suffice; evening dosing increases the risk of next morning hypoglycemia and usually is not needed unless the patient is receiving peritoneal dialysis.
4. For patients with T1D receiving hemodialysis, reduced doses of glargine/detemir and rapid-acting insulin or CSII basal-bolus settings are recommended.
5. For critically ill patients with diabetes and ESRD, the BG target for intravenous insulin infusion should be set at 160–200 mg/dL to reduce the risk of hypoglycemia.
6. For patients with diabetes receiving inpatient continuous peritoneal dialysis, NPH BID and rapid-acting analog with meals are recommended. The relative doses of NPH should be based on the relative dextrose concentrations of the different dialysis exchanges, and titrated in response to changes in the dialysate.
7. Hypoglycemia in insulin-treated patients occurs most frequently between 2 and 7 A.M., a time window largely regulated by the dose of basal insulin.
   a. Decrease the dose of long-acting or basal insulin (if using CSII) every day by at least 20% if the 6 A.M. BG level is <100 mg/dL.
   b. Avoid the temptation to give "correction" doses of rapid-acting insulin at bedtime if the BG is elevated.
   c. Recheck BG at 2 A.M. in patients with bedtime BG <100 mg/dL.
   d. Reduce the dose of basal insulin by 25% on hemodialysis days in ESRD.
8. Discharge recommendations for patients with end-stage renal disease and T2D: the role of inpatient HbA_{1c}.
   a. When HbA_{1c} <8% in a patient with T2D and ESRD, discontinue sulfonylurea therapy because of the increased risk of hypoglycemia.
   b. When HbA_{1c} <7% in a patient with T2D and ESRD discontinue rapid-acting insulin.
   c. When HbA_{1c} <6% in a patient with T2D and ESRD discontinue all antidiabetic therapy.
   d. When HbA_{1c} >8% and antidiabetic therapy is needed, pioglitazone, DPP-4 inhibitors, or low-dose NPH/basal insulin are the safest choices.

BG, blood glucose; CSII, continuous subcutaneous insulin infusion; DPP-4, dipeptidyl peptidase-4; eGFR, estimated glomerular filtration rate; ESRD, end-stage renal disease; T1D, type 1 diabetes; T2D, type 2 diabetes.

REFERENCES

1. Moen MF, Zhan M, Hsu VD, Walker LD, Einhorn LM, Seliger SL, Fink JC. Frequency of hypoglycemia and its significance in chronic kidney disease. *Clin J Am Soc Nephrol* 2009;4:1121–1127

2. Umpierrez GE, Hellman R, Korytkowski MT, Kosiborod M, Maynard GA, Montori VM, Seley JJ, Van den Berghe G. Management of hyperglycemia in hospitalized patients in non-critical care setting: an Endocrine Society clinical practice guideline. *J Clin Endocrinol Metab* 2012;97:16–38

3. Mak RH. Impact of end-stage renal disease and dialysis on glycemic control. *Semin Dial* 2000;13:4–8

4. Cano N. Bench-to-bedside review: glucose production from the kidney. *Crit Care* 2002;6:317–321

5. Iglesias P, Díez JJ. Insulin therapy in renal disease. *Diabetes Obes Metab* 2008;10:811–823

6. Gerich JE, Campbell PJ. Overview of counterregulation and its abnormalities in diabetes mellitus and other conditions. *Diab Metab Rev* 1988;4: 93–111

7. Cersosimo E, Garlick P, Ferretti J. Renal substrate metabolism and gluconeogenesis during hypoglycemia in humans. *Diabetes* 2000;49:1186–1193

8. Haviv YS, Sharkia M, Safadi R. Hypoglycemia in patients with renal failure. *Ren Fail* 2000:22(2):219–223

9. Ricks J, Molnar MZ, Kovesdy CP, Shah A, Nissenson AR, Williams M, Kalantar-Zadeh K. Glycemic control and cardiovascular mortality in hemodialysis patients with diabetes: a 6-year cohort study. *Diabetes* 2012;61:708–715

10. Kalantar-Zadeh K. A critical evaluation of glycated protein parameters in advanced nephropathy: a matter of life or death: A1C remains the gold standard outcome predictor in diabetic dialysis patients. *Diabetes Care* 2012;35:1625–1628

11. Rhee CM, Leung AM, Kovesdy CP, Lynch KE, Brent GA, Kalantar-Zadeh K. Updates on the management of diabetes in dialysis patients. *Semin Dial* 2014;27:135–145

12. Biesenbach G, Raml A, Schmekal B, Eichbauer-Sturm G. Decreased insulin requirement in relation to GFR in nephropathic type 1 and insulin-treated type 2 patients with diabetes. *Diabet Med* 2003;20:642–645

13. Park J, Lertdumrongluk P, Molnar MZ, Kovesdy CP, Kalantar-Zadeh K. Glycemic control in diabetic dialysis patients and the burnt-out diabetes phenomenon. *Curr Diab Rep* 2012;12:432–439

14. Rave K, Heise T, Pfützner A, Heinemann L, Sawicki PT. Impact of diabetic nephropathy on pharmacodynamic and pharmacokinetic properties of insulin in type 1 patients with diabetes. *Diabetes Care* 2001;24:886–890

15. Baldwin D, Zander J, Munoz C, Raghu P, Delange-Hudec S, Lee H, Emanuele MA, Glossop V, Smallwood K, Molitch M. A randomized trial of two weight-based doses of insulin glargine and glulisine in hospitalized subjects with type 2 diabetes and renal insufficiency. *Diabetes Care* 2012;34: 1970–1974

16. Sandler V, Misiasz MR, Jones J, Baldwin D. Reducing the risk of hypoglycemia associated with intravenous insulin: experience with a computerized insulin infusion program in 4 adult intensive care units. *J Diabetes Sci Technol* 2014;8:923–929

17. Kazempour-Ardebili S, Lecamwasam VL, Dassanyake T, Frankel AH, Tam FW, Dornhorst A, Frost G, Turner JJ. Assessing glycemic control in maintenance hemodialysis patients with type 2 diabetes. *Diabetes Care* 2009;32: 1137–1142
18. Sobngwi E, Enoru S, Ashuntantang G, Azabji-Kenfack M, Dehayem M, Onana A, Biwole D, Kaze F, Gautier JF, Mbanya JC. Day-to-day variation of insulin requirements of patients with type 2 diabetes and end-stage renal disease undergoing maintenance hemodialysis. *Diabetes Care* 2010;33:1409–1412
19. Burkart J. Metabolic consequences of peritoneal dialysis. *Semin Dial* 2004;17:498–504
20. Li PKT, Cullerton BF, Ariza A, Do J, Johnson DW, Sanabria M, Shockley TR, Story K, Vatazin A, Verrelli M, Yu AW, Bargman JM. Randomized controlled trial of glucose-sparing peritoneal dialysis in patients with diabetes. *J Am Soc Nephrol* 2013;24:1889–1900
21. Korsatko S, Ellmerer M, Schaupp L, Mader JK, Smolle K, Tiran B, Plank J. Hypoglycemia coma due to falsely high point of care glucose measurements in an ICU patient with peritoneal dialysis. *Intensive Care Med* 2009;35: 571–572
22. Quellhorst E. Insulin therapy during peritoneal dialysis: Pros and cons of various forms of administration. *J Am Soc Nephrol* 2001;13:S92–S96
23. Almalki MH, Altuwaijri MA, Albehthel MS, Sirrs SM, Singh RS. Subcutaneous versus intraperitoneal insulin for patients with diabetes mellitus on continuous ambulatory peritoneal dialysis: meta-analysis of non-randomized clinical trials. *Clin Invest Med* 2012;35:E132–E143

Chapter 15

Insulin Resistance in Patients Treated with Therapeutic Hypothermia and in Patients with Severe Burns

Boris Draznin, MD, PhD,[1] Kathleen Dungan, MD,[2] and Stacey Seggelke, RN, MS, CDE[1]

Insulin resistance is a common feature of many patients with obesity, type 1 diabetes, and type 2 diabetes,[1,2] resulting in varying degrees of insulin resistance among hospitalized patients with diabetes or other risk factors for hyperglycemia who are exposed to illness or therapies that are known to incite hyperglycemia.[3] Severe insulin resistance is defined as requiring either >2 units/kg of body weight of insulin or >200 units/day to control glycemia.[4,5] Some clinicians use the term "extreme insulin resistance" to characterize patients with diabetes whose daily insulin requirement exceeds 3 units/kg of body weight.[5] When patients with severe and extreme insulin resistance are hospitalized, they present challenging therapeutic dilemmas.

Table 15.1 enumerates the most common clinical situations resulting in severe insulin resistance in hospitalized individuals. It is not surprising to encounter severe insulin resistance in patients treated as outpatients with U-500 insulin (see Chapter 16) and in individuals with various syndromes of severe insulin resistance who might be hospitalized for any other medical reasons.[6] On the other hand, numerous situations drastically impair insulin sensitivity in patients with diabetes or hyperglycemia. For example, administration of steroids or adrenergic medications can precipitously increase insulin requirements. Similar detrimental effects on glycemia can be observed in patients receiving large amounts of dextrose, in uremic individuals, and in patients receiving HIV therapy and highly active antiretroviral therapy (HAART).[3,4] Patients without a prior history of diabetes but who have underlying risk factors such as increasing age, insulin resistance, or obesity may be more likely to develop hyperglycemia in conjunction with these factors.

A variety of circumstances that markedly increase insulin resistance among hospitalized patients are discussed in detail elsewhere in this book. This chapter discusses the pathogenesis and therapeutic approach to patients with severe insulin resistance induced by therapeutic hypothermia and by severe burns.

[1]Division of Endocrinology, Diabetes and Metabolism, Department of Medicine, University of Colorado Anschutz Medical Campus, Aurora, CO. [2]Division of Endocrinology, Diabetes and Metabolism, The Ohio State University Wexner Medical Center, Columbus, OH.

DOI: 10.2337/9781580406086.15

Table 15.1—Causes of Severe Insulin Resistance in Hospitalized Patients

- Patients treated with U-500 insulin as outpatients
- Syndromes of severe insulin resistance
- Administration of steroids or adrenergic medications
- Administration of large amounts of dextrose (e.g., parenteral or enteral nutrition)
- Uremia
- HIV therapy and HAART
- Therapeutic hypothermia
- Severe burns or trauma

THERAPEUTIC HYPOTHERMIA

Therapeutic hypothermia (also called targeted temperature management) is used widely in patients with in- or out-of-hospital cardiac arrest. Therapeutic hypothermia significantly improves neurological deficits and survival in these patients.[7] Duration of cooling varies considerably, ranging from 2–3 days to up to 10 days. Body temperature can be lowered to 34–35.9°C, 32–33.9°C, or 30–31.9°C, for mild, moderate, or moderate-deep hypothermia, respectively.[8] Deep hypothermia (<30°C) is rarely used as it is associated with a much greater risk for severe side effects. In fact, a recent international, multicenter, randomized trial suggested that a temperature <36°C (targeted at 33°C) did not confer any additional benefit.[9]

When the core temperature drops to 32°C, the metabolic rate decreases to 50–65% of normal, and oxygen consumption and CO_2 production decrease by the same percentage. At the same time, the levels of free fatty acids, ketones, and lactate increase.[10]

Another important consequence of hypothermia is decreased insulin secretion and moderate to severe insulin resistance leading to hyperglycemia, particularly in patients with diabetes.[11,12] The mechanism of severe insulin resistance in hypothermia is not well understood, but diminished insulin binding to its receptor as well as diminished signal transduction and human glucose transporter (GLUT-4) function (recruitment of glucose transporters to the plasma membrane and their subsequent internalization) certainly play a significant role.[12] All steps involved in mediating insulin action on glucose transport and intracellular metabolism are significantly diminished by lower temperature. Undoubtedly, vasoconstriction and possible changes in adrenergic tone might contribute as well. Furthermore, hypothermia may induce accumulation of lactate and mild acidosis, which diminishes insulin sensitivity.

At the same time, impaired insulin release also could contribute to hyperglycemia.[11] The mechanism of this impairment is hypothesized to include diminished intracellular metabolism of glucose and slower rates of fusion and fission of insulin-containing secretory vesicles in the pancreatic β-cells under hypothermic conditions.

As a result, in some patients, particularly in those with diabetes, hyperglycemia can be extreme, approaching or exceeding 1,000 mg/dL (55.6 mM/L). The insulin requirement is greatly increased, and frequently intravenous (IV) insulin infusion at the rate of 20 to 30 units/h may be insufficient to control hyperglycemia.

Clinical implications of the temperature dependence of insulin action become particularly important in the rewarming phase. With the core temperature rising, both insulin release and insulin action improve dramatically and, with large quantities of exogenous insulin on board, hypoglycemia may ensue precipitously. The insulin infusion rate must be decreased aggressively in the rewarming phase to avoid hypoglycemia. In practical terms, the danger of hypoglycemia during the rewarming phase is the most important point to remember during the management of glycemia in patients with therapeutic hypothermia. A concomitant infusion of D10% may be needed in addition to a reduction in the insulin infusion rate to stabilize glycemia and prevent hypoglycemia in the rewarming phase.

Overall, early involvement of an endocrinologist or a specialist in the inpatient management of diabetes may prevent disastrous hypoglycemia in the rewarming stage of therapeutic hypothermia.

SEVERE BURNS

Hyperglycemia and insulin resistance are frequently seen in patients with severe trauma and especially in those with severe burns.[13–15] Severe burns typically are accompanied by a period of stress and hyperinflammation.[16] One study in 242 severely burned children found that a hypermetabolic state strongly correlated with significantly elevated glucose levels and insulin concentrations,[17] defining the presence of insulin resistance.

At least three different mechanisms are working in concert to induce a hypermetabolic state and to elevate blood glucose levels in patients with severe burns: release of catecholamines, glucocorticoids, and cytokines.[18] Catecholamines increase glycogenolysis, lipolysis, and proteolysis with release of glucose, glycerol, free fatty acids, and amino acids. Stress-induced elevations in glucocorticoids lead to enhanced gluconeogenesis and peripheral insulin resistance. Cytokines such as tumor necrosis factor-α (TNFα), interleukin-6 (IL-6), and IL-18 cause severe insulin resistance by increasing serine phosphorylation of insulin receptor substrate-1 (IRS-1),[19] thus reducing intracellular signal transduction to phosphatidylinositol 3-kinase and downstream mediators of insulin action. Although release of catecholamines and glucocorticoids are increased 2- to 10-fold, the levels of cytokines and inflammatory mediators rise up to 100-fold and remain elevated for long periods of time. The pediatric literature suggests that insulin resistance remains prominent for months or even years postburn.[20]

Hyperglycemia in severely burned patients has been shown to impair wound healing and increase the incidence of infections and skin graft loss as well as mortality.[17] Most outcomes data among severely burned patients are derived from observational studies. A randomized controlled trial of 239 pediatric burn patients demonstrated, however, that intensive insulin therapy (targeting a glucose range of 80–110 mg/dL) decreased the incidence of infection and sepsis, and improved organ function and measures of inflammation and catabolism compared with standard care (glucose target 140–180 mg/dL).[21] However, the incidence of hypoglycemia was increased (the incidence of severe hypoglycemia was 26% in the intensive versus 9% in the control group, $P < 0.05$). The study was not powered to detect differences in mortality. Therefore, further study is needed in larger populations, with a focus on methods that minimize severe hypoglycemia.

Most patients with severe burns are admitted to specialized burn intensive care units (ICU) and also undergo frequent surgeries. IV insulin infusion is the best method of controlling hyperglycemia in ICU patients and in the operating room. Virtually every hospital has developed and refined protocols for IV insulin infusion. Most protocols are run by the nursing staff and take into consideration both the actual blood glucose levels and changes in glycemic values. It is not uncommon to raise the insulin infusion rate to double digits in diabetic patients who have sustained severe burns.

Critically ill patients with severe burns frequently receive parenteral nutrition or enteral nutrition to compensate for energy needs consumed by this catabolic condition. These nutrient mixtures provide large amounts of dextrose that further aggravate severe insulin resistance and hyperglycemia (see Chapter 6). Inclusion of the registered dietitian nutritionist on the patient care team is critical to achieving positive outcomes for the patient and reducing hospital length of stay.

Because insulin resistance in patients with severe burns lasts for many weeks and even months, the danger of hypoglycemia usually is low even though the doses of insulin required to control hyperglycemia in these patients greatly exceed their preburn home insulin requirement. The risk of hypoglycemia can be further minimized by aggressive decreases of insulin doses when patients' insulin sensitivity begins to return to preburn state with time of healing.

The problem with selecting initial appropriate insulin doses may arise when a patient with severe burns is unconscious and unaccompanied by someone who knows his or her therapeutic regimen at home. The first task of the managing team is to estimate the total daily dose of insulin (TDDI). Without the benefit of knowing how much insulin the patient administered at home, one approach to estimating the TDDI is based on the patient's weight and body mass index (BMI). For a patient with type 1 diabetes, 0.15–0.25 units/kg of body weight of insulin for basal needs may be needed. For patients with type 2 diabetes, initial doses in the range of 0.3–0.6 units/kg of body weight might be appropriate. Assuming mealtime boluses are approximately equal to total basal insulin, one might estimate TDDI as double of that for basal needs.

The alternate calculations can be based on the amount of carbohydrate the patient receives from enteral nutrition via tube feeding (TF) or with total parenteral nutrition (TPN). Insulin coverage for both TF and TPN is described elsewhere in this book. When either TF or TPN is discontinued and oral intake resumed, most patients can return to their home insulin regimen.

CONCLUSION

Many hospitalized patients with diabetes treated with therapeutic hypothermia and those admitted with severe burns can display extreme insulin resistance. These patients may require high doses of insulin given either intravenously or subcutaneously. Although aggressive reduction in insulin doses must accompany the warming process posthypothermia to avoid hypoglycemia, patients with severe burns remain hyperglycemic for weeks and months after acute presentation. Successful treatment of hyperglycemia in patients with severe burns results in better outcome and most patients are able to return to their preburn diabetes regimen.

REFERENCES

1. Olefsky, LM, Revers RR, Prina M, Henry RR, Garvey WT, Scarlett JA, et al. Insulin resistance in non-insulin dependent (type II) and insulin dependent (type I) diabetes mellitus. *Adv Exp Med Biol* 1985;189:176–205
2. Nadeau KJ, Zeitler PS, Bauer TA, Brown MS, Dorosz JL, Regensteiner JG, Draznin B, Reusch JE. A unique phenotype of insulin resistance in adolescents with type 1 diabetes: implications for cardiovascular function. *J Clin Endocrinol Metab* 2010;95:513–521
3. Ovale F. Clinical approach to the patient with diabetes mellitus and very high insulin requirements. *Diab Res Clin Pract* 2010;90:231–242
4. Larsen J, Goldner W. Approach to the hospitalized patient with severe insulin resistance. *J Clin Endocrinol Metab* 2011;96:2652–2662
5. Lane WS, Cochran EK, Jackson JA, Scism-Bacon JL, Corey IB, Hirsch IB, et al. High-dose insulin therapy: is it time for U-500 insulin? *Endocr Pract* 2009;15:71–79
6. Semple RK, Williams RM, Dungert DB. What is the best management strategy for patients with severe insulin resistance? *Clin Endocrinol* 2010;73:286–290
7. Polderman KH, Herold I. Therapeutic hypothermia in the intensive care unit: practical considerations, side effects, and cooling methods. *Crit Care Med* 2009;37:1101–1120
8. Polderman KH. Mechanisms of action, physiological effects, and complications of hypothermia. *Crit Care Med* 2009;37(Suppl.):S186–S202
9. Nielsen N, Wetterslev J, Cronberg T, Erlinge D, Gasche Y, Hassager C, et al. Targeted temperature management at 33°C versus 36° C after cardiac arrest. *New Eng J Med* 2013;369:2197–2206
10. Aoki M, Nomura F, Stromski ME, Tsuji MK, Fackler JC, Hickey PR, Holtzman DH, Jonas RA. Effects of pH on brain energetics and hypothermic circulatory arrest. *Ann Thorac Surg* 1993;55:1093–1103
11. McClenaghan N, Berts A, Dryselius S, Grapengiesser E, Saha S, Hellman B. Induction of a glucose-dependent insulin secretory response by the nonmetabolizable amino-acid alpha-aminoisobutyric acid. *Pancreas* 1997;14:65–70
12. Haring HU, Biermann E, Kemmler W. Coupling of insulin binding and insulin action on glucose transport in fat cells. *Am J Physiol* 1981;240:E556–E565
13. McCowen KC, Malhotra A, Bistrian BR. Stress-induced hyperglycemia. *Crit Care Clin* 2001;17:107–124

14. Xin-Long C, Zhao-Fan X, Dao-Feng B, Jian-Guang T, Duo W. Insulin resistance following thermal injury: an annual study. *Burns* 2007;33:480–483
15. Jeschke MG, Finnerty CC, Herndon DN, Song J, Boehning D, Tompkins RG, Baker HV, Gauglitz GG. Severe injury is associated with insulin resistance, endoplasmic reticulum stress response, and unfolded protein response. *Ann Surg* 2012;255:370–378
16. Gaudlitz GG, Herndon DN, Kulp GA, Meyer WJ, III, Jeschke MG. Abnormal insulin sensitivity persists up to three years in pediatric patients post-burn. *J Clin Endocrinol Metab* 2009;94:1656–1664
17. Jeschke MG, Chinkes DL, Finnerty CC, Kulp G, Suman OE, et al. Pathophysiologic response to severe burn injury. *Ann Surg* 2008;248:387–401
18. Hart DW, Wolf SE, Mlack R, Chinkes DL, Ramzy PI, Obeng MK, Ferrando AA, Wolfe RR, Herndon DN. Persistence of muscle catabolism after severe burn. *Surgery* 2000;128:312–319
19. Morino K, Petersen KF, Shulman GI. Molecular mechanisms of insulin resistance in humans and their potential links with mitochondrial dysfunction. *Diabetes* 2006;55(Suppl. 2):S9–S15
20. Cree MG, Fram RY, Barr D, Chinkes D, Wolfe RR, Herndon DN. Insulin resistance, secretion and breakdown are increased 9 months following severe burn injury. *Burns* 2009;35:63–69
21. Jeschke MG, Kulp GA, Kraft R, Finnerty CC, Mlcak R, Lee JO, Herndon DN. Intensive insulin therapy in severely burned pediatric patients: a prospective randomized trial. *Am J Respir Crit Care Med* 2010;182:351–349

Chapter 16

Inpatient Management of Patients with Extreme Insulin Resistance Receiving U-500 Insulin

Amy Diesburg-Stanwood, DNP, FNP-BC,[1] Neda Rasouli, MD,[1,2] and Boris Draznin, MD, PhD[2]

INTRODUCTION

Insulin resistance (IR) is a central feature of many patients with obesity and type 2 diabetes (T2D).[1,2] It is estimated that >90% of people with T2D are overweight and insulin resistant to varying degrees. Approximately 30% of diabetics are using 60 units or more of basal insulin per day.[3,4] Not infrequently, clinicians encounter patients with severe IR requiring supraphysiologic doses of insulin. These doses exceed the capacity of the U-100 syringe and require large volumes of insulin altering the pharmacokinetics and interfering with absorption of the insulin. In these cases, concentrated insulin such as U-500 regular is an alternative option for glucose management. Patients treated with large doses of insulin and those receiving U-500 insulin in the outpatient setting are admitted to the hospital frequently for problems unrelated to diabetes. Once in the hospital, they present a challenge to the inpatient team. The transition between home and hospital insulin regimens, including types and concentrations of insulin, present a safety challenge for clinicians and hospital staff. By implementing a multidisciplinary approach, it is possible to create a safe environment for insulin-resistant patients on high-dose insulin regimens in the hospital setting.

INSULIN RESISTANCE

IR is a pathophysiological condition in which peripheral insulin target tissues, such as adipose tissue, skeletal muscle, and liver, fail to respond to the normal action of insulin, resulting in greater concentrations of insulin to maintain normoglycemia. As long as the pancreas can compensate for the IR by an increased secretion of insulin, patients maintain normoglycemia or exhibit glucose intolerance without overt diabetes. When the pancreas can no longer keep up with the increasing demands of the peripheral tissues for insulin, patients develop T2D. Because of the progressive loss of β-cell function over time, most patients with T2D require increasing amounts of exogenous insulin in an attempt to achieve good glycemic control. Clinically, a subgroup of patients with diabetes and IR present with hyperglycemia despite large doses of exogenous insulin. This is either

[1]Denver VA Medical Center, Denver, CO. [2]University of Colorado Anschutz Medical Campus, Aurora, CO.

DOI: 10.2337/9781580406086.16

due to consuming large quantities of carbohydrate or syndromes of severe IR, such as insulin receptor defects and type A or type B severe insulin resistance (SIR),[5–8] to name a few (see Chapter 15 for more details). In clinical practice, patients with SIR often require >200 units/day of insulin or a dose >2 units/kg of body weight.

In 1997, in an effort to manage the increasing insulin requirements of patients with diabetes and SIR, Eli Lilly & Co developed the first concentrated insulin known as U-500.[9] In contrast to U-100 (100 units/mL), U-500 is five times more concentrated and contains 500 units/mL. U-500 allows patients to give subcutaneous (SQ) injections of large doses of insulin in a reasonable volume with less injection pain, better absorption, and increased patient satisfaction.[10,11]

U-500 has been available for years targeting patients with SIR. In 2015, the U.S. Food and Drug Administration (FDA) approved three new concentrated insulins: U-200 lispro[12] U-200 degludec,[13] and U-300 glargine.[14]

SAFETY OF CONCENTRATED INSULIN

The use of concentrated insulin such as U-500 in the hospital setting can lead to confusion and errors among providers and requires a systematic protocol that includes layers of double-checking.[15,16] U-500 insulin is differentiated from U-100 by bottle size and color; U-500 is a larger vial with bold diagonal orange stripes (Figure 16.1). Dosing this insulin is complicated because a dedicated U-500 syringe failed usability testing.[17] Instead, clinicians must convert into one of two delivery options when ordering U-500 insulin. U-500 "syringe units" are calculated by dividing the total daily dose (TDD) by 5 for delivery in a U-100 syringe. Alternatively, the TDD can be divided by 500 and converted to volume for injection via a tuberculin syringe. Misinterpretation occurs often when using a U-100 syringe because the patient believes they are on "20 units of insulin" as drawn up in the syringe, but they actually are on "20 syringe units," which is equivalent to 100 units of insulin (Table 16.1). Ongoing confusion led the Institute of Safe Medical Practices (ISMP) to implement guidelines when prescribing U-500 insulin, recommending that clinicians "use extreme caution when expressing or interpreting doses of U-500 insulin. Consistent use of a tuberculin syringe with U-500 insulin is recommended, with total doses expressed in terms of both units and volume to be injected."[15]

Adding three new insulins to the market has the potential to lead to provider confusion, but unlike U-500, the newer concentrated insulins require no conversion. They are available only in a pen, which has simplified the prescribing process. The actual units of insulin are visible in the pen window, but the volume of delivered insulin is less and hidden in the pen casing (see Figure 16.2). For example if the patient is on 20 units of U-200 lispro, and it wasn't available in the hospital, they would be converted to 20 units of U-100 lispro (it would just be more volume).

PHARMACOKINETICS

HUMULIN REGULAR U-500

There are significant pharmacokinetic differences between U-100 regular insulin and U-500 regular insulin. U-100 insulin has an onset of within 30 min and

Table 16.1—Dose Conversion for Humulin R U-500 Insulin When Using a U-100 Syringe or a Tuberculin Syringe

Humulin R U-500 dose (units)	U-100 insulin syringe (unit markings)	Tuberculin syringe (volume in mL)
25	5	0.05
50	10	0.1
75	15	0.15
100	20	0.2
125	25	0.25
150	30	0.3
175	35	0.35
200	40	0.4
225	45	0.45
250	50	0.5
275	55	0.55
300	60	0.6
325	65	0.65
350	70	0.7
375	75	0.75
400	80	0.8
425	85	0.85
450	90	0.9
475	95	0.95
500	100	1.0

Source: Eli Lilly & Co.[9]

typical duration of 4–6 h, whereas U-500 has a greater time to peak insulin concentration (1.75–8.5 h) and a longer duration of action (6–24 h),[18-20] Although U-500 is considered regular insulin, its pharmacokinetics more closely mimics NPH insulin allowing it to be dosed twice a day.[21–23] Dosing recommendations for U-500 are based largely on clinical experience; there are no randomized controlled trials to guide dosing decisions for clinicians. Many providers split the insulin dosing based on the TDD of insulin (Table 16.2),[8] whereas others find twice daily dosing sufficient.[11] In 2014, de la Pena et al.[24] studied the pharmacokinetics and pharmacodynamics of U-500 by administering a total daily dose of 500 units given in different frequencies (once, twice, or three times daily). Their findings revealed that doses given twice or three times daily provide 24-h basal insulin coverage in contrast to once daily dosing, which was the most variable (Figure 16.3).[24]

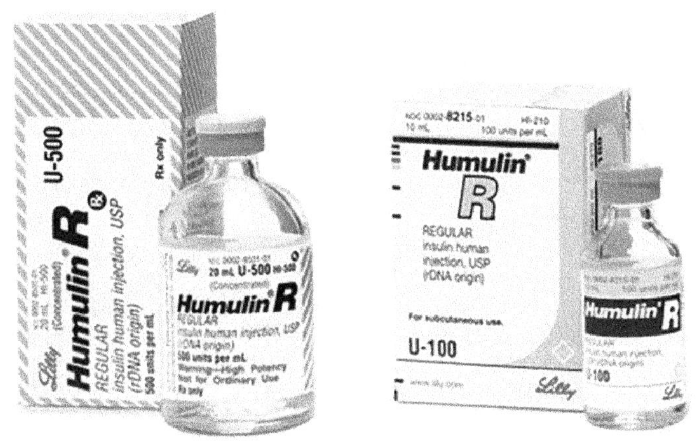

Figure 16.1—Appearance of U-500 insulin and U-100 insulin vials and boxes. Differentiating features of U-500 insulin include 20-mL vial size, black and white labeling with red lettering of drug warning, orange/brown stripes, and gray flip top.

Source: Segal et al.[43]

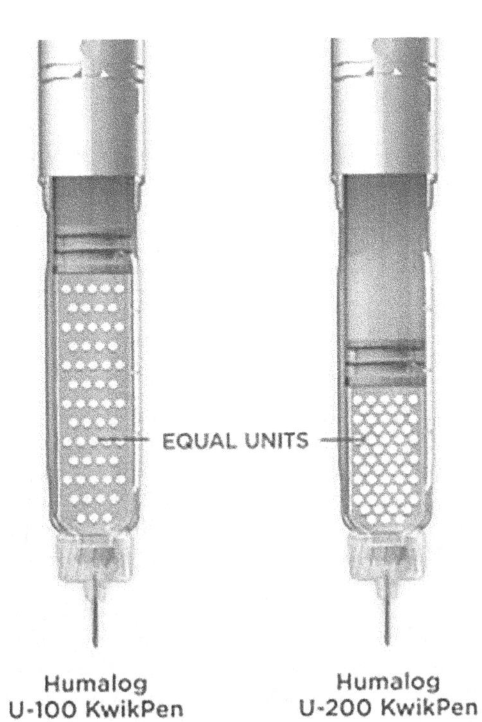

Figure 16.2—Delivered volume of insulin in U-100 Humalog KwikPen versus U-200 Humalog KwikPen.

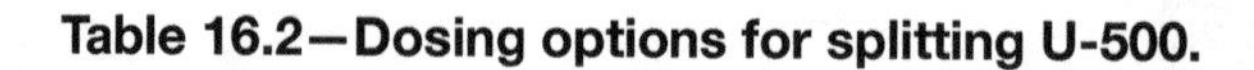

Table 16.2—Dosing options for splitting U-500.

- <200 units of insulin daily
  - Use U-100 insulin preparations (U-500 not recommended)
- 200–300 units of insulin daily
  - Split into twice daily doses
  - 50% before breakfast and 50% before dinner
- 300–600 units of insulin daily
  - Split into three times daily doses
  - 33% before breakfast, 33% before lunch, 33% before dinner
- >600 units of Insulin Daily
  - Split into four daily doses
  - 30% before breakfast, 30% before lunch, 30% before dinner and 10% before bedtime

Source: Cochran et al.[8]

U-200 lispro KwikPen is the first concentrated mealtime insulin analog to be approved. In a bioequivalence and pharmacodynamics study, U-200 lispro demonstrated bioequivalence when compared to U-100 lispro (Figure 16.4).[25] This new formulation delivers the same dose as U-100 lispro but in half the volume. The U-200 lispro KwikPen contains a total of 600 units per pen versus 300 units in a traditional U-100 pen and will dial in 1-unit increments up to 60 units per plunge.

U-100 glargine was the first long-acting insulin analog on the market. Predominantly used as basal insulin, the insulin action profile of glargine is relatively constant without a pronounced peak.[26] U-200 degludec is a long-acting concentrated insulin that is delivered in soluble multihexamers at the injection site. Monomers then separate and are slowly absorbed. This mechanism of action is what allows it to last >40 h.[27] In studies, the hemoglobin A_{1C} reduction and rates of hypoglycemia were similar when compared to U-100 glargine, but the rate of

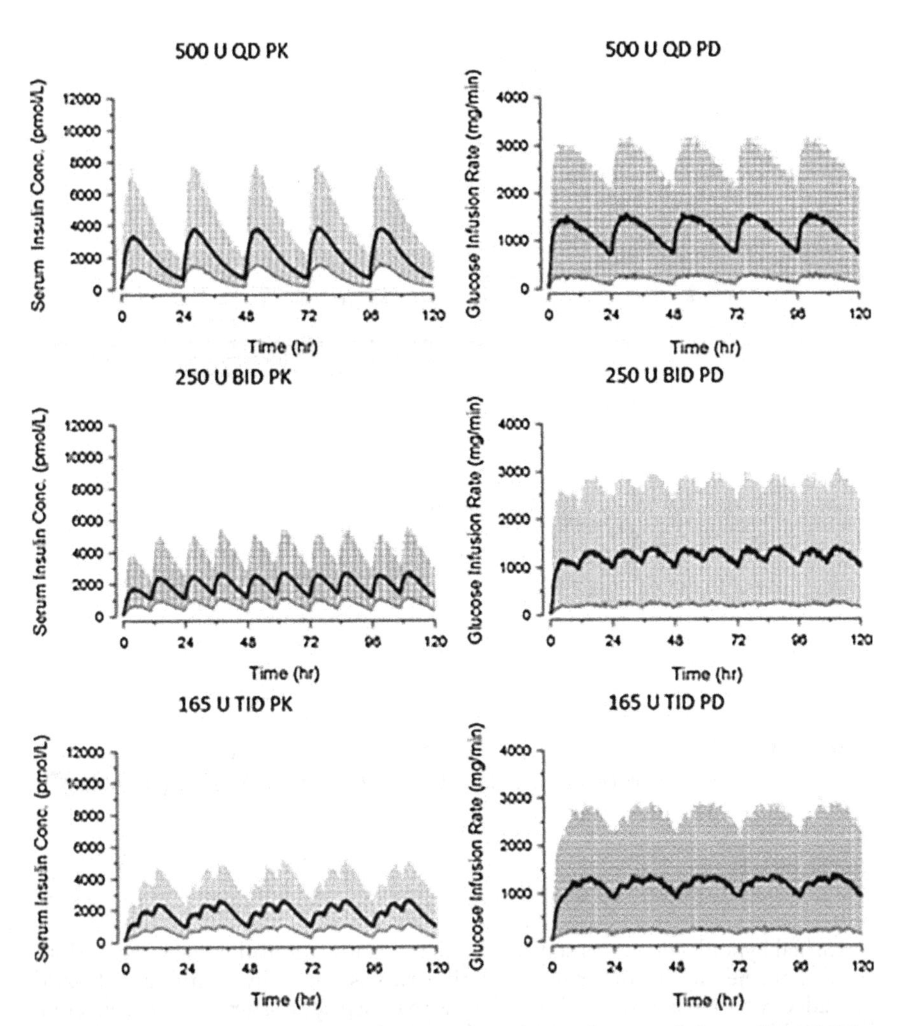

Figure 16.3—Phamacokinetics/pharmacodynamics modeling of U-500R doses at steady-state: 500-U QD, 250-U BID, 165-U TID. QD doses were administered at 7 A.M., BID doses at 7 A.M. and 6 P.M., and TID doses at 7 A.M., 12 noon, and 6 P.M.. The hatched area represents the 90th prediction interval from the model; the thicker line represents the median.

Source: de la Pena et al.[24]

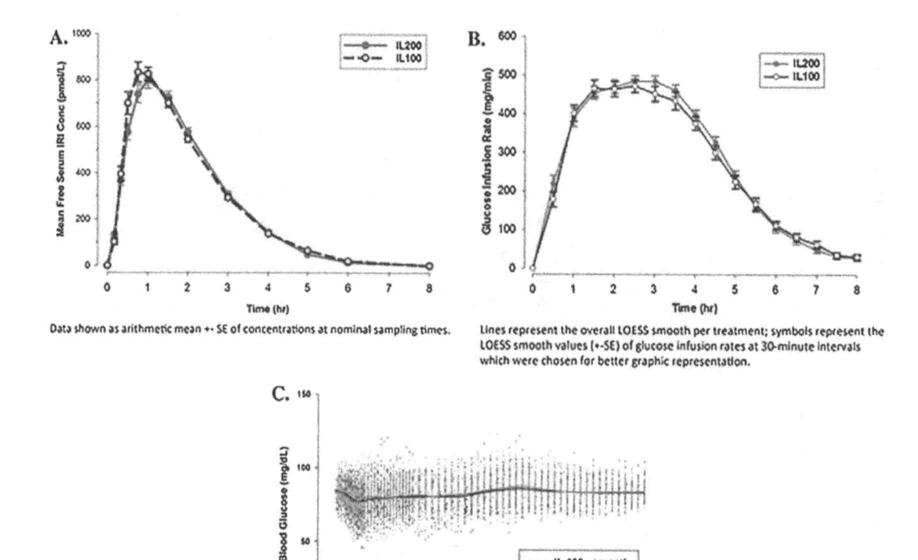

Figure 16.4—Bioequivalence and comparative pharmacodynamics of insulin lispro 200 units/mL relative to insulin lispro (Humalog®) 100 units/mL.

Source: de la Pena[25]

nocturnal hypoglycemia was statistically significant with insulin degludec.[28] More studies are needed to determine whether this is clinically significant. U-200 degludec comes in a flexpen with a window that displays the actual units delivered. The U-200 degludec flexpen delivers doses in 2-unit increments up to 160 units per plunge. Again, this insulin is a unit per unit conversion to a U-100 long-acting preparation, so if a patient was taking 60 units of U-200 degludec, they would be converted to 60 units of U-100 glargine.

U-300 GLARGINE

Recently, a new concentrated U-300 glargine was approved by the FDA for use in patients with type 1 diabetes and T2D. The advantage U-300 glargine over U-100 glargine is that the absorption of the smaller volume per injection is less variable and extends blood glucose control beyond 24 h.[29] U-300 glargine demonstrates "peakless" insulin action with a flat pharmacokinetic profile, resulting in a lower risk of nocturnal hypoglycemia compared with the U-100 formulation.[29] U-300 is

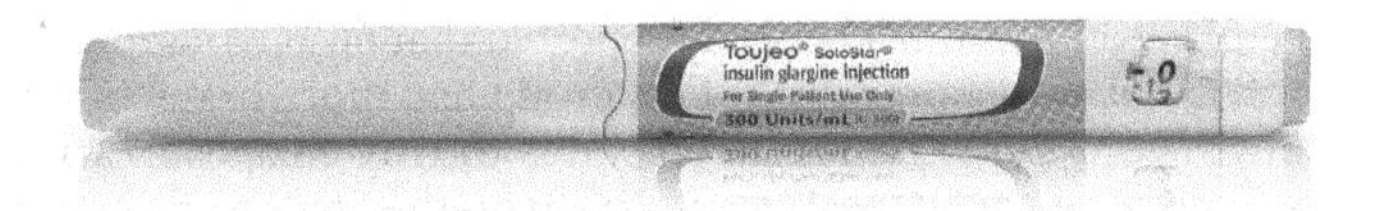

Figure 16.5—U-300 glargine insulin pen.

intended for severely insulin-resistant patients and for patients at risk for nocturnal hypoglycemia with U-100 formulations.[30,31] U-300 glargine is dispensed in a disposable SoloSTAR prefilled pen that contains a total of 450 units/1.5 mL. The current pen will deliver up to 80 units per injection (Figure 16.5).[14] In clinical trials, U-300 glargine had a flatter profile with a longer duration of action as compared to U-100 glargine and less nocturnal hypoglycemia.[30–32]

INPATIENT GLYCEMIC GOALS

The American Diabetes Association (ADA) and the American Association of Clinical Endocrinologists (AACE) recommend that blood glucose concentrations be maintained between 140 and 180mg/dL in critically ill hospitalized patients using insulin. For noncritically ill hospitalized patients, the ADA, AACE, and the Endocrine Society recommend premeal glucose concentrations be <140 mg/dL and randomly tested glucoses not to exceed 180 mg/dL.[33–35] Patients with high-dose insulin requirements are not an exception.

CONCENTRATED INSULIN IN THE HOSPITAL SETTING

When patients who are using concentrated insulin are admitted to the hospital, the first step is to determine whether they should continue on this type of insulin. Many hospitals do not carry U-300 or U-500 on their formulary, so a transition to U-100 insulin (traditionally, a basal-bolus regimen) is often required. Insulin requirements in hospitalized patients vary dramatically from home requirements. An adjustment of 15–20% of the TDD may be necessary based on concomitant illness, infection, or variances from the usual nutritional intake or meal pattern.

OPTION 1: CONTINUE U-500 INSULIN

Inpatient use of U-500 insulin in the hospital setting presents several challenges that might lead to potential medication errors.[15] As recommended by the Institute for Safe Medication Practices, all U-500 doses should be administered with a tuberculin syringe, regardless of the type of syringe the patient uses at home.[15] In 2015, Tripathy and Lansang[36] published a retrospective review of patients who used U-500 insulin at home and were admitted to the hospital between 2001 and 2011. Patients either continued on U-500 in the hospital or were converted to a conventional insulin regimen (long-, intermediate-, short-, or fast-acting insulin). Those that remained on U-500 tended to have higher insulin doses at home and were more likely to be on steroids during the hospitalization. The main reason for switching to a conventional regimen was either admission for surgical procedures or hypoglycemia at admission. The study reported that 66% of patients remained on U-500 at 85% of their home dose. This group had more frequent hypoglycemic days and severe hyperglycemic episodes during hospitalization.[38] The researchers attributed the increased rate of hypoglycemia to frequent insulin adjustments needed to correct steroid-induced hyperglycemia as well as higher insulin requirements (exceeding 0.6 units/kg). Doses at and above this ratio increase the risk of hypoglycemia because of the prolonged action of the U-500.[24]

Attempts by hospitals to standardize U-500 administration have met mixed results. A 500-bed community hospital developed an inpatient policy to address safety concerns for patients continuing U-500 during hospitalization.[37] One year after implementing the policy, they reported on the results of 12 patients treated with U-500 insulin after admission. Despite attempting to meticulously follow the protocol, nursing associates were often unaware of their responsibilities and did not notify the certified diabetes educator (CDE) that a patient on U-500 was admitted. The order set led to confusion among physicians, nurses, and pharmacists and often did not meet the needs of patients when corrective doses were used.[37]

The most successful inpatient transition protocol to date was published by Deal and Tobin[42] in a 1,200-bed academic medical center that reported an improvement in hypoglycemia rates among patients treated with U-500. Before the policy, the rate of hypoglycemia was 85.7%. Postpolicy, only 39% ($P = 0.009$) of patients experienced a blood glucose value <70 mg/dL. Rates of severe hypoglycemia (<40 mg/dL) were reduced from 57.1% to 5.6% ($P = 0.002$).[42] The components of their protocol and multidisciplinary inpatient policy are summarized as follows:

1. An endocrine/inpatient diabetes management consult is mandatory.
2. All doses of U-500 insulin are ordered in milliliters and corresponding units (Table 16.1).
3. All U-500 doses are measured by the pharmacy department, drawn up in tuberculin syringes, and dispensed to the inpatient unit.
4. Doses are provided in packages that label the product as concentrated insulin and the electronic medical record highlights the same precautions.
5. All patients are educated during their stay by a CDE who collaborates with the treating team for transition of care to home.

Some additional considerations include the following:

1. Decrease all outpatient U-500 doses by 15–20% upon admission unless clinical judgment recognizes a further decrease is necessary because of low blood glucoses and or low A_{1C} before admission.
2. Continue the frequency of the insulin administration as prescribed at home (e.g., twice daily, three times daily, or four times daily).
3. For twice-daily dosing, titrate the morning U-500 dose based on the predinner blood glucose and titrate the evening U-500 dose based on the morning fasting blood glucose.
4. For three times a day dosing, titrate the morning dose of U-500 based on the lunch blood glucose, titrate the lunch dose based on the predinner blood glucose, and titrate the dinner dose based on the bedtime and overnight fasting blood glucose.

5. For four times a day dosing, titrate the morning dose of U-500 based on the lunch blood glucose, titrate the lunch dose based on the predinner blood glucose, titrate the dinner dose based on the bedtime and overnight fasting blood glucose, and titrate the bedtime dose based on the overnight and fasting blood glucose.

OPTION 2: CONVERT TO NPH INSULIN

If the hospital does not have U-500 on formulary or for medical reasons the patient would be better served off U-500, a transition to NPH insulin may be appropriate. As mentioned, the pharmacokinetic profile of U-500 mimics that of NPH insulin. When converting a patient from U-500 regular to NPH, twice-daily dosing is recommended. It is critical that this conversion is done using the total units of insulin the patient takes at home, *not* "syringe units" because this will significantly underdose the patient (Table 16.3).

OPTION 3: CONVERT TO BASAL-BOLUS THERAPY

If it is determined that the patient should be on basal-bolus therapy (long-acting insulin with the addition of fast-acting insulin for meals), it is critical that this conversion be done based on the total units of insulin the patient takes at home, *not* "syringe" units because this will significantly underdose the patient. The TDD of insulin should be calculated and then divided equally between long-acting and short-acting insulin (Table 16.4).

A recent informal poll of endocrinologists engaged in inpatient management of diabetes revealed a preference for *not* using U-500 insulin in the hospital setting. According to the poll, these providers felt that >95% of patients on U-500 insulin in the outpatient setting could be managed successfully in the hospital with U-100 insulin.

U-200 AND U-300 IN THE HOSPITAL SETTING

These insulins were approved in 2015. At the time of this publication, there were no data on their use in the hospital setting. Because they are administered via a pen, the dosing is much simpler and can be carried over to the inpatient setting without dose conversion or confusion. The units displayed on the dosing window of the pen

Table 16.3—Example Conversion of U-500 to NPH Insulin

1) Calculate the current TDD of U-500
   25 "syringe units" of U-500 twice daily
   25x5 = 125 units twice daily or TDD of 250 units
2) Consider a 20% dose reduction
   0.80 x 250 = 200 units
3) Convert this to a dose of NPH Insulin
   100 units twice daily

Table 16.4—Example Conversion of U-500 to Basal-Bolus Therapy

A patient is admitted on 40 "syringe units" of U-500 three times a day using a U-100 syringe

1) Calculate the current TDD of U-500
   40 "syringe units" of U-500 three times daily
   40 x 5 (concentration) = 200 units three times daily = TDD of 600 units of insulin
2) Consider a 20% dose reduction
   0.80 x 600 = 480 units
3) Put 50% into U-100 long acting insulin
   480/2 = 240 units – most likely 120 units twice daily
4) Put remaining 50% into bolus insulin or correction factor
   240/3 = 80 units three times daily

are the actual units the patient will receive. U-200 degludec and U-300 glargine are used as basal insulins, and rapid-acting insulin meal coverage should be continued or added depending on patient presentation. The conversion of U-300 glargine to a U-100 insulin is not necessary because the units delivered by the pen are equivalent to the units delivered via syringe, but the volume is different (Table 16.5).

CONVERTING INPATIENT DOSES TO OUTPATIENT DOSES

When a patient is ready for discharge from the hospital, it may be difficult to predict the dose of insulin needed at home because of changes in food intake and physical activities. The insulin regimen in the hospital should be compared with the preadmission home regimen and adjusted based on the condition of the patient and their anticipated appetite and activity at home. For safety reasons, it is safer to discharge them on their current hospital dose and recommend a close follow-up by their primary care provider or endocrinologist within 1–2 weeks for titration of their insulin (see Chapter 30).

ADMINISTRATION OF U-500 INSULIN BY CONTINUOUS SQ INSULIN INFUSION

A small subset of patients use U-500 insulin in their insulin pump.[39–42] The largest pump reservoir holds 300 units of U-100 insulin and is changed every 3 days.

Table 16.5—Example Conversion of U-300 to Basal-Bolus Therapy

A patient is admitted on 40 units of U-300 glargine with aspart 10 units three times a day

1) Convert the basal U-300 into a dose of long acting U-100. This is a unit to unit conversion
   40 units of U-100 glargine
2) No dose reduction necessary in most cases
3) Order aspart
   10 units three times a day with meals with corrections per your hospital protocol

When doses of U-100 insulin exceed 200 units/day, patients are forced to change their set and reservoir daily, increasing the cost of pump supplies. Insulin pumps deliver units of insulin, not volumes. When the decision is made to transition from U-100 insulin to U-500, the pump settings will need to be adjusted to allow for the concentrated insulin. Using U-500, each "pump unit" will deliver 5 units of insulin.

When a patient using continuous SQ insulin infusion (CSII) and U-500 insulin presents to the inpatient setting, we recommend the following:

1. An endocrine or glucose management team consult is mandatory.
2. Discontinuation of the pump if the patient is severely ill in the intensive care unit, has evidence of disorientation or confusion or is receiving medications known to impair judgment.
    a. Patient should be transitioned to a long-acting as well as short- or rapid-acting U-100 preparation with a correction factor. The TDD of U-500 insulin is not apparent on the pump or in the reservoir. The TDD can be obtained from the pump by accessing the pump history, but this is generally facilitated by the endocrine consultants, glucose management team, or CDE.
3. Refer to Chapter 24 for information regarding the use of CSII in the inpatient setting.

CONCLUSION

Concentrated insulin is efficacious for patients who have SIR and require >200 units/day of insulin. As more concentrated insulins enter the market, providers will encounter these patient situations more often. There is some concern over using U-500 insulin in the hospital setting because of the increased potential for medication errors and risk of hypoglycemia.[15–16,37] For these reasons, many experts in the field do not recommend routine use of U-500 insulin in the hospital setting. Institutions that use U-500 insulin must implement strict protocols for its use. When the hospital staff is well educated on the use of U-500 insulin, extra measures are taken to ensure safety, and a multidisciplinary approach is supported, U-500 can be used successfully. Ultimately, recommendations are limited by lack of randomized controlled trials comparing different methods of inpatient diabetes management in patients with SIR. In our experience the biggest limitation to safe use of U-500 insulin is lack of sufficient knowledge and experience among hospital staff.

REFERENCES

1. Olefsky JM, Revers RR, Prince M, et al. Insulin resistance in non-insulin dependent (type II) and insulin dependent (type I) diabetes mellitus. *Adv Exper Med Biol* 1985;189:176–205

2. Nadeau KJ, Regensteiner JG, Bauer TA, et al. Insulin resistance in adolescents with type 1 diabetes and its relationship to cardiovascular function. *J Clin Endocrinol Metab* 2010;95(2):513–521

3. Rodbard HW, Gough S, Lane W, et al. Reduced risk of hypoglycemia with insulin degludec vs insulin glargine in patients with type 2 diabetes requiring high doses of basal insulin: meta-analysis of five randomized trials. *Endoc Pract* 2014;20(4):285–292
4. Chiu HK, Tsai EC, Juneja R, et al. Equivalent insulin resistance in latent autoimmune diabetes in adults (LADA) and type 2 diabetic patients. *Diabetes Res Clin Pract* 2007;77(2):237–244
5. Arioglu E, Andewelt A, Diabo C, Bell M, Taylor SI, Gorden P. Clinical course of the syndrome of autoantibodies to the insulin receptor (type B insulin resistance): a 28-year perspective. *Medicine* 2002;81(2):87–100
6. Flier JS, Kahn CR, Jarrett DB, Roth J. Characterization of antibodies to the insulin receptor: a cause of insulin-resistant diabetes in man. *J Clin Invest* 1976;58(6):1442–1449
7. Kahn CR, Flier JS, Bar RS, et al. The syndromes of insulin resistance and acanthosis nigricans. Insulin-receptor disorders in man. *New Engl J Med* 1976;294(14):739–745
8. Cochran E, Musso C, Gorden P. The use of U-500 in patients with extreme insulin resistance. *Diabetes Care* 2005;28(5):1240–1244
9. Humulin R regular U-500 (concentrated insulin human injection USP rDNA origin) [package insert]. Indianapolis, IN, Eli Lilly & Co., 2010
10. Dailey AM, Williams S, Taneja D, Tannock LR. Clinical efficacy and patient satisfaction with U-500 insulin use. *Diabetes Res Clin Pract* 2010;88(3):259–264
11. Ballani P, Tran MT, Navar MD, Davidson MB. Clinical experience with U-500 regular insulin in obese, markedly insulin-resistant type 2 diabetic patients. *Diabetes Care* 2006;29(11):2504–2505
12. Humalog U-200 (insulin Lispro injection) [package insert]. Lily and Co, Indianapolis, Indiana, 2015
13. Tresiba (insulin degludec injection) [package insert]. Lily and Co, Indianapolis, Indiana, 2015
14. U-300 Glargine (TOUJEO - insulin glargine injection, solution) [package insert]. U.S. S-A, ed, Sanofi Pasteur, Lion, France, 2014
15. Cohen MR. ISMP medication error report analysis: extra caution needed with U-500 regular insulin. *Hosp Pharm.* 2001; 36:616.16
16. Hellman R. A systems approach to reducing errors in insulin therapy in the inpatient setting. *Endoc Pract* 2004;10(Suppl. 2):100–108
17. Abraham K, Patail B, Wurth D. Usability testing of a U-500 insulin syringe: a human factors approach. *Patient Safety & Quality Healthcare* 2013. Available from http://psqh.com/usability-testing-of-a-u-500-insulin-syringe-a-human-factors-approach. Accessed 6 May 2015
18. Kahn M, Lee Y-Y. The pharmacokinetics and pharmacodynamics of regular U500 insulin in healthy non-obese subjects [article online], 2007. Available

from http://connection.ebscohost.com/c/articles/25821596/pharmacokinetics-pharmacodynamics-regular-u500-insulin-health-non-obese-subjects. Accessed January 2016

19. Khan MI, Sarabu B. The pharmacokinetic and pharmacodynamic properties of regular U-500 insulin in healthy non-obese subjects (abstract). *Diabetes* 2007;569(Suppl.):P–1294

20. Davidson MB, Navar MD, Echeverry D, Duran P. U-500 regular insulin: clinical experience and pharmacokinetics in obese, severely insulin-resistant type 2 diabetic patients. *Diabetes Care* 2010;33(2):281–283

21. Galloway JA, Spradlin CT, Nelson RL, et al. Factors influencing the absorption, serum insulin concentration, and blood glucose responses after injections of regular insulin and various insulin mixtures. *Diabetes Care* 1981;4(3): 366–376

22. Binder C, Lauritzen T, Faber O, Pramming S. Insulin pharmacokinetics. *Diabetes Care* 1984;7(2):188–199

23. Jorgensen KH, Hansen AK, Buschard K. Five fold increase of insulin concentration delays the absorption of subcutaneously injected human insulin suspensions in pigs. *Diabetes Res Clin Pract* 2000;50(3):161–167

24. de la Pena A, Ma X, Reddy S, Ovalle F, Bergenstal RM, Jackson JA. Application of PK/PD modeling and simulation to dosing regimen optimization of high-dose human regular U-500 insulin. *J Diabetes Sci Technol* 2014;8(4): 821–829

25. de la Pena A. Bioequivalence and comparative pharmacodynamics of insulin lispro 200 U/ml relative to insulin lispro (Humalog) 100 U/ml. *Clin Parmacol Drug Devel* 2016;5:69–75

26. Lucidi P, Porcellati F, Rossetti P, et al. Pharmacokinetics and pharmacodynamics of therapeutic doses of basal insulins NPH, glargine, and detemir after 1 week of daily administration at bedtime in type 2 diabetic subjects: a randomized cross-over study. *Diabetes Care* 2011;34(6):1312–1314

27. Jonassen I, Havelund S, Hoeg-Jensen T, Steensgaard DB, Wahlund PO, Ribel U. Design of the novel protraction mechanism of insulin degludec, an ultra-long-acting basal insulin. *Pharm Res* 2012;29(8):2104–2114

28. Zinman B, Philis-Tsimikas A, Cariou B, et al. Insulin degludec versus insulin glargine in insulin-naive patients with type 2 diabetes: a 1-year, randomized, treat-to-target trial (BEGIN Once Long). *Diabetes Care* 2012;35(12):2464–2471

29. Becker RH, Dahmen R, Bergmann K, Lehmann A, Jax T, Heise T. New insulin glargine 300 Units/mL-1 provides a more even activity profile and prolonged glycemic control at steady state compared with insulin glargine 100 Units/mL-1. *Diabetes Care* 2015;38(4):637–643

30. Jax T, Heisel T, Dahmen R, Bergmann K, Lehmann A, Tillner J, Becker RJH. New insulin glargine formulation has a flat and prolonged steady state profile in subjects with type 1 diabetes [abstract]. *Diabetologia* 2013;56(Suppl. 1): A1029

31. Jax T, Bergmann K, Lauer T, Dahmen R, et al. Euglycemia single dose clamp profile of new insulin glargine formulation in subjects with type 1 diabetes is flat and prolonged [abstract]. *Diabetologia* 2013;56(Suppl. 1):A1033
32. Riddle MC, Bolli GB, Ziemen M, Muehlen-Bartmer I, Bizet F, Home PD. New insulin glargine 300 units/mL versus glargine 100 units/mL in people with type 2 diabetes using basal and mealtime insulin: glucose control and hypoglycemia in a 6-month randomized controlled trial (EDITION 1). *Diabetes Care* 2014;37(10):2755–2762
33. Handelsman Y, Mechanick JI, Blonde L, et al. American Association of Clinical Endocrinologists Medical Guidelines for Clinical Practice for developing a diabetes mellitus comprehensive care plan. *Endoc Pract* 2011;17(Suppl. 2):1–53
34. Moghissi ES, Korytkowski MT, DiNardo M, et al. American Association of Clinical Endocrinologists and American Diabetes Association consensus statement on inpatient glycemic control. *Diabetes Care* 2009;32(6):1119–1131
35. Umpierrez GE, Hellman R, Korytkowski MT, et al. Management of hyperglycemia in hospitalized patients in non-critical care setting: an Endocrine Society clinical practice guideline. *J Clin Endocrinol Metab* 2012;97(1):16–38
36. Tripathy PR, Lansang MC. U-500 regular insulin use in hospitalized patients. *Endoc Pract* 2015;21(1):54–58
37. Samaan KH, Dahlke M, Stover J. Addressing safety concerns about U-500 insulin in a hospital setting. *AJHP* 2011;68(1):63–68
38. Deal EN, Tobin GS. Policy implementation for inpatient management of U-500 insulin resulting in lower incidence of hypoglycemia. *Endoc Pract* 2011;17(3):521
39. Lane WS, Weinrib SL, Rappaport JM, Przestrzelski T. A prospective trial of U-500 insulin delivered by Omnipod in patients with type 2 diabetes mellitus and severe insulin resistance. *Endoc Pract* 2010;16(5):778–784
40. Reutrakul S, Brown RL, Koh CK, Hor TK, Baldwin D. Use of U-500 regular insulin via continuous subcutaneous insulin infusion: clinical practice experience. *J Diabetes Sci Technol* 2011;5(4):1025–1026
41. Schwartz FL. A caution regarding U-500 insulin by continuous subcutaneous infusion. *Endoc Pract* 2004;10(2):163–164
42. Lane WS. Use of U-500 regular insulin by continuous subcutaneous insulin infusion in patients with type 2 diabetes and severe insulin resistance. *Endoc Pract* 2006;12(3):251–256
43. Segal AR, Brunner JE, Burch FT, Jackson JA. Use of concentrated insulin human regular (U-500) for patients with diabetes. *AJHP* 2010;67(18):1526–1535

Chapter 17

Management of Patients Postpancreatectomy

Sarah Kim, MD,[1] Boris Draznin, MD, PhD,[2] and Robert J. Rushakoff, MD[3]

INTRODUCTION

According to the National Inpatient Sample, a database of ~7 million annual hospital discharges in the U.S., there were 102,417 pancreatectomies performed between 1998 and 2006. Approximately half were for treatment of a malignant neoplasm and a third was for the treatment of nonmalignant conditions, including pancreatitis and cystic disease.[1] In the past 5 to 10 years, pancreatic surgery has been frequently and successfully performed on an elective basis for a variety of pancreatic disorders. There are several types of pancreatectomy, including the Whipple procedure (pancreaticoduodenectomy), distal pancreatectomy, segmental pancreatectomy, and total pancreatectomy. A common complication after pancreatic resection is new or worsened diabetes, a consequence of the surgical removal of insulin-producing β-cells. Pancreatic resections vary widely in the percent of parenchyma removed (Table 17.1) and, as such, the rate of new onset diabetes after pancreatectomy varies widely, from 24 to 100%.[2–5] Interestingly, the prevalence of diabetes preoperatively in these cases is also higher than average (20–80%) presumably because of underlying pancreatic disease for which surgery is indicated.[6]

Pancreatogenic diabetes, also known as type 3c diabetes, is due to disease or resection of the pancreas,[7] and is distinct from both type 1 and 2 diabetes in that in addition to the lack of adequate insulin secretion, there is a concomitant loss of glucagon secretion by α-cells. The lack of glucagon and its counterregulatory effects, especially in those with total pancreatectomy, results in an increased risk of iatrogenic hypoglycemia with the use of insulin. In addition, those with near-total or total pancreatectomy will experience protein and fat malabsorption, further complicating insulin replacement.[8] Generally, it may be difficult to achieve good glycemic control in patients following total pancreatectomy, but fear of diabetes should not preclude surgery when total pancreatectomy is indicated. Because

[1]Assistant Professor of Medicine, Division of Endocrinology and Metabolism, University of California, San Francisco, San Francisco General Hospital, San Francisco, CA. [2]Director, Adult Diabetes Program, University of Colorado Denver School of Medicine, Anschutz Medical Campus, Aurora, CO. [3]Director, Inpatient Diabetes, Professor of Medicine, Division of Endocrinology and Metabolism, University of California, San Francisco, CA.

DOI: 10.2337/9781580406086.17

Table 17.1—Percent of Pancreas Resected Following Different Pancreatic Procedures

Procedure	Pancreas resected (%)
Total pancreatectomy	100
Near-total pancreatectomy	80–95
Pancreaticoduodenectomy	50–80
Distal pancreatectomy	40–80

Source: Adapted from Slezak et al.[5]

there are no published data or systematic approaches for management of these patients, the following recommendations are based on the authors' knowledge of this underlying pathophysiology and extensive personal experience.

PREOPERATIVE MANAGEMENT

As discussed, preoperatively, patients with pancreatic diseases have a high incidence of diabetes. For most of these patients, the issue will be insulinopenia and an impaired insulin response to meals. Patients may have gastrointestinal symptoms, experience weight loss, and be in a catabolic state. They may have been treated previously with metformin, but for most, this medication will not be effective and may worsen their gastrointestinal symptoms, worsen anorexia, and decrease needed nutrient intake.

For some patients, particularly following partial pancreatectomy, an insulin secretagogue may be effective, but from our experience, the combination of likely underlying pancreatic inflammation and unpredictable eating patterns often renders this medication group useless or will place the patient at risk for hypoglycemia. Thus, for most patients with pancreatogenic diabetes, insulin treatment (generally premeal and basal) will be required.

A preoperative consultation with a diabetologist or a certified diabetes educator (CDE) is becoming a common procedure in most centers for patients undergoing pancreatic surgery. At this time, patients are given information about potential diabetes, receive explanations about treatment options, and are taught home glucose-monitoring techniques. In our experience, these preoperative consultations have been extremely helpful for postoperative care of diabetes.

INPATIENT AND POSTOPERATIVE MANAGEMENT

Descriptions of intravenous (IV) insulin therapy, transition from IV insulin to subcutaneous (SQ) insulin, and SQ insulin management are discussed in detail in other chapters of this book. Only specific details for patients undergoing pancreatectomy are discussed here.

Postoperative glucose management following pancreatectomy depends in part on the extent of pancreas removed as well as age, obesity, family history of diabetes, and the nature of the pancreatic disease. For patients who have undergone total or near-total pancreatectomy, both basal and prandial insulin will be required long term to achieve adequate glucose levels, although the doses of insulin required will be lower because of the lack of glucagon secretion. In fact, patients with type 3c diabetes are sensitive to insulin and avoidance of hypoglycemia becomes a critically important element of their treatment. In these cases, insulin infusion should begin perioperatively and continue 1–2 h after the first injection of basal insulin is received. Prandial insulin should be administered when the patient begins eating, although cautiously, as gastrointestinal malabsorption may result in hypoglycemia. The dosing of prandial and basal insulin can be based on the IV insulin infusion. Alternatively, from our experience, a weight-based calculation of 0.2 units/kg/day total (50% basal, 50% bolus) often is sufficient. For patients who have a more complicated postoperative course (i.e., requiring total parenteral nutrition or enteral feedings), basal insulin should be continued and nutritional dosing should be added for the feeding as appropriate (see Chapter 6 for details on enteral and parenteral nutrition). Again, as these patients are insulin sensitive, small doses often are required.

In the past, we observed that because these patients were on low rates of IV infusions, or because the interoperative and immediate postoperative levels of glycemia were not significantly elevated, these patients mistakenly were placed only on sliding-scale insulin. Glucose levels would then become high and labile. Again, from our experience, if IV insulin is used until the patient is stable and then basal-bolus insulin immediately instituted, glucoses can be controlled easily.

For those with lesser degrees of pancreatic loss, the ideal insulin regimen will vary. In patients without preexisting diabetes or prediabetes and pancreatic resection of <44%,[2] little or no long-term insulin may be required. As the postoperative course is often unpredictable and pancreatic manipulation and inflammation leads to continued decreased insulin production, the initial postoperative management plan is the same as that described for patients undergoing total pancreatectomy. As the patient stabilizes with reliable nutritional intake, however, a secretagogue often may be tried. We frequently use meglitinides initially as they are short acting, and patients can be educated to not take the medication if they will not be eating, limiting their risk for hypoglycemia. In addition, some patients will need only small doses taken just for high-carbohydrate meals.

When using mealtime insulin boluses, the insulin-to-carbohydrate ratio can be beneficial to calculate the insulin dose. Because these patients are insulin sensitive, a ratio of 1 unit of rapid-acting insulin to 20 or 25 g of carbohydrate may be a good starting point. Frequently, an accurate estimate of insulin requirement in postpancreatectomy patients cannot be made until after discharge from the hospital. Thus, inpatient diabetes education and a timely referral to a diabetologist postdischarge are of great importance for adequate and safe long-term management of these patients.

REFERENCES

1. Simons JP, et al. National complication rates after pancreatectomy: beyond mere mortality. *J Gastrointest Surg* 2009;13(10):1798–1805
2. Shirakawa S, et al. Pancreatic volumetric assessment as a predictor of new-onset diabetes following distal pancreatectomy. *J Gastrointest Surg* 2012;16(12):2212–2219
3. Hirata K, et al. Predictive factors for change of diabetes mellitus status after pancreatectomy in preoperative diabetic and nondiabetic patients. *J Gastrointest Surg* 2014;18(9):1597–1603
4. Park JW, et al. Effects of pancreatectomy on nutritional state, pancreatic function and quality of life. *B J Surg* 2013;100(8):1064–1070
5. Slezak LA, Andersen DK. Pancreatic resection: effects on glucose metabolism. *World J Surg* 2001;25(4):452–460
6. Parsaik AK, et al. Metabolic and target organ outcomes after total pancreatectomy: Mayo Clinic experience and meta-analysis of the literature. *Clin Endocrinol* 2010;73(6):723–731
7. Diagnosis and classification of diabetes mellitus. *Diabetes Care* 2011;34 (Suppl. 1):S62–S69
8. Cui Y, Andersen DK. Pancreatogenic diabetes: special considerations for management. *Pancreatology* 2011;11(3):279–294

Chapter 18

Inpatient Management of Patients with Diabetes after Bariatric Surgery

Sara Alexanian, MD,[1] and Ildiko Lingvay, MD, MPH, MSCS[2]

BACKGROUND

Bariatric surgery is a well-established therapy for achieving long-term weight loss in the morbidly obese. Along with weight loss, these patients experience improvement in multiple other medical comorbidities postoperatively including diabetes.[1,2] Although many of these improvements are due to weight loss and are therefore gradual, it has been noted with much interest that glucose homeostasis improves within days after surgery, before substantial weight loss occurs.[3] This rapid change in glycemic status, coupled with the specific changes in the meal plan and nutritional needs following surgery, poses particular therapeutic challenges during the inpatient period as well as in the selection of a suitable and safe antihyperglycemic therapeutic regimen upon discharge. Inclusion of a registered dietitian nutritionist (RD or RDN) on the bariatric team is critical to ensure patient understanding of the necessary changes in nutritional intake and will enable positive short- and long-term outcomes. This chapter reviews the major weight loss procedures, explains the main metabolic changes that occur after surgery, discusses the care of the patient with diabetes in the days immediately after bariatric surgery, and addresses discharge considerations.

BARIATRIC SURGERY TYPES AND OUTCOMES

It is estimated that nearly 180,000 bariatric procedures are completed yearly in the U.S.[4] Bariatric procedures traditionally were classified as "restrictive" or "malabsorptive," but as our knowledge of their specific metabolic effects has expanded, it is recognized that this simple mechanistic classification may be incomplete. The four most common bariatric procedures currently performed are presented in Figure 18.1. Laparoscopic adjustable gastric banding (LAGB; Figure 18.1*A*) had a tremendous gain in popularity starting in 2001 when the first-generation Lap-Band® was approved. In this procedure, a fillable band is

[1]Assistant Professor, Department of Endocrinology, Diabetes, Nutrition and Weight Management, Director, Inpatient Diabetes Program, Boston Medical Center, Boston, MA. [2]Associate Professor, Department of Internal Medicine/Endocrinology, UT Southwestern Medical Center, Dallas, TX.

DOI: 10.2337/9781580406086.18

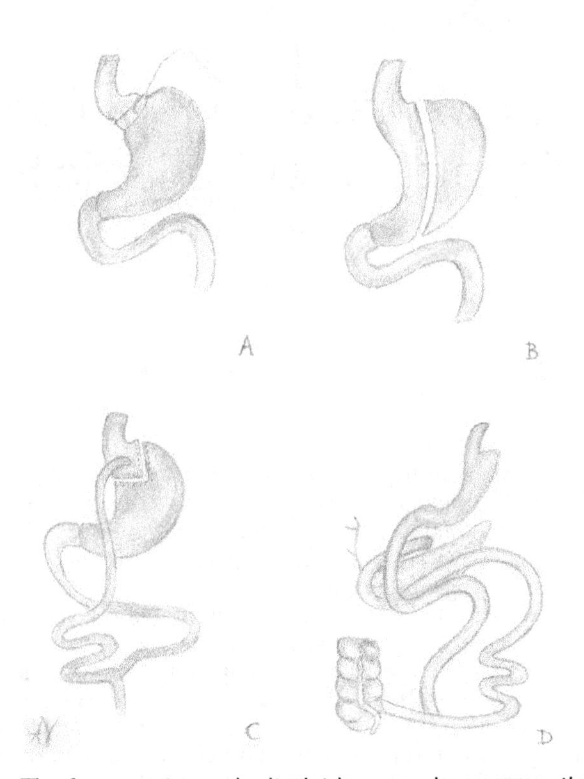

Figure 18.1—The four most popular bariatric procedures currently performed in the U.S. *A*: Laparoscopic adjustable gastric banding (LAGB). *B*: Sleeve gastrectomy (SG). *C*: Roux-en-Y gastric bypass (RYGB). *D*: Biliopancreatic diversion with duodenal switch (BPD-DS).

placed around the upper part of the stomach creating a pouch that can hold only a small amount of food and therefore limits caloric intake. As the long-term risk-benefit ratio is now better understood and other more durable procedures have been perfected, the popularity of the LAGB is rapidly decreasing. Roux-en-Y gastric bypass (RYGB; Figure 18.1*C*) has been the gold standard bariatric procedure in the U.S. It involves the surgical formation of a small stomach pouch (<30 mL). The small intestine is divided about 75 cm distally from the ligament of Treitz and the Roux (or alimentary) end is connected to the newly created small stomach pouch that functions to drain food. The upper small intestine is then attached about 125 cm distal to this gastrojejunostomy and channels gastric juices, bile, and pancreatic endocrine products. The effect of this procedure is to change the transport of nutrients through the upper gastrointestinal tract such that food enters a small stomach and passes directly into the jejunum where it travels approximately 125 cm before mixing with digestive juices in a common channel. Biliopancreatic diversion (BPD) with or without duodenal switch (DS) involves a more extreme nutrient rerouting (via a shorter common channel) and a partial gastrectomy (Figure 18.1*D*). Although the results are dramatic, the short- and long-term complications, including severe nutritional deficiencies, are common, leading to its low popularity except in the superobese. Sleeve gastrectomy (SG), in which the greater curvature of the stomach is removed and a tubular stomach is created (Figure 18.1*B*), was used in the past to promote weight loss in superobese patients and to serve as a bridge to other procedures. It now, however, has been found to be quite effective even in isolation, which coupled with its beneficial long-term safety profile and relative surgical ease has made it an increasingly popular choice with patients and surgeons alike.[5]

The effectiveness of surgery in terms of weight loss and resolution of diabetes varies significantly among the different procedures. It is estimated that within 1–2 years following surgery, patients lose on average of 46% excess body weight following LAGB, 60% after RYGB, 64% after BPD/DS, and 61% after SG.[2,6] The percentage of patients with resolution of type 2 diabetes (T2D) 2 years after surgery is estimated as follows: LAGB: 58%, RYGB: 71%, BPD/DS: 96%, SG: 68%.[2,6] Reports of glycemic "improvement" in type 1 diabetes (T1D) and T2D after surgery are higher than rates of remission and are 100% in most studies of RYGB and BPD.[7] It is worth noting that there have been controversies regarding the definitions of partial and complete diabetes remission. One study showed that applying more stringent diabetes resolution criteria based on the American Diabetes Association 2009 definition of diabetes resulted in a rate of diabetes resolution of 41% after RYBG versus 58% when older criteria are used.[8] Regardless, bariatric surgery has been shown to be a more effective treatment in controlling diabetes than any other intervention, including intensive lifestyle changes coupled with pharmacologic therapy.[9,10] Several factors have been associated with an increased likelihood of diabetes remission after surgery, including shorter duration of diabetes, no insulin need before surgery, low HbA_{1c}, higher preoperative BMI, and a larger percentage of excess body weight loss.[11,12] These patient characteristics should be evaluated closely to ensure proper patient selection, to guide the decision regarding the appropriate surgical procedure, and when counseling patients preoperatively regarding the anticipated results of the surgery. These characteristics could serve as the basis for a patient-centered decision regarding the need for continued antihyperglycemic therapy upon hospital discharge.

METABOLIC CHANGES AFTER SURGERY

Many factors are thought to play a role in the rapid and ongoing improvement in glycemia after surgery,[7,13] and we are far from having a full understanding of the mechanisms behind the observed effects. Patients who undergo a purely restrictive procedure such as LAGB do not manifest any acute metabolic changes[14] and diabetes improvement mainly parallels with long-term weight loss. All other procedures (RYGB, BPD/DS, SG) produce alterations in the enteroendocrine axis, leading to their designation as metabolic surgeries. Much attention has focused on the postoperative changes in glucagon-like peptide 1 (GLP-1), a hormone that is secreted by the L-cells in the small intestine. GLP-1 promotes insulin secretion, slows gastric emptying, reduces hunger, and inhibits glucagon secretion, and therefore it is a logical mediator of the observed effects.[15–17] Although a number of studies have confirmed postprandial GLP-1 elevations, recent studies have put in question the magnitude of the contribution of this hormonal alteration to glycemic changes.[18,19] Other hormones have been studied and overall the findings to date are most consistent with increases in the anorexic hormone peptide YY (PYY) and lower levels of leptin and ghrelin.[16] Another key mechanism that plays a role in glycemic improvement is calorie restriction and weight loss. It is known that acute and significant calorie restriction will improve glycemia and insulin resistance in the liver.[20] Yet, significant weight loss takes weeks to ensue, and therefore calorie restriction is likely the biggest contributor to glycemic improvement and remission of diabetes in the acute postoperative period.[21] On the basis of the totality of the available evidence, it is likely that many different mechanisms, some yet to be discovered, contribute to the observed satiety and glycemic improvement following these metabolic surgeries, with the relative contribution of each being different in the immediate postoperative period versus the first few months versus years after the procedure.[13] We suspect that caloric restriction is a primary contributor to the rapid resolution in T2D noted within days of the metabolic surgeries,[21] which has significant impact on the therapeutic decisions regarding management of glycemia during this period of rapid transition.

IMMEDIATE POSTOPERATIVE NUTRITION AND GLYCEMIC MANAGEMENT

The following discussion primarily relates to the care of patients after metabolic bariatric surgeries. LAGB is usually an outpatient procedure, and the glycemic changes occurring after this procedure are more gradual and track with the weight loss. In these patients, we recommend a gradual decrease in the dose of the antihyperglycemic agents tailored to the improvements observed based on frequent self-monitoring of blood glucose.

Metabolic bariatric procedures typically are followed by a 2–4 day inpatient stay, occasionally longer if perioperative complications occur. After the procedure, most patients will be admitted to the general surgical ward, with <30% of patients requiring a short admission to the intensive care unit (ICU). The nutrition program for these patients involves extremely limited caloric intake in the immediate postoperative period. Although there is no official published protocol, most institutions employ a similar routine to that described here. As mentioned earlier, it is critical that the RDN is included as a member of the bariatric team or is consulted to enable patient understanding of the changes in meal planning and nutritional needs following surgery. Patients do not ingest anything orally in the first 12–24 h. Some institutions await radiographic confirmation of an intact anastomosis before initiating oral intake. On the first postoperative day, patients begin a clear liquid diet (such as water, ice chips, and crystal light) restricted in volume to 30 cc/h. Over the next couple of days, the volume restriction gradually increases to 120 cc/h as tolerated by the patient. Once this volume is tolerated, a gradual substitution to calorie-containing protein-based liquids occurs. During the first 2 weeks postoperatively, it is estimated that caloric intake is approximately 400–800 calories/day, increasing to 800–1,000 calories/day thereafter. Figure 18.2 shows the average daily caloric intake of 10 patients with T2D who underwent an uncomplicated RYGB procedure and were followed in an inpatient setting for 7 days postoperatively (authors' data, adapted from Lingvay et al.[21]). Of note, the total caloric intake for the entire first postoperative week was approximately 1,750 calories, representing the significant caloric restrictions these patients undergo postoperatively.[21] An additional challenge posed by this feeding regimen is the frequent (up to every 15 min while awake) but limited caloric intake, making traditional premeal glucose monitoring and mealtime insulin coverage impossible. Figure 18.2 also shows the daily average of the six capillary blood glucose determinations in the 10 patients noted previously. The slight initial increase in glycemia in the first few postoperative days likely is related to surgery-induced systemic stress; this quickly improved to reach below-baseline levels by postoperative day 7. This represents the rapid changes in glycemia and therapeutic needs that occur in the days following the surgery. Most patients are discharged on postoperative days 2 to 4, a time that coincides with the fastest decline in glucose level and the time of highest risk of hypoglycemia if medical management decisions are not aligned.

No studies specifically address the optimal glycemic targets in this patient population while hospitalized postsurgery, and therefore the guidelines use extrapolated data from other surgical patients and recommend a target glucose level of 140–180 mg/dL.[22] Some institutions may employ a lower (80–140 mg/dL)

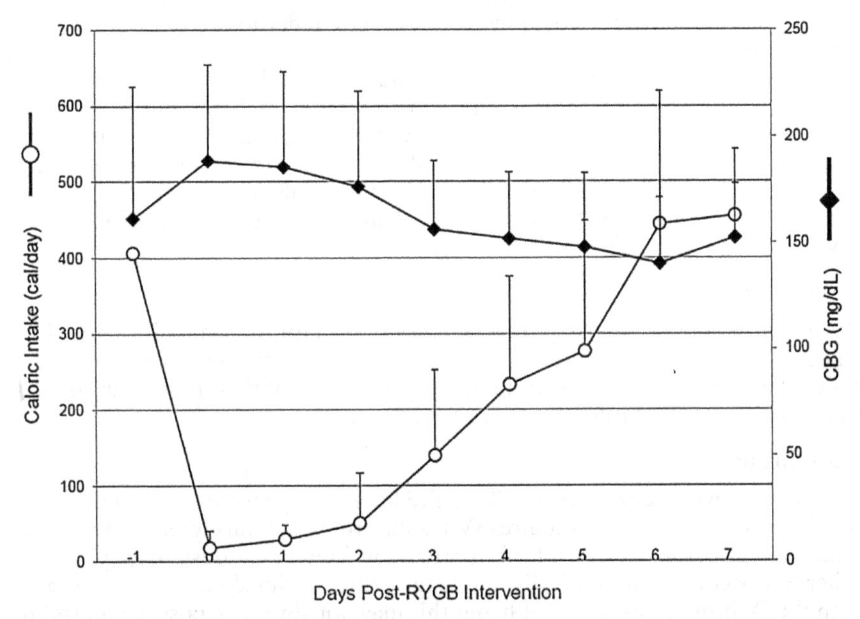

Figure 18.2—Glycemic profile and caloric intake in 10 patients with type 2 diabetes who underwent RYGB on day 0. CBG, capillary blood glucose, calculated as the average of 6 daily readings performed 4 h apart.

Source: Data extracted from Lingvay et al.[21]

target while the patients are in the ICU. In practice, we monitor the patients' glucose levels upon arrival for the procedure and perioperatively. Patients who exceed the treatment threshold either in the operating room or while in an ICU setting are initiated on a continuous regular insulin intravenous (IV) infusion according to the local institutional protocol. This treatment offers the advantage of a quick onset, the ability to titrate the infusion rate frequently to the individual patient's need, and the ability to stop treatment with a quick offset. Additionally, steady-state infusion rates can be used to estimate the ongoing need for basal insulin.

Few studies have examined inpatient medical management of hyperglycemia in this population. Oral antihyperglycemic agents are not recommended during the hospital stay because of practical limitations in oral intake (patients cannot swallow pills, even crushed), the potential side effects, and the longer-lasting effect in the setting of rapidly changing glycemic status. Therefore, insulin is the only antihyperglycemic agent used, but there is no consensus or clear guidelines regarding an optimal regimen. In one study, patients randomized to subcutaneous (SQ) once-daily glargine insulin dosed at 0.3 units/kg/day were found to have improved control compared with patients using sliding-scale SQ regular insulin every 6 h.[23] The total insulin dose in the glargine group was nearly four times higher than in the sliding-scale regular insulin group (179 vs. 44 units); therefore, the difference in outcome could mainly be due to underdosing of insulin in the sliding-scale group.

Given the lack of studies in this area, it may be useful to look at the separate elements of an insulin management program (nutritional, basal, and correction) and address them individually. Note that the following considerations are based on experience, and further research would be required to support the development of evidence-based guidelines. The following discussion is in general consistent with guidelines published by the American Association of Clinical Endocrinologists and The Obesity Society.[22]

Prandial Insulin

Patients will not consume any substantial calories until immediately before discharge, so prandial insulin rarely is needed during the hospital stay. Providers should familiarize themselves with the diet progression at their particular institution to be aware when calories will be introduced.

Basal Insulin

Determining whether a patient will require long-acting insulin can be challenging. In general, if a patient requires IV insulin treatment during or immediately after the operation, we consider initiating a weight-based dose of glargine or other long-acting insulin. Ideally, the long-acting insulin should be overlapped with the IV insulin infusion by 4 h, but this may not always be possible if insulin infusions are not allowed on the general medical ward and a discharge from the intensive care or postoperative care unit is imminent. We initiate glargine insulin at a dose of 0.2–0.25 units/kg/day, using lower doses for patients at increased risk for hypoglycemia such as those with renal insufficiency or elderly patients. On subsequent days, we reassess for ongoing need and adjust this dose daily based on the capillary glucose measurements. As the duration of calorie restriction lengthens, the hyperglycemia generally will improve. For patients who do well postoperatively and have glucose levels below the upper threshold of the goal (180 mg/dL), we prophylactically decrease basal insulin by 10–30% on subsequent postop days.

Correction Insulin

All patients who undergo bariatric surgery should have a correction insulin scheme in place to address the hyperglycemia that occurs either due to preexistent diabetes or due to postsurgical stress in patients with no prior diagnosis. Typically correction insulin is scheduled every 4 or 6 h and initiated if the preestablished glycemic target is crossed (usually 140 mg/dL) and escalated based on the capillary glucose readings. The repeat need for correction insulin administration during a 24-h period indicates that either initiation or uptitration of scheduled basal insulin may be necessary.

Not all patients who undergo bariatric procedures have T2D. All patients on insulin should have a review of their diabetes history to assess type of diabetes and current treatment regimen. Patients with T1D should not have any interruption in their insulin treatment, although it is expected that they will require a significant dose reduction in both their basal as well as mealtime insulin, adjustments that will continue past the hospital discharge.

CONSIDERATIONS FOR DISCHARGE

Evidence to guide clinical care upon discharge is also lacking. We use individual safety considerations, diabetes history, medication characteristics, and patient glucose trend data during the hospital stay to tailor the discharge regimen to the individual patient's characteristics and needs. Many patients with diabetes do not require a continuation of any pharmacologic treatment at the time of discharge. Patients with long-standing, insulin-treated, or uncontrolled diabetes are more likely to continue to require ongoing therapy. It is important to identify the most appropriate treatment regimen to avoid hypoglycemia in the face of rapidly changing glycemic status.

Sulfonylureas and meglitinides are not recommended after bariatric surgery because of the high risk of hypoglycemia.[22] Metformin may be continued postoperatively (if no specific contraindications exist) at least until prolonged clinical diabetes resolution is demonstrated.[22] The large pill size can be a challenge in the immediate postoperative period. Patients may need to crush the pills, or use the liquid form, but the liquid form is not routinely carried by many pharmacies. Use of thiazolidinediones following bariatric surgery have no specific safety concern, yet their propensity for weight gain makes them less desirable for this patient population, and they seldom are continued in practice after surgery. α-Glucosidase inhibitors have gastrointestinal side effects that could be intolerable in this setting, specifically in the immediate postoperative period. These agents have been used with some success in treating postprandial hypoglycemia, which is a relatively common complication after bariatric surgery. Incretin-based therapies, including GLP-1 agonists and dipeptidyl peptidase-4 (DPP-4) inhibitors, in theory are superfluous because natural postmeal GLP-1 levels rise significantly after surgery. There are no reported studies and little clinical experience using these agents after bariatric surgery but available data suggest no contraindications and a possible beneficial effect, especially to boost metabolic improvements once a steady-state is reached following surgery. In the acute postoperative period, however, these also would be discontinued. Sodium-glucose linked transporter (SGLT-2) inhibitors are a newer class of antihyperglycemic agents, and evidence regarding their use in this setting is lacking. These agents promote diuresis, at least in the first few weeks after initiation, and therefore, they should be used with caution, if at all, in the first few weeks after surgery when the risk of dehydration is high because of limited volume intake. These agents, however, are associated with a modest weight loss effect and therefore could be considered should additional antihyperglycemic effects be needed and if the noted risks are mitigated.

Patients taking insulin before surgery need to be reevaluated at discharge to assess whether continued use is warranted. We consider continuing basal insulin only if the patient demonstrates a significant basal insulin need while in the hospital. This may happen in patients with long-standing or poorly controlled diabetes. We use the glycemic response to insulin during the postoperative period to guide dosing recommendations, but recommend a preemptive substantial decrease (usually 30–50%) upon discharge to avoid hypoglycemia. In our experience, the typical dose of basal insulin at discharge is 0.1–0.15 units/kg/day. Prandial insulin is not usually resumed after surgery as it is unlikely to be necessary, but also the meal pattern is of such nature (very small intake every 15–30 min) that timing mealtime insulin correctly is a big challenge. Should prandial insulin prove to be necessary, it is better to introduce it after a few weeks when the patient is tolerating mashed and solid foods and to use the shortest-acting formulation available. Pre-mixed insulin is not recommended after bariatric surgery, especially in the first few months, because of the high risk of hypoglycemia.

Monitoring the glucose level after discharge is important to ensure glycemic control and to identify early any need to adjust therapy. Patients who are discharged without any antihyperglycemic treatment are asked to check glucose levels at least daily in the first couple of weeks after surgery, primarily to ensure that they are controlled and there is indeed no need to restart therapy. If glucose levels continue to be normal, they can decrease or even stop their home monitoring. Conversely, patients discharged on any hypoglycemic agents are asked to check blood glucose three to four times per day for safety reasons and titration purposes. Patients are instructed to halve their medication dose if their glucose levels are consistently <100 mg/dL. If they experience any low blood glucose (<70 mg/dL), we advise them to hold their hypoglycemic therapy and contact their physician for further recommendations. The risk of iatrogenic hypoglycemia following discharge is high, and therefore patients should receive counseling about how to appropriately prevent and manage hypoglycemia after surgery.

Patients may undergo several medication changes and receive many instructions upon discharge, so it is important to ensure that the patient understands how to manage their diabetes in the immediate postoperative period and appropriately manage expectations. Patients should be given clear instructions about the following aspects: which medications to continue, any dose adjustments that will be made upon discharge, how often to monitor blood glucose level, when to call a provider, and hypoglycemia treatment. We encourage patients to see their outpatient provider within a week of discharge to assess their progress and therapeutic regimen.

CONCLUSION

Bariatric surgery can provide dramatic and durable improvements in diabetes and reduce or eliminate the need for medications in many patients, although over subsequent years, diabetes may recur. Alterations in glucose homeostasis begin within days following metabolic procedures, necessitating close monitoring and antihyperglycemic therapy adjustments during the hospital stay. Understanding these changes and the postoperative dietary program is important to providing safe and effective inpatient care and when deciding on a safe and appropriate discharge regimen. Few clinical studies are available to guide acute diabetes management in these patients. We hope the coming years will bring more data to further elucidate postoperative alterations in the enteroendocrine axis as well as provide a prospective literature to inform optimal management targets and strategies in the immediate weeks after surgery.

REFERENCES

1. Poires WJ, Macdonald KG Jr, Morgan EJ, Sinha MK, Dohm GL, et al. Surgical treatment of obesity and its effect on diabetes: 10-y follow-up. *Am J Clin Nutr* 1992;55:S582–S585
2. Buchwald H, Estok R, Fahrback K, Banel D, Jensen MD, et al. Weight and type 2 diabetes after bariatric surgery: systematic review and meta-analysis. *Am J Med* 2009;122(3):248–256
3. Wickremesekera K, Miller G, Naotunne TD, Knowles G, Stubbs RS. Loss of insulin resistance after Roux-en-Y gastric bypass surgery: a time course study. *Obes Surg* 2005;15(4):474–481
4. American Society for Metabolic and Bariatric Surgery. http://asmbs.org/resources/estimate-of-bariatric-surgery-numbers. Accessed 16 January 2015
5. Buchwald H, Oien DM. Metabolic/bariatric surgery worldwide 2011. *Obes Surg* 2013;23(4):427–436
6. Jimenez A, Casamitjana R, Flores L, et al. Long-term effects of sleeve gastrectomy and Roux-en-Y gastric bypass surgery on type 2 diabetes mellitus in morbidly obese subjects. *Ann Surg* 2012;256(6):1023–1029
7. Mingrone G, Castagneto-Gissey L. Mechanisms of early improvement/resolution of type 2 diabetes after bariatric surgery. *Diabetes Metab* 2009;35 (6 Pt. 2):518–523
8. Pournaras DJ, Aasheim ET, Sovik TT, Andrews R, Mahon D, et al. Effect of the definition of type 2 diabetes remission in the evaluation of bariatric surgery for metabolic disorders. *Br J Surg* 2012;99(1):100–103
9. Schauer PR, Bhatt D, Kirwan JP, Wolski K, Bethauer SA, et al. Bariatric surgery versus intensive medical therapy for diabetes – 3 year outcomes. *N Engl J Med* 2014;370(21)2002–2013

10. Mingrone G, Panunzi S, De Gaetono A, et al. Bariatric surgery versus conventional medical therapy for type 2 diabetes. *N Engl J Med* 2012;366(17):1577–1585
11. Hayes MT, Hunt LA, Foo J, Tychinskaya Y, Stubbs RS. A model for predicting the resolution of type 2 diabetes following Roux-en-Y gastric bypass surgery. *Obes Surg* 2011;21(7):910–916
12. Dixon JB, Chuang ML, Chong SC, Lambert GW, Straznicky NE, et al. Predicting the glycemic response to gastric bypass surgery in patients with type 2 diabetes. *Diabetes Care* 2013;36(1):20–26
13. Knop FK, Taylor R. Mechanism of metabolic advantages after bariatric surgery. *Diabetes Care* 2013;36(Suppl. 2):S287–S291
14. Usinger L, Hansen KB, Kristiansen VB, Larsen S, Holst JJ, et al. Gastric emptying of orally administered glucose solution and incretin hormone responses are unaffected by laparoscopic adjustable gastric banding. *Obes Surg* 2011;21(5):624–632
15. Jorgensen NB, Dirksen C, Bojsen-Moller KN, Jacobsen SH, Worm D, et al. Exaggerated glucagon-like peptide 1 response is important for improved beta-cell function and glucose tolerance after Roux-en-Y gastric bypass in patients with type 2 diabetes. *Diabetes Care* 2013;62(9):3044–3052
16. Beckman LM, Beckman TR, Earthman CP. Changes in gastrointestinal hormones and leptin after Roux-en-Y gastric bypass procedure: a review. *J Am Diet Assoc* 2010;110(4):571–584
17. Nannipieri M, Baldi S, Mari A, Colligiani D, Guarino D, Camastra S, et al. Roux-en-Y gastric bypass and sleeve gastrectomy: mechanisms of diabetes remission and role of gut hormones. *J Clin Endocrinol Metab* 2013;98(11):4391–4399
18. Jimenez A, Casamitjana R, Flores L, et al. GLP-1 and the long-term outcome of type 2 diabetes mellitus after Roux-en-Y gastric bypass surgery in morbidly obese subjects. *Ann Surg* 2013:257(5):849–849
19. Mokadem M, Zechner JF, Margolskee RF, Drucker DJ, Aguirre V. Effects of Roux-en-Y gastric bypass on energy and glucose homeostasis are preserved in two mouse models of functional glucagon-like peptide-1 deficiency. *Mol Metab* 2013:3(2):191–201
20. Lim EL, Hollingsworth KG, Aribisala BS, Chen MJ, Mathers JC, Taylor R. Reversal of type 2 diabetes: normalization of beta cell function in association with decreased pancreas and liver triacylglycerol. *Diabetologia* 2011;54(10):2506–2514
21. Lingvay I, Guth E, Islam A, Livingston E. Rapid improvement in diabetes after gastric bypass surgery: is it the diet or surgery? *Diabetes Care* 2013;36(9):2741–2747
22. Mechanick JI, Youdim A, Jones DB, Garvey WT, Hurley DL, et al. Clinical practice guidelines for the perioperative nutritional, metabolic, and nonsurgical support of the bariatric surgery patient – 2013 update: cosponsored by American Association of Clinical Endocrinologists, The Obesity Society, and American Society for Metabolic and Bariatric Surgery. *Obesity* 2013;21(Suppl. 1):S1–S27
23. Datta S, Qaadir A, Villaneuva G, Baldwin D. Once-daily insulin glargine versus 6-hour sliding scale regular insulin for control of hyperglycemia after a bariatric surgical procedure: a randomized clinical trial. *Endocr Pract* 2007;13(3):225–231

Chapter 19

Emergency Department Management of Diabetes Patients with Non-crisis Hyperglycemia

Michelle F. Magee, MD,[1] Carine M. Nassar, MS, RD, CDE,[2] John J. Reyes-Castano, MD,[3] and Marie E. McDonnell, MD[4]

MAKING THE CASE FOR PROACTIVE DIABETES MANAGEMENT IN THE EMERGENCY DEPARTMENT

Annually in the U.S., adults over 18 years of age with diabetes accrue over 12 million visits to hospital emergency departments (EDs). Although the primary reason for the majority of these visits is not glycemic control, the ED setting presents an opportunity to intervene in and initiate evidence-based care for the patient with either known or previously unrecognized diabetes. Such interventions have the potential to affect both short- and long-term health-related clinical, behavioral, and economic outcomes, including resources utilization, and will be the main focus of this chapter.

The ED is a common setting for the initial diagnosis and management of diabetes. Patients presenting with hyperosmolar hyperglycemic state (HHS) or diabetic ketoacidosis (DKA) will require hospital admission or care in a program designed to manage mild to moderate DKA expediently in the ED or in specially created ED observation units (EDOUs)[1,2] or diabetes treatment units (DTU),[3] and are not the focus of this chapter (see Chapter 22). Patients who present without HHS or DKA usually are not admitted for glycemic management alone and the decision to admit will be based on the acuity of other underlying comorbid conditions. Each of these groups of diabetes patients is at a high risk for recurrent ED visits or hospital admission if not treated and followed-up appropriately. Unfortunately, such repeat acute care encounters are not uncommon because of overburdened health systems in which outpatient follow-up may not occur in a timely fashion or may not occur at all.

Regardless of the precipitating reason for a given ED visit, the ED is well positioned to identify patients with previously unrecognized or previously diagnosed but uncontrolled diabetes based on blood glucose (BG) measures or hemoglobin A_{1c} (HbA_{1c}) levels obtained during the encounter. This setting provides an

[1]Georgetown University School of Medicine, MedStar Washington Hospital Center, MedStar Health Diabetes and Research Institutes, Washington, DC. [2]MedStar Health Diabetes and Research Institutes, Washington, DC. [3]Section of Endocrinology, MedStar Washington Hospital Center and Georgetown University, Washington, DC. [4]Division of Endocrinology, Diabetes and Hypertension, Harvard Medical School, Brigham and Women's Hospital, Boston, MA.

DOI: 10.2337/9781580406086.19

opportunity to initiate evidence-based diabetes care to intervene in the overall management of uncontrolled or previously undiagnosed diabetes. Usual ED care for hyperglycemia coincident to other conditions is variable and may include intravenous (IV) hydration, treatment with rapid-acting insulin, the addition to or adjustment of doses of antihyperglycemic medications, and a recommendation for timely follow-up with primary care. The principles of the Model of the Clinical Practice of Emergency Medicine[4] support a more comprehensive approach, including prescribing antihyperglycemic oral or injectable agents, initiating an effort to address deficits in diabetes self-care management knowledge, providing skills training in the use of a glucose monitor and in self-administration of injectables for pharmacotherapy, and effecting a smooth transition to an appropriate primary medical home. Accomplishing these tasks within the workflow of a busy ED, however, presents challenges.

This chapter provides an overview of strategies for diabetes care delivery and self-management education in the ED and postdischarge. It focuses on the patient who presents for any reason who has uncontrolled hyperglycemia and will be discharged to the outpatient setting.

DIABETES IN THE ED: THE SCOPE OF THE PROBLEM

ED visits among patients with uncontrolled diabetes pose a burden on the U.S. health-care system are an important health quality measure and a national target for cost reduction, and these visits have been shown in some circumstances to be avoidable through specific interventions.[5,6] Fully 12% of ED visits in the U.S. were incurred by patients with diabetes in 2012.[7] Among this population, health resource use was attributed to diabetes itself in 5% of visits, to chronic diabetes complications in 26% of visits, and to general medical conditions in 68% of visits. The cost accrued to the health-care system for these visits was $15.3 million, representing 11.5% of the total $176 billion annual burden in direct medical costs for diabetes. These statistics make diabetes the third most costly chronic disease treated in the ED behind cardiovascular and renal disease.[7] Furthermore, analysis of readmission data suggests that hyperglycemia is rarely the chief complaint or primary diagnosis in the ED, or for the subsequent admission, even if uncontrolled diabetes is the primary condition being treated at that time.[8,9]

Among the 12,128,00 Americans making diabetes-related visits to the ED in 2010, the U.S. Health-Care Cost and Utilization Project demographics data reveal that women made diabetes-related ED visits more commonly than men (55.3% compared with 44.7%). ED visit rates increase by age, being highest among those >65 years (1,307 per 10,000 U.S. population) compared with 45- to 64-year-olds (584 per 10,000) and 18- to 44-year-olds (183 per 10,000), and by income level, being higher among those from the lowest income communities (526 per 10,000 U.S. population) than from the highest income communities (236 per 10,000). Other characteristics correlated with higher rates of diabetes-related ED visits are area of residence, with large metropolitan areas having the highest rates, and region of the country, with rates being markedly higher in the South compared with other regions of the country and lowest in the West.[10]

High rates of ED utilization among patients with diabetes may be attributed to a number of patient and provider variables. Patient-related variables include absence of a primary care provider or lack of same-day access to primary care, deficits in self-care management knowledge and skills, lack of understanding of the principles of diabetes self-management education (DSME), inability to adhere to recommended lifestyle behaviors or medication regimens, lack of access to healthy food and physical activity choices, limited resources to obtain prescribed medications, and the presence of diabetes-related complications.[11] In addition, one study found that individuals with low socioecomonic status often prefer the ED over primary care services because of perceived ease and high value.[12]

A significant portion of diabetes-related ED visits are likely ambulatory-care sensitive and could be prevented with improved access to primary care centers and appropriate DSME.[13] In one report of 86 patients making ED visits to an urban tertiary care ED, 42% stated that the reason for the visit was that they were unable to get a same-day appointment with a primary care provider and another 10% that they were sent to the ED by their primary care provider.[14] A 2012 study conducted in a large, urban, adult ED reported that 28.2% (n = 227) of patients with a history of diabetes denied having a primary care provider. The study also found that patients claiming to have a primary care provider had significantly lower HbA_{1c} levels.[15] Among provider variables contributing to uncontrolled diabetes, however, clinical inertia in advancement of the antihyperglycemic medication regimen remains common.[16,17].

ED OPPORTUNITIES FOR IDENTIFICATION AND MANAGEMENT OF PATIENTS AT RISK OR WITH DIABETES

The ED presents a novel setting for diabetes screening, affording an opportunity to identify patients diabetes, and those with previously unrecognized or suboptimally controlled diabetes. Identification will allow initiation of appropriate lifestyle or medication management and DSME to enable glycemic control, prevent recurrent acute care visits for uncontrolled hyperglycemia, and prevent long-term diabetes complications. Recognition, communication, and management of hyperglycemia in the ED, however, are suboptimal.[18]

Hyperglycemic patients presenting to the ED may have a known diagnosis of diabetes, previously unrecognized diabetes, prediabetes or stress- and illness-related hyperglycemia. On presentation, it may not be clear whether the patient meets the formal diagnostic criteria for diabetes and pre-diabetes. BG levels are commonly obtained during an ED admission and often are relied on in the absence of an HbA_{1c} level. The pragmatic approach shown on Table 19.1 may be useful to guide action to be taken. This approach acknowledges the American Diabetes Association (ADA) classification of diabetes and prediabetes based on BG levels: prediabetes as a fasting BG of 100–125mg/dL or a 2-h post-75-gm oral glucose tolerance test result of >140–199 mg/dL and of diabetes based on a fasting BG of >126 mg/dL or a casual plasma glucose of >200 mg/dL with symptoms of hyperglycemia.[19] Of note, only glucoses measured in the laboratory should be relied on for diagnostic purposes and unless BG is >200 mg/dL and symptoms of

Table 19.1—Pragmatic Approach to Elevated Blood Glucose Levels in the ED*

BG (mg/dL)	Action
126–139 (fasting)	BG not completely normal. Possible diabetes, prediabetes, or stress hyperglycemia. See PCP for follow-up fasting BG within 2 weeks.
140–199 (random)	Probable diagnosis of diabetes, prediabetes, or stress hyperglycemia. See PCP for follow-up BG within 2 weeks or sooner if symptoms of hyperglycemia.
>200	
Without symptoms of hyperglycemia	If modest elevation, likely diagnosis of diabetes. Consider pharmacotherapy based on BG level and clinical picture. Timely follow-up postdischarge with PCP.
With symptoms of hyperglycemia	Inform patient of diagnosis of diabetes. Initiate pharmacotherapy as appropriate per BG level and refer to PCP for follow-up and DSME.

BG, blood glucose; DSME, diabetes self-management education; PCP, primary care provider.
*Use laboratory analyzed glucose values only unless BG is >200mg/dL and symptoms of hyperglycemia are present. Glucose testing for diagnostic classification purposes must be repeated in the ambulatory care setting.
Source: Adapted from Magee and Nassar[20]

hyperglycemia are present. The formal diagnostic criteria for diabetes-glucose testing for diagnostic purposes must be repeated in the ambulatory care setting.

HbA_{1c} testing, when available, also may be used to inform the DM-related diagnosis or may be used in conjunction with the BG level at the time of ED admission to assess the degree of glycemic control during the 2–3 months preceding the ED visit.[20,21] Point-of-care (POC) HbA_{1c} testing used in conjunction with the clinical presentation of the patient and the BG at admission also may be used to inform pharmacotherapy decisions (see the management section). The A1CNow® by PTS system, which uses a 5 mL fingerstick sample and provides a result in 5 min is an option for obtaining an HbA_{1c} level during the ED visit. The upper limit of the A1CNow® assay is 13%.[22] The test is National Glycohemoglobin Standardization Program certified, Clinical Laboratory Improvement Amendments waived, and International Federation of Clinical Chemistry certified.

Once patients are known or suspected to have diabetes by simple screening procedures, appropriate transition and follow-up may not be supported by standard ED processes. A retrospective cohort study of patients with an initial serum glucose >140 mg/dL in the ED of an urban, academic institution examined recognition and management of diabetes, including communication of abnormal BG results. Patients were selected randomly from consecutive ED visits that had at least one serum glucose result charted during a 1-year period. Of the 27,688 initial ED BG results, 13% were in the 140–199 mg/dL range and 8% were >200 mg/dL.

Overall, 107 (55%) of patients with BG 140–199 mg/dL and 31 (16%) patients with BG >200 mg/dL had no prior diabetes-related diagnosis. Only 61 (16%) received insulin in the ED for their hyperglycemia, and hyperglycemia was charted as a diagnosis in only 36 (9%) cases.[18] Inpatient or ED discharge instructions informed just 36 (10%) of these patients of their hyperglycemia and 23 (6%) provided a plan for further evaluation and management. These data indicate that ED patients have a relatively high prevalence of previously undiagnosed diabetes. Additionally, recognition, communication, and management of ED hyperglycemia to establish a diagnosis of DM or pre-DM post-discharge were clearly suboptimal, representing missed opportunities to affect clinical care and outcomes.

RATIONALE, FEASIBILITY, AND STRATEGIES FOR INITIATION OF DELIVERY OF DSME IN THE ED

Although for some patients the ED is the primary point of contact with the health-care system, it has been hypothesized that the ED presents a chaotic environment that may not be conducive to patient education. Compounding the challenge of delivering DSME in the ED, crowding has become a significant problem with the number of ED visits increasing by 26% between 1994 and 2004, despite a decrease in the total number of EDs by 9%.[23] Further arguments against education in the ED include patients' potentially anxious mental state, limited staffing, unpredictable census, and lack of sufficient expertise among the ED staff to provide patient education for the vast array of medical conditions they treat.[25]

Nonetheless, despite the challenges noted for educating patients in the ED, success has been achieved in improving outcomes for other chronic, complex medical conditions, including asthma and heart failure patients.[26–28] Characteristics of these successful programs have included interactive one-on-one teaching as well as follow-up and continued education after the ED encounter.[29] As demonstrated with asthma and heart failure patients, flexibility and customization of patient education materials to address literacy and cultural sensitivities are important given the diversity of the diabetes patient population of the ED.[29]

Survival skills education has been suggested as a short-term approach for teaching the topics essential to ensure a safe discharge from the acute care setting.[30,31] The American Diabetes Association and the Joint Commission for Accreditation of Healthcare Organizations (the Joint Commission) delineate key education content that should be communicated to the patient before discharge from hospital settings to the outpatient setting.[19,32] In a recent report, Lewis et al.[33] evaluated the impact of DSME provided in a large urban ED by a certified diabetes educator (CDE) utilizing a learner-centered approach based on the individual needs, skills, and interests of the patient. Baseline diabetes-related knowledge and skills were assessed in the ED and patients were asked to demonstrate meter and insulin injection techniques. Survival skills education was provided to adults presenting to the ED with uncontrolled type 2 diabetes. Education focused on identified gaps in knowledge and skills and incorporated an opportunity for the patient to exercise control in the treatment process. At a 12–72-h post-ED follow-up outpatient visit, a significant increase in diabetes knowledge test scores was shown. In addition, significantly fewer patients required BG meter reinstruction and none required further insulin injection instruction. The latter findings indicate successful conveyance of survival skills DSME during the ED visit and retention of these self-management skills in the short term following ED discharge. These results provide evidence that supports the effectiveness of learner-centered DSME to impart critical knowledge and skills to patients with diabetes in this setting[33] and supports the importance of using education strategies that are flexible and customized.

Patient attrition is a challenge for DSME programs initiated in any setting. In the Lewis et al. study,[33] although 8 of 51 patients (15.7%) did not return for follow-up education, 43 patients (84%) attended the first short-term post-ED visit follow-up appointment. The authors contend that these results support the importance of initiating the DSME process in the ED and that ED visits offer a timely opportunity to engage the patient in learning recommended diabetes self-care behaviors.[34]

Some have suggested that DSME be delivered only by CDEs. In most institutions, however, these educators may not be readily available after usual daytime work hours. As will be discussed, the surge in EDOUs of the past decade, and development of disease-specific practice EDOU guidelines that include education,[34,35] may alter the landscape of DSME administration in the acute care setting.[36,37] With more time available within a 24–48-h directed short stay, there is theoretically more opportunity to deliver DSME to an individual patient. ED or other hospital-based or ambulatory care center staff (e.g., doctor of pharmacy or nurse practitioner) also could be trained to deliver DSME and prescribe an appropriate discharge diabetes medication regimen. A careful cost analysis would be required to determine whether there is clear benefit to the required staff training in addition to the extended acute-care stay, when compared with a model focused on rapid follow-up for specialty-level education and management.

EVIDENCE AND BEST PRACTICES FOR MANAGEMENT OF UNCONTROLLED DIABETES PRESENTING TO THE ED

ACUTE GLYCEMIC MANAGEMENT IN THE ED

Emergency medicine has become highly protocol and pathway driven. As a result, individual institutions often develop and employ hyperglycemic emergency triage strategies and protocols. Part of this triage procedure involves determining which patients meet the criteria for DKA or HHS, which patients require specific care for severe hypoglycemia, and which patients have noncrisis hyperglycemia, often termed "marked hyperglycemia." As noted, this latter patient category is the focus of this chapter. The mainstay of therapy for hyperglycemia of all degrees of severity is IV fluids administered for the goal of volume resuscitation. Beyond IV fluids in the noncrisis patient, the most important therapy is subcutaneous insulin.

Few studies have evaluated the treatment of hyperglycemia in the ED. In a pilot study, 54 patients with a history of diabetes and glucose >200 mg/dL were treated with insulin aspart dosed by weight every 2 h until BG was <200 mg/dL and were then compared with an historical control group (Figure 19.1). In the intervention group, the mean blood glucose at the end of the ED visit was 158

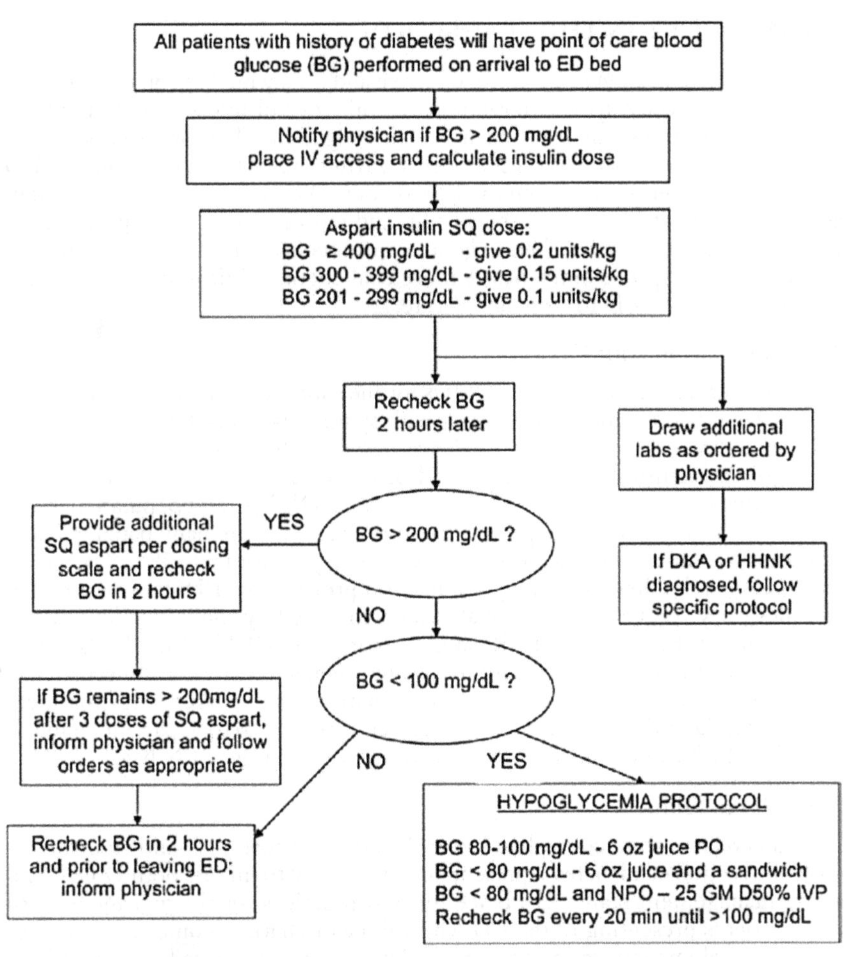

Figure 19.1—Rush emergency department hyperglycemia intervention protocol.

versus 242 mg/dL ($P < 0.001$) among control subjects, of which only 35% received insulin therapy. There was no difference in associated hospitalization rates between groups.[38] In a follow-up randomized control study ($n = 175$), these investigators evaluated the impact of a unique protocol that included rapid initiation of a detemir-aspart insulin protocol for patients who were being admitted to the hospital. The intervention resulted in lower BG levels in the ED without prolonging ED stay or hospital stay and, among hospitalized patients, the intervention patients had better glycemic control measured by patient-day weighted mean BG when compared with controls (163 vs. 202 mg/dL, respectively).[39] These studies support the use of standardized subcutaneous insulin protocols in the ED regardless of planned disposition.

MANAGEMENT IN THE TRANSITION

Methodology to facilitate delivery of effective and timely medication management and DSME for type 2 diabetes targeting glycemic control across acute and chronic care delivery settings is an evolving area of investigation. There are two significant transition points for patients with diabetes leaving the ED, namely, from the ED to the inpatient setting and from the ED to home. As reviewed earlier, few studies address this diabetes "handoff" specifically, and most focus on the hyperglycemic crisis. Data show, however, that, in general, protocolized insulin therapy starting in the ED can improve outcomes. A more challenging clinical scenario is in the transition from the ED to ambulatory care.

The Observation Unit Option

Many hospitals have established EDOUs for the short-term acute management of specific conditions. Patients presenting with symptomatic insulin deficiency provide an opportunity to introduce evidence-based insulin practices using subcutaneous basal insulin in the background of both nutritional and correctional rapid-acting insulins. Protocols applied to the non-DKA patient population, however, were not designed for rapid glucose correction and, in many patients, these protocols may not reliably achieve glucose <180 mg/dL for up to 48 h.[40] It may be more reasonable, then, to employ a transition protocol for EDOU patients that includes early frequent correctional insulin followed by the initiation of basal insulin, such as that used by the Rush University group.[38] The EDOU also presents an opportunity for individualized insulin therapy for specific clinical scenarios, such as the patient receiving corticosteroids experiencing postmeal hyperglycemia or the patient with hyperglycemia related to total parenteral nutrition (TPN) who would benefit from receiving insulin in the TPN bag.

From ED to Home

ED visits related to uncontrolled hyperglycemia in those with known or previously unrecognized diabetes represent an opportunity to initiate both DSME and a care management plan.[41] Evidence for best practices for the management of these patients presenting to the ED who will be discharged home and strategies for their implementation are emerging. Best practice published guidelines[7] for outpatient type 2 diabetes management and medication management algorithms can be used to guide ED discharge diabetes management recommendations. Three major unknowns make it challenging for a provider to select a specific therapeutic approach at the time of discharge from the ED. The first is the potential for limitations in the patient's ability to self-manage the condition and the second is the delay in accessing appropriate disease-focused follow-up once discharged. Both of these factors are known to affect the postdischarge outcome. For the newly identified patient with diabetes, the third unknown is the type of diabetes (type 1 vs. type 2 diabetes or severe progressive insulin deficiency vs. transient insulin deficiency) and the potential urgency for insulin therapy to be started quickly to prevent a subsequent hyperglycemic crisis.

Despite evidence that DSME reduces HbA_{1c}, ED visits, and hospital admissions,[42–44] <55% of all diabetes patients in the U.S. receive any DSME during the course of their illness[45,46] and <7% receive this in the first year of diagnosis.[47]

Survival skills DSME has been introduced to focus teaching on imparting basic knowledge, including meal planning, safe medication administration, blood glucose monitoring, and hypoglycemia treatment along with the skills required to enable safe self-management until further education can be provided.[48]

Antihyperglycemic Medication Management and Transition to Primary Care

Discharge diabetes regimens vary across different ED settings and also between ED practitioners. Initiation of insulin therapy[7] usually is recommended when severe hyperglycemia is present (BG >300 mg/dL) or A1C is >10%. Initiating insulin therapy in the ED, however, can be difficult due to the time and training required to provide appropriate education in insulin self-administration and glucose monitoring. For this reason, many ED physicians rely on the use of oral anti-diabetic medications such as sulfonylureas as the preferred diabetes regimen upon discharge, with little or no attention given to providing DSME.

Few reported studies have specifically assessed short-term outpatient pharmacotherapeutic strategies for type 2 diabetes in patients presenting with BG >200–300 mg/dL. A small number of studies have specifically assessed short-term outpatient pharmacotherapeutic strategies for type 2 diabetes presenting with BG >200–300 mg/dL. Two early reports, although not specific to the ED setting, suggested that maximal doses of a sulfonylurea are safe and effective for such patients and could avoid the need for hospital admission.[49,50] A more recent randomized study found that a sulfonylurea (glipizide XL 10 mg daily) with or without 10 units of insulin glargine (Lantus) daily improved glucose levels in patients with type 2 diabetes who were discharged from the ED. This study provided DSME at the initial ED visit with no drug dose changes allowed after randomization.[51]

The drawback of these general approaches to hyperglycemia in the ED is the lack of individualization for the individual patient and diabetes subtypes. Moreover, evidence is lacking that routine efforts to obtain disease-focused primary care follow-up are effective in preventing ED recidivism and improving clinical outcomes.[52] For example, data suggest that the design of medical home practices likely affects the success of follow-up regardless of whether or not there are open-access clinics.[53] At a hospital in Boston, an analysis of patients who presented to the ED with glucose >300 mg/dL and were subsequently discharged showed that, of those patients who returned to the ED within 30 days, the mean time to primary care follow-up appointment was 26 days.[54]

Rapid Follow-Up to Outpatient Specialty Care

Rapid access to ambulatory specialty care from the ED is an alternative that is being explored. Early results of an Emergency Department Diabetes Rapid-Referral Program (EDRP) indicate feasibility and reduced recidivism. The EDRP is a hospital-funded program designed to determine the cost effectiveness of open-access, direct referral to an outpatient diabetes center within 24 business hours from discharge from an ED visit. During a nonrandomized pilot study of this program, the ED referred 469 subjects to an outpatient diabetes center via direct electronic booking. If patients were sent to the center on the same day as discharge from the ED, 100% came to the visit, but when looking at all referrals including those for subsequent days, the overall show rate was 65%. The 1-year unadjusted hospitalization rate among patients accessing the clinic was approximately half the rate of the no-show group (18% vs. 40%, $P < 0.001$). Patients who arrived at the visit incurred less total health-care costs over 1 year of follow-up despite greater costs accrued to ambulatory care.[54]

This model has the advantage of providing patients with survival skills education without the need to train ED staff or deploy diabetes educators and diabetes care providers to the ED. Additionally, care is individualized by a specialty interdisciplinary team of providers and educators before a patient transitions back to primary care. Not all patients, however, are captured in this model and not all centers have access to such a resource at this time.

Table 19.2*A*—STEP-Diabetes Algorithm for Initiation or Titration of Antihyperglycemic Medications before Discharge from the Emergency Department

<table>
<tr><th colspan="2">No prior antihyperglycemic agent therapy*</th><th rowspan="2">Definitions and diagnostic criteria</th></tr>
<tr><th>BG (mg/dL)</th><th>Action</th></tr>
<tr><td>126–139 (fasting)</td><td>Follow-up BG with MD within 2 weeks. BG is not completely normal. Possible prediabetes or diabetes.</td><td rowspan="3">Prediabetes:
Fasting BG 100–125 mg/dL
2-h 75 gm OGTT >140 mg/dL
Diabetes:
Fasting BG >126 mg/dL (confirmed by repeat testing)
Casual plasma glucose >200 mg/dL with symptoms of hyperglycemia 2-h 75 gm OGTT >200 mg/dL</td></tr>
<tr><td>140–199 (random)</td><td>Follow-up BG with MD within 2 weeks. Sooner if symptoms of hyperglycemia. Probable diagnosis of diabetes or prediabetes.</td></tr>
<tr><td>200–250</td><td>Inform patient of DM diagnosis.
Start metformin 500 mg po bid
OR low-dose sulfonylurea if metformin contraindicated</td></tr>
<tr><td>251–300</td><td colspan="2">Metformin 500 mg po bid PLUS starting dose sulfonylurea (see Table 19.2B, General Principles),
OR basal insulin: glargine (or detemir) 10 units SQ once daily,
OR NPH (or 70/30) 5 units twice daily (with breakfast and dinner).</td></tr>
<tr><td>301–350</td><td colspan="2">Correction dose of rapid-acting insulin analog in ED (see Table 19.2C, Correction Dose Insulin Algorithm)
Basal insulin: glargine (or detemir) 10 units SQ once daily or 0.2 units/kg/day OR NPH (or 70/30) 5 units twice daily, first dose given in ED.</td></tr>
<tr><td>350–400</td><td colspan="2">Correction dose of rapid-acting insulin analog in ED (see Table 19.2C, Correction Dose Insulin Algorithm)
Basal insulin: glargine (or detemir) 0.2 units/kg/day. First dose given in ED.
May use NPH or 70/30, but split dose to bid.</td></tr>
<tr><td>>400</td><td colspan="2">Treat with IV fluids and correction dose of rapid-acting insulin analog (see Table 19.2C). Observe for 2–4 h. If patient responds with a decrease in BG, start basal insulin as noted for BG 350–400.</td></tr>
</table>

continued

Table 19.2A—STEP-Diabetes Algorithm for Initiation or Titration of Antihyperglycemic Medications before Discharge from the Emergency Department *(continued)*

Preexisting diabetes on oral antihyperglycemic agents*				
BG (mg/dL)	**1 agent**			**2–3 oral agents**
	On metformin	**On sulfonylurea**	**On other agent**	
80–139	No change. Follow up with MD.			
140–199	<1,000 mg daily: Titrate dose upward >1,000 mg daily: Add sulfonylurea	Add metformin ***OR*** titrate sulfonylurea dose upward	Add metformin (or sulfonylurea if metformin contraindicated)	Titrate to higher or maximal dose(s).
200–300	Titrate to higher or maximal dose ***AND/OR*** add second agent ***OR*** add basal insulin: glargine (or detemir) 10 units SQ daily. If not already on metformin, add 500 mg po bid.			Basal insulin: glargine (or detemir) 0.2 units/kg/day. If not already on metformin, add 500 mg po bid. Discontinue third agent.
301–400	Correction dose of insulin in ED (see Figure 19.1). Basal insulin: glargine (or Detemir) 0.2 units/kg/day. If not already on metformin, add 500 mg po bid.			
>400	Treat with IV fluids and correction dose of rapid acting insulin analog in ED (see Table 19.2C). Observe for 2–4 h. If patient responds, start basal insulin as noted.			
Preexisting diabetes on insulin (with or without oral agents)*				
BG (mg/dL)	**Action**			
Fasting >120 (morning)	Increase basal dose (daily glargine/detemir or **evening** dose of NPH) by 10%. If patient is on a premixed regimen (70/30), increase predinner dose by 10%.			
Premeal >140 (lunch, dinner)	Increase glargine or detemir dose by 10% ***IF*** **morning** fasting BG is also elevated—***UNLESS*** overnight hypoglycemia is suspected (history of insomnia, night sweats, nightmares), in which case, decrease basal glargine dose by 10–20% Increase **morning** dose of NPH or pre-mix insulin by 10-20% Decrease **evening** doses of NPH or pre-mix ***IF*** **overnight** hypoglycemia suspected or **fasting** hypoglycemia is present			

BG, blood glucose; ED, emergency department; IV, intravenous; MD, medical doctor; OGTT, oral glucose tolerance test; SQ, subcutaneous.
Source: Adapted from ADA and EASD Consensus Statement. *Diabetes Care* 2006;29:1963–1972

Survival Skills DSME Plus Specialty Management Delivered in the ED with Rapid Follow-Up

The ideal follow-up model would incorporate both survival skills DSME and evidence-based medical management in a treatment strategy that could feasibly be delivered in the ED. Magee et al.,[13] reported the results of a pilot study in which patients presenting to the ED with BG >200 mg/dL (11.1 mmol/L) received

Table 19.2*B*—General Principles of Antihyperglycemic Therapy in the Emergency Department

General principles*	Agent	Dosing		Comments
		Start	**Maximum recommended**	
First-line agent	**Metformin** (unless contraindicated)	500 mg twice daily	1,000 mg two times daily	Contraindicated if serum creatinine >1.4 mg/dL (female), >1.5 mg/dL (male), CHF, and/or liver disease. Mild upper-GI discomfort or loose stools usually resolve in 2–3 weeks.
Second- and/or third-line agents	**Sulfonylurea**			
	Glipizide	10 mg daily	40 mg divided	Do not use if sulfa allergy. Decrease dose for chronic kidney disease or elderly patients. Hypoglycemia education. May cause mild GI upset and/or rash.
	Glipizide XL (Glucotrol XL)	5 mg daily in the morning	20 mg daily	
	Glimepiride (Amaryl)	1–2 mg daily	8 mg daily	
	Insulin glargine or detemir	10 units once daily at bedtime or in the morning	Maximum recommended starting dose for ED: 0.2 units/kg/day	Insulin shot instruction and hypoglycemia education.
Other	TZD (Pioglitazone) *not recommended* for initial Rx from the ED as 2–3 weeks to onset of action. **α-Glucosidase inhibitors, meglitinides, DPP-4 inhibitors, GLP-1 analogs** may be considered at follow-up with PCP or endocrinologist.			
Dose titration	If hyperglycemic and already on oral agent(s), increase dose(s) step-wise to upper range of maximum dose(s), as noted.			
Combinations	Add another oral agent with *synergistic action* when previously prescribed agent(s) are at or above half maximum recommended dose. ***Consider Adding Insulin*** when at maximum doses of two oral agents. ***Add Insulin*** when at maximum doses of three oral agents. ***Add Insulin*** if marked (BG >250–300 mg/dL) or symptomatic hyperglycemia.			

continued

Table 19.2*B*—General Principles of Antihyperglycemic Therapy in the Emergency Department *(continued)*

BG, blood glucose, CHF, congestive heart failure; DPP-4, dipeptidyl peptidase-4; ED, emergency department; GI, gastrointestinal; GLP-1, glucagon-like peptide 1; TZD, thiazolidinediones.
*Algorithms and general principles for initiation and management of Type 2 diabetes in nonpregnant adults adapted from ADA and EASD Consensus Statement. *Diabetes Care* 2006; 29:1963–1972. **Type 1 diabetes must always be managed using insulin to avoid DKA.** Dosing recommendations for anti-hyperglycemic agents have been adjusted to assure patient safety after ED discharge. Individual patient dosing requirements will vary. Caution is advised with patients who are elderly, have chronic kidney disease, liver dysfunction, or low body mass. All patients must be provided with diabetes survival skills education and advised to follow-up with their doctor.
Source: Magee et al.[13]

Table 19.2*C*—Correction Dose Insulin Algorithm

Use subcutaneous rapid-acting insulin analog (lispro, aspart, or glulisine) to treat hyperglycemia in the ED; *do not give correction dose insulin more frequently than every 2 h.*

Low dose: <40 units of total insulin/day, weight <70 kg		**Medium dose:** 40–100 units of total insulin/day, weight 70–125 kg		**High dose:** >100 units of total insulin/day, weight >125 kg	
BG (mg/dL)	**Dose**	**BG (mg/dL)**	**Dose**	**BG (mg/dL)**	**Dose**
150–199	1 unit	150–199	1 unit	150–199	2 units
200–249	2 units	200–249	3 units	200–249	4 units
250–299	3 units	250–299	5 units	250–299	7 units
300–349	4 units	300–349	7 units	300–349	10 units
>349	5 units	>349	8 units	>349	12 units

pharmacotherapy for type 2 diabetes using a medication algorithm that took into account presenting BG and use of prior diabetes medications, if any (Tables 19.2*A*, 19.2*B*, and 19.2*C*). Basal insulin therapy was initiated if BG was >300 mg/dL (16.6 mmol/L). Survival skills DSME also was provided (Table 19.3). Significant reductions in BG and HbA_{1c} were observed. No hypoglycemic episodes were reported in the first 24 h following the ED visits, demonstrating preliminary safety of the medication management algorithm and feasibility of initiating the intervention in the ED setting.[13,20]

A subsequent randomized, controlled trial further evaluated the impact of the STEP-Diabetes mellitus care model on glycemic outcomes and medication adherence when initiated in the ED and continued postdischarge. The results demonstrate that ED visits made by adults with uncontrolled type 2 diabetes can clearly be used to initiate a focused intervention providing timely titration of diabetes medications and survival skills DSME. Algorithm-based diabetes medications initiation and titration (Table 19.2), survival skills DSME, and navigation to outpatient services for patients presenting with BG >200 mg were delivered by an endocrinologist-supervised CDE.

Table 19.3—Patient Information Sheet: Diabetes Survival Skills

KNOW YOUR DIABETES NUMBERS:

Target blood glucose for MOST people with diabetes:

- In the morning before eating (fasting) and before meals should be between **80** and **140** mg/dL
- 2 h after eating should be < **180** mg/dL

WHAT BLOOD GLUCOSE IS TOO LOW (also called hypoglycemia)?

- <**70** mg/dL

WHAT BLOOD GLUCOSE IS TOO HIGH (also called hyperglycemia)?

- >**180** mg/dL: Talk to your doctor at the next visit
- >**300** mg/dL for two or more readings over 12–24 h: Call your doctor at his/her office
- >**500** mg/dL, "HI" or "HHH" on your meter: Call your doctor right away or go to the emergency room

WHEN TO CHECK YOUR BLOOD GLUCOSE:

- Always check: Every day when you wake up in the morning, and at least one more time during the day.
- If you take pills for your diabetes: check before breakfast and 2 h after your biggest meal of the day, usually this will be 2 h after dinner.
- If you take insulin for your diabetes: check before each meal and bedtime.
- Your doctor may ask you to check your blood glucose at other times as well.
- Check ***any*** time you feel like your blood glucose might be too high or too low.

HOW DO YOU FEEL IF YOUR BLOOD GLUCOSE IS LOW (hypoglycemia)?

- Sweaty
- Shaky
- Fast heartbeat
- Dizzy
- Headache
- Not thinking clearly
- Hungry
- Tired
- Blurry vision
- Confused
- Moody or angry

HOW TO TREAT LOW BLOOD GLUCOSE (hypoglycemia):

- **First**, drink or eat 15 g of easy-to-swallow carbohydrate, such as the following:
  - ½ cup of juice
  - ½ cup of regular (*not* diet) soda
  - 1 cup of milk (skim is best)
  - 1 tablespoon of honey or sugar
  - 1 small tube of gel mate cake frosting
- Then, test your blood sugar
- Test your blood sugar *again* in 15 min
  - If sugar is not >70 mg/dL, drink or eat another 15 g of carbohydrate
- Eat some protein and carbohydrate as soon as you can to stop from going low again. Try eating:
  - Half of a sandwich (with meat, cheese, or peanut butter)
  - Your next meal or the meal you missed

continued

Table 19.3—Patient Information Sheet: Diabetes Survival Skills *(continued)*

HOW DO YOU FEEL IF YOUR GLUCOSE IS HIGH (hyperglycemia)?

- Increased urination
- Increased thirst
- Tired
- Blurred vision
- Dry skin/dry mouth

WHAT TO DO IF YOU THINK YOU HAVE HIGH BLOOD GLUCOSE:

- Check your blood glucose as soon as you can

EATING: WHAT TO DO UNTIL YOU GET A MEAL PLAN OR SEE A REGISTERED DIETITIAN NUTRITIONIST (RD or RDN):

Here are some tips to help keep your blood glucose under control before you learn more meal planning for diabetes.*

- Eat three meals a day
- Eat your main meals 4–5 h apart
- Do not skip meals
- Eat less food overall
- Do not eat second servings
- Do not snack between meals
- Do not drink fruit juice, regular sodas, or sweet tea
- Instead, drink calorie-free liquids such as diet soda, Crystal Light, crystal unsweetened tea, coffee or water
- Stay away from foods that are nutrient sparse and refined or processed carbohydrates, such as cake, pie, doughnuts, sweetened cereal, honey, jam, and jelly
- Limit addition of caloric sweeteners to your foods
- Consider using nonnutritive sweeteners; use sugar substitutes like Equal, Sweet 'n Low, Splenda, or Stevia instead

WHEN TO CALL YOUR DOCTOR OR GO TO THE EMERGENCY ROOM:

- Blood glucose is >300 mg/dL two or more times over 12–24 h
- More than two low blood glucose readings (<70 mg/dL) in 1 day
- Vomiting or diarrhea for more than 6 h
- Moderate or large urine ketones (if you have type 1 diabetes)
- Other medical problem that requires immediate attention

*The tips presented are framed as survival skills nutrition education content for adults with uncontrolled type 2 diabetes, as utilized in a study by Magee et al.[13] The 2014 ADA Nutrition therapy recommendations for the management of adults with diabetes contains guidance on nutrition strategies for all people with diabetes.[59]

Source: Magee et al.[13]

Glycemic outcomes (BGs and HbA_{1c}) and medication adherence improved. Hypoglycemia rates, the main safety outcome, were low overall and no severe hypoglycemia was reported. Basal insulin was dosed conservatively at a starting dose of 0.2 units/kg/day to minimize the possibility of post-ED discharge hypoglycemia, a key concern of the ED physicians. Among the participants started on insulin, it was commonly necessary to increase the dose of basal insulin during follow-up to enable further improvement in glycemic control. These data provide further evidence that once-daily basal insulin can be started safely at low doses in the ED.

DSME including diabetes survival skills allows patients to make informed decisions regarding their diabetes care on a daily basis, offering the possibility of better overall control.[7,55] A CDE can successfully deliver the intervention DSME, algorithm-driven diabetes medications management, and navigation to primary care. Evidence that medication management by trained nurse case managers and pharmacists can improve glycemic management outcomes has been reported.[56–58] The STEP-Diabetes study has generated evidence that ED visits made by adults with uncontrolled type 2 diabetes can be used to initiate a focused intervention providing timely titration of antihyperglycemic medications and survival skills DSME. The intervention improved medication adherence and short-term glycemic outcomes, without increasing risk for hypoglycemia. This study provided evidence that a trained, endocrinologist-supervised CDE can safely and effectively make diabetes medication adjustments using a guideline-based algorithm (Table 19.1) in a structured program, thus interrupting prior clinical inertia in the advancement of diabetes medications, significantly improving glycemic outcomes. In the absence of standardized guidelines, however, diabetic discharge medications will continue to vary depending on the ED physician and the ED setting.

CONCLUSION

Specific care strategies for the patient with noncrisis hyperglycemia presenting to the ED has substantial potential to affect clinical outcomes in the short and long term. Best practices for management of the markedly hyperglycemic patient presenting to the ED and strategies for their implementation are beginning to emerge. A small number of studies have specifically assessed short-term outpatient pharmacotherapeutic strategies for patients with type 2 diabetes presenting with BG >200 mg/dL. Early outcomes from clinical programs that deliver timely survival skills DSME during or directly following ED visits indicate improved glycemic control and reduced expenditures in the weeks to months following the index encounter. More controlled studies are needed in this area to determine the cost effectiveness of different strategies in the short and long term.

REFERENCES

1. Benaiges D, Chillarón JJ, Carrera MJ, et al. Efficacy of treatment for hyperglycemic crisis in elderly diabetic patients in a day hospital. *Clin Interv Aging* 2014;9:843–9. doi: 10.2147/CIA.S60581.eCollection 2014. PubMed PMID: 24868152; PubMed Central PMCID: PMC4027922

2. Chojnicki M, Koen M, Hamdy O. Treatment of mild DKA in the emergency department. EVADE protocol. OR:F11C Presented at American Association of Diabetes Educators (AADE), August 8, 2014, Orange County, CA

3. Maldonado MR, D'Amico S, Rodriguez L, Iyer D, Balasubramanyam A. Improved outcomes in indigent patients with ketosis-prone diabetes: effect of a dedicated diabetes treatment unit. *Endocr Pract* 2003;9(1):26–32. PubMed PMID: 12917089

4. ABEM, ACEP, CORD, EMRA, RRC-EM, SAEM. Model of the clinical practice of emergency medicine, 2013. Available from http://www.acep.org/uploadedFiles/ACEP/Practice_Resources/policy_statements/2013%20EM%20Model%20-%20Website%20Document(1).pdf. Accessed 19 December 2015

5. Mitchell SE, Gardiner PM, Sadikova E, Martin JM, Jack BW, Hibbard JH, Paasche-Orlow MK. Patient activation and 30-day post-discharge hospital utilization. *J Gen Intern Med* 2014;29(2):349–55. doi:10.1007/s11606-013-2647-2. Epub 2013 Oct 4. PubMed PMID: 24091935

6. Hansen LO, Young RS, Hinami K, Leung A, Williams MV. Interventions to reduce 30-day rehospitalization: a systematic review. *Ann Intern Med* 2011;155(8):520–528. doi: 10.7326/0003-4819-155-8-201110180-00008. Review

7. American Diabetes Association. Economic costs of diabetes in the U.S. in 2012. *Diabetes Care* 2013;36(4):1033–1046

8. Pennsylvania Health Care Cost Containment Council, April 2012. Available from http://hcupnet.ahrq.gov/HCUPnet.jsp. Accessed 4 March 2015

9. Rubin DJ, Donnell-Jackson K, Jhingan R, Golden SH, Paranjape A. Early readmission among patients with diabetes: a qualitative assessment of contributing factors. *J Diabetes Complications* 2014;28(6):869–873. PubMed PMID: 25087192

10. Washington RE, Andrews RM, Mutter R. Emergency department visits for adults with diabetes, 2010. Statistical Brief No. 167, Healthcare Cost and Utilization Project HCUP, November 2013. Available from https://www.hcup-us.ahrq.gov/reports/statbriefs/sb167.jsp. Accessed 24 March 2015

11. Rubin DJ. Hospital readmission of patients with diabetes. *Curr Diab Rep* 2015;15(4):584. doi: 10.1007/s11892-015-0584-7. PubMed PMID: 25712258

12. Kangovi S, et al. Understanding why patients of low socioeconomic status prefer hospitals over ambulatory care. *Health Aff (Millwood)* 2013;32(7):1196–1920

13. Magee MF, Nassar CM, Copeland J, Fokar A, Sharrets JM, Dubin JS, Smith MS. Synergy to reduce emergency department visits for uncontrolled hyperglycemia. *Diabetes Educ* 2013;39:354–364

14. Weinick RM, Burns RM, Mehrotra A. Many emergency department visits could be managed at urgent care centers and retail clinics. *Health Aff* 2010;29:1630–1636

15. Horwitz DA, Schwarz ES, Scott MG, Lewis LM. Emergency department patients with diabetes have better glycemic control when they have identifiable primary care providers. *Acad Emerg Med* 2012;19(6):650–655

16. Shah BR, Hux JE, Laupacis A, et al. Clinical inertia in response to inadequate glycemic control: do specialists differ from primary care physicians? *Diabetes Care* 2005;28:600–606

17. Griffith M, Boord J, Eden S, et al. Clinical inertia of discharge planning among patients with poorly controlled diabetes mellitus. *J Clin Endocrinol Metab* 2012;97:2019–2026

18. Ginde AA, Savaser DJ, Camargo CA, Jr. Limited communication and management of emergency department hyperglycemia in hospitalized patients. *J Hosp Med* 2009;4(1):45–49

19. American Diabetes Association. Standards of medical care in diabetes–2015. *Diabetes Care* 2015;38(Suppl. 1):S4–S85

20. Magee MF, Nassar C. Hemoglobin A1C testing in an emergency department. *J Diabetes Sci Technol* 2011;5:1437–1443

21. Ginde A, Cagliero E, Nathan D, Camargo CA. Point-of-care glucose and hemoglobin A1C in emergency department patients without known diabetes: implications for opportunistic screening. *Acad Emerg Med* 2008;15:1241–1247

22. A1CNow®+ System. PTS Diagnostics. Available from http://www.ptsdiagnostics.com/a1cnow.html. Accessed 7 April 2015

23. Kellermann AL. Crisis in the emergency department. *N Engl J Med* 2006;355(13):1300–1303

24. Wei HG, Camargo CA. Patient education in the emergency department. *Acad Emerg Med* 2000;7(6):710–717

25. Mainous AG, Koopman RJ, Gill JM, Baker R, Pearson WS. Relationship between continuity of care and diabetes control: evidence from the Third National Health and Nutrition Examination Survey. *Am J Public Health* 2004;94(1):66–70

26. Kelso TM, Self TH, Rumbak MJ, Stephens MA, GarrettW AK. Educational and long-term therapeutic intervention in the ED: effect on outcomes in adult indigent minority asthmatics. *Am J Emerg Med* 1995;13:632–637

27. Emond SD, Reed CR, Graff LG IV, Clark S, Camargo CA Jr. Asthma education in the emergency department. *Ann Emerg Med* 2000; 36:204-211

28. Rich MW, Beckham V, Wittenberg C, Leven CL, Freedland KE, Carney RM. A multidisciplinary intervention to prevent the readmission of elderly patients with congestive heart failure. *N Engl J Med* 1995;333:1190–1195

29. Wei HG, Camargo CA. Patient education in the emergency department. *Acad Emerg Med* 2000;7(6):710–717

30. Nettles AT. Patient education in the hospital. *Diabetes Spectr* 2005;18:44–48

31. Magee MF, Khan NH, Desale S, Nassar CM. Diabetes to go: knowledge- and competency-based hospital survival skills diabetes education program improves postdischarge medication adherence. *Diabetes Educ* 2014;40:344–350

32. Joint Commission. Advanced certification in inpatient diabetes. Available from http://www.jointcommission.org/certification/inpatient_diabetes.aspx. Accessed 8 April 2013

33. Lewis VR, Benda N, Nassar C, Magee M. Successful patient diabetes education in the emergency department. *Diabetes Educ* 2015 [Epub ahead of print]. Available from http://tde.sagepub.com/cgi/reprint/0145721715577484v1.pdf?ijkey=xapX4xXDdewbIyz&keytype=finite. Accessed 25 March 2015

34. Gucciardi E, DeMelo M, Offenheim A, Grace SL, Stewart DE. Patient factors associated with attrition from a self-management education programme. *BMC Health Serv Res* 2008;8:33

35. Peacock F, Beckley P, et al. Recommendations for the evaluation and management of observation services: a consensus white paper: the Society of Cardiovascular Patient Care. *Crit Pathway Cardiol* 2014;13(4):163–198

36. Wiler JL, Ginde AA. 440: National study of emergency department observation services. *Ann Emerg Med* 2010;56(3):S142

37. Carpentier F, Guignier M, Eytan VL. Short emergency hospitalization. *Therapie* 2001;56:151

38. Munoz C, Villanueva G, Fogg L, Johnson T, Hannold K, Agruss J, Baldwin D. Impact of a subcutaneous insulin protocol in the emergency department: Rush Emergency Department Hyperglycemia Intervention (REDHI). *J Emerg Med* 2011;40(5):493–498. doi: 10.1016/j.jemermed.2008.03.017. Epub 2008 Oct 1. PubMed PMID: 18829205

39. Bernard JB, Munoz C, Harper J, Muriello M, Rico E, Baldwin D. Treatment of inpatient hyperglycemia beginning in the emergency department: a randomized trial using insulins aspart and detemir compared with usual care. *J Hosp Med* 2011;6(5):279–284. doi: 10.1002/jhm.866. PubMed PMID: 21661100

40. Umpierrez GE, Smiley D, Zisman A, Prieto LM, Palacio A, Ceron M, Puig A, MejiaR. Randomized study of basal-bolus insulin therapy in the inpatient management of patients with type 2 diabetes (RABBIT 2 trial). *Diabetes Care* [Epub 2007 May 18] 2007;30(9):2181–2186

41. Charfen MA, Ipp E, Kaji AH, Saleh T, Qazi MF, Lewis RJ. Detection of undiagnosed diabetes and prediabetic states in high-risk emergency department patients. *Acad Emerg Med* 2009;16:394–402

42. Norris S, Lau J, Smith SJ, Schmid CH, Engelgau MM. Self-management education for adults with type 2 diabetes. *Diabetes Care* 2002;25:1159–1171

43. Mühlhauser I, Bruckner I, Berger M, Cheţa D, Jörgens V, Ionescu-Tîrgovişte C, Scholz V, Mincu I. Evaluation of an intensified insulin treatment and teaching programme as routine management of type 1 (insulin-dependent) diabetes. The Bucharest-Düsseldorf Study. *Diabetologia* 1987;30:681–690

44. Boren S, Fitzner K, Panhalkar P, Specker J. Costs and benefits associated with diabetes education: a review of the literature. *Diabetes Educ* 2009;35;72–96

45. American Association of Diabetes Educators. Diabetes education fact sheet. Available from https://www.diabeteseducator.org/export/sites/aade/resources/pdf/research/DiabetesEducationFact_Sheet09-10.pdf. Accessed 19 December 2015

46. Ali MK. Achievement of goals in U.S. diabetes care, 1999–2010. *N Engl J Med* 2013;368:1613–1624

47. Li R, Shrestha SS, Lipman R, Burrows NR, Kolb LE, Rutledge S, Centers for Disease Control and Prevention (CDC). Diabetes self-management education and training among privately insured persons with newly diagnosed diabetes—United States, 2011–2012. *Morb Mortal Wkly Rep* 2014;63(46): 1045–1049. PubMed PMID: 25412060

48. AADE Position Statement. Diabetes inpatient management. *Diabetes Educ* 2012;38:142–146

49. Davidson MB. Successful treatment of markedly symptomatic patients with type II diabetes mellitus using high doses of sulfonylurea agents. *W J Med* 1992;157:199–200

50. Peters AJ, Davidson MB. Maximal dose glyburide therapy in markedly symptomatic patients with type 2 diabetes: a new use for an old friend. *J Clin Endocrinol Metab* 1996;81:2423–2427

51. Babu A, Mehta A, Guerrero P, et al. Safe and simple emergency department discharge therapy for patients with type 2 diabetes mellitus and severe hyperglycemia. *Endocr Pract* 2009;15(7):696–704

52. Weinberger M, Oddone EZ, Henderson WG. Does increased access to primary care reduce hospital readmissions? Veterans Affairs Cooperative Study Group on Primary Care and Hospital Readmission. *N Engl J Med* 1996;334(22):1441–1447. PubMed PMID: 8618584

53. Bojadzievski T, Gabbay RA. *Diabetes Care* 2011;34(4):1047–1053

54. McDonnell M, Palermo, N, et al. Direct access to acute diabetes clinic reduces hospitalizations and cost at one year. ADA Meeting, Boston, MA 2014;63:A23

55. Haas L, Maryniuk M, Beck J, Cox C, Duker P, Edwards L, Fisher EB, Hanson L, Kent D, Kolb L, Mclaughlin S, Orzeck E, Piette JD, Rhinehart AS, Rothman R, Sklaroff S, Tomky D, Youssef G. National standards for diabetes self-management education and support. *Diabetes Care* 2013;36(Suppl. 1):S100–S108

56. Fanning EL, Selwyn BJ, Larme AC, DeFronzo RA. Improving efficacy of diabetes management using treatment algorithms in a mainly Hispanic population. *Diabetes Care* 2004;27:1638–1646

57. Davidson MB, Ansari A, Karlan VJ. Effect of a nurse-directed diabetes disease management program on urgent care/emergency room visits and hospitalizations in a minority population. *Diabetes Care* 2007;30:224–227

58. Cranor CW, Bunting BA, Christensen DB. The Asheville project: long term clinical and economic outcomes of a community pharmacy diabetes care program. *J Am Pharm Assoc* 2003;43:173–184

59. Evert AB, Boucher JL, Cypress M, Dunbar SA, Franz MJ, Mayer-Davis EJ, Neumiller JJ, Nwankwo R, Verdi CL, Urbanski P, Yancy WS, Jr. Nutrition therapy recommendations for the management of adults with diabetes. *Diabetes Care* 2014;37(Suppl. 1):S120–S143. doi: 10.2337/dc14-S120

Chapter 20

Diabetic Gastroparesis: Update with Emphasis on Inpatient Management

Jorge Calles-Escandón, MD,[1] Kenneth L. Koch, MD,[2] Boris Draznin, MD, PhD,[3] and Andjela Drincic, MD[4]

INTRODUCTION

When gastroparesis (GP) afflicts patients with type 1 diabetes (T1D) or type 2 diabetes (T2D), the consequences are particularly severe. Symptoms associated with GP such as early satiety, prolonged fullness, nausea, and vomiting of undigested food not only reduce the quality of life but also compound difficulties in controlling blood glucose levels.

GP is defined as a delay in the empting of ingested food in the absence of mechanical obstruction of the stomach or duodenum.[1] In patients with diabetes complicated by GP, ingested food is not emptied in a predictable time period; thus, the anticipated nutrient absorption is unpredictable. Consequently, the selected dose and timing of insulin therapy to control postprandial glucose may be inappropriate.

In many patients with GP, erratic postprandial glucose levels result in swings from hypoglycemia to severe hyperglycemia and even ketoacidosis.[2] Hyperglycemia itself elicits gastric dysrhythmias and slows gastric emptying.[3,4] Patients with GP frequently are seen in emergency rooms for low glucose, severe hyperglycemia, or ketoacidosis.

EPIDEMIOLOGY

The estimates of prevalence of GP in DM vary widely. Although in tertiary centers, up to 40% of patients with T1D are reported to have GP, surveys in Olmsted County, Minnesota, indicated a prevalence of 5% in T1D and 1% in T2D.[5] Our own data from an analysis of more than 40 million medical records is much closer to the Olmsted County estimate supporting a prevalence of GP in diabetes of <5%.[6] Thus, GP in diabetes is not so common, but it has a large negative impact

[1]Professor of Internal Medicine, Chief, Section on Endocrinology, MetroHealth Regional, Case Western Reserve University School of Medicine, Cleveland, OH. [2]Professor of Internal Medicine, Chief, Section on Gastroenterology, Wake Forest School of Medicine, Winston-Salem, NC. [3]The Celeste and Jack Grynberg Professor of Medicine, Director, Adult Diabetes Program, University of Colorado Anschutz Medical Canpus, Aurora, CO. [4]Associate Professor of Medicine, Division of Diabetes, Endocrinology and Metabolism, Medical Director, The Nebraska Medical Center Diabetes Center, Omaha, NE.

DOI: 10.2337/9781580406086.20

on the lifestyle of patients and intensively increases the use of hospital resources by these patients. Although good control of glycemia prevents or delays many of the chronic complications of T1D,[7] the effect of good glucose control on the onset or progression of GP in DM is unknown. Compared with T2D, T1D patients with GP are younger, thinner, and tend to have more severe delays in gastric emptying.[8] Obesity in patients with T2D is a risk factor for GP.[9] Mortality is increased in patients with diabetes when they develop GP and usually is related to cardiovascular events.

NORMAL POSTPRANDIAL GASTRIC NEUROMUSCULAR ACTIVITY

The normal stomach performs a series of complex neuromuscular activities in response to the ingestion of solid foods.[10] First, the fundus relaxes to accommodate the volume of ingested food (Figure 20.1). Normal fundic relaxation requires an intact vagus nerve and is mediated by enteric neurons containing nitric oxide.

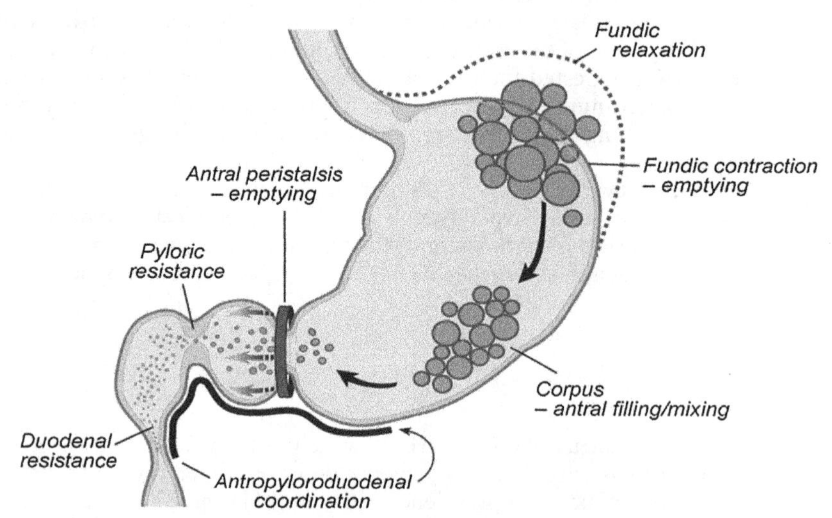

Figure 20.1—Gastric neuromuscular responses to the ingestion of solid food. The fundus, corpus, antrum, pylorus, and duodenum are shown. The fundus relaxes to accommodate the ingested solid food. The fundus presses the food into the corpus-antrum, the "mixing chambers" of the stomach. Recurrent peristaltic waves triturate the solids into 1- to 2-mm particles (termed chyme), which are emptied from the antrum through the pylorus into the duodenum. The sequence requires antral-pyloro-duodenal coordination.

Source: Modified from Koch.[8]

The relaxation of the fundus allows food to be accommodated without excess stretch on the fundic walls.

Second, the corpus and antrum produce recurrent peristaltic waves that mix or triturate the ingested solids into fine particles termed chyme.

Third, emptying of chyme into the duodenum begins when the ingested solid foods are sufficiently triturated. The peristaltic waves empty aliquots of chyme through the pylorus into the duodenum (Figure 20.1). In the normal condition, the number of calories emptied per minute is consistent at about 5 calories/min in humans.[11] The emptying of food from the stomach is altered by the nature of the constituents (carbohydrate, protein, and fat) and the fiber and indigestible components. Carbohydrates are emptied faster than proteins, which are emptied faster than fats and fiber.[12] Finally, normal postprandial neuromuscular activity is associated with a sense of comfortable fullness. In contrast, in patients with diabetes with GP, the ingestion of food elicits early satiety, nausea, and epigastric discomfort or pain.

PATHOPHYSIOLOGY OF DIABETIC GASTROPARESIS

Full-thickness biopsies of the gastric corpus from patients with T1D and T2D and GP indicate the disease is primarily a disease of gastric enteric neurons and interstitial cells of Cajal (ICC).[13,14] Interestingly, these neurons are surrounded by an immune infiltrate composed primarily of type 2 macrophages, suggesting a role for the immune system. The pathophysiological alterations in stomach function in GP include the following:

- **Abnormal fundic relaxation** (Figure 20.2).[15] Due to dysfunction of the ICCs, which also are stretch receptors.[16]
- **Poor contractility and gastric dysrhythmias of the corpus-antrum.** The depletion of ICCs and presence of abnormal enteric neurons are the mechanisms of gastric neuromuscular dysfunction associated with the presence of gastric dysrhythmias and loss of the normal myoelectrical rhythm.[17,18]
- **Abnormal pyloric relaxation.** The pyloric sphincter also regulates gastric emptying. Relaxation of the pyloric sphincter to allow flow is mediated by nitric oxide released from enteric neurons. In a subset of patients with diabetic GP, pylorospasm (failure of pyloric relaxation in coordination with antral peristaltic waves) results in GP.[19,20]

CLINICAL PRESENTATION

Symptoms associated with diabetic GP are early satiety, prolonged fullness, bloating, nausea and vomiting, and abdominal discomfort and pain. These are nonspecific symptoms. Approximately 20% of patients develop these symptoms acutely. Nausea is the most bothersome and predominant symptom in patients with diabetes with GP. Vomitus frequently contains previously ingested and nondigested food. Prolonged stomach fullness and vague epigastric discomfort are common. Symptoms are similar in patients with T1D and T2D, although T2D patients tend

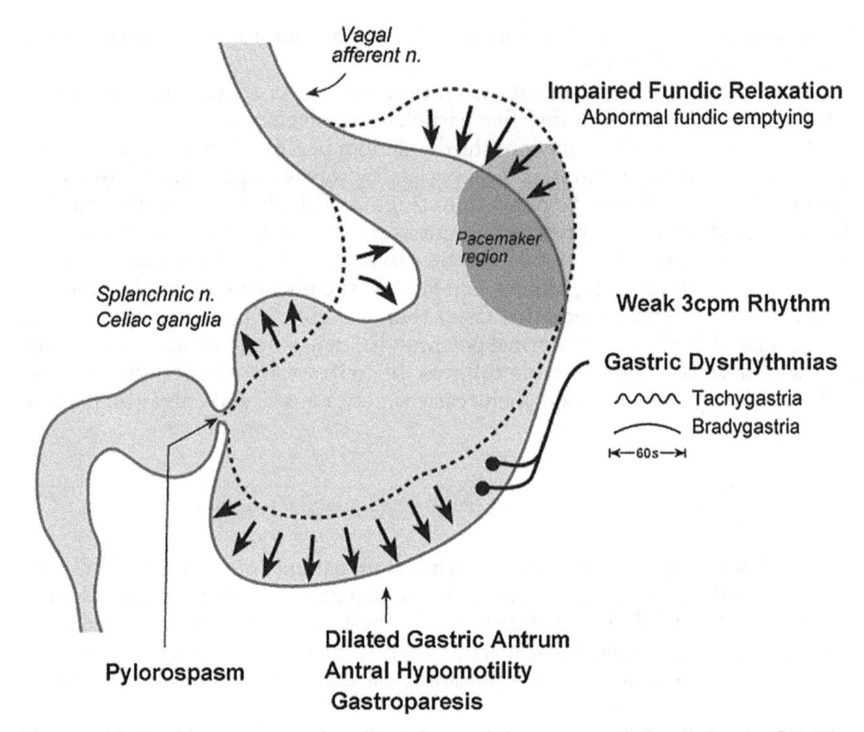

Figure 20.2—Neuromuscular disorders of the stomach in diabetic GP. The fundus fails to relax normally to accommodate food. The gastric electrical rhythm is abnormal because of the loss of ICCs, resulting in weak or absent 3 cpm activity and tachygastria and bradygastria. The antrum may dilate and antral contractions are weak and uncoordinated, all of which leads to delayed gastric emptying. In a subset of patients with GP, 3 cpm myoelectrical activity is present, but GP occurs because of pyloric dysfunction. Abnormalities of vagal afferent nerve or splanchnic nerve innervation may also be present in patients with diabetic GP.

Source: Modified from Koch.[9]

to have more fullness and bloating. In a minority of patients (20%) with GP, abdominal pain is the predominant symptom.[21] Physical examination may be normal or reveal obesity or undernutrition, retinopathy, neuropathy, or signs of vitamin deficiency (cheilosis). Abdominal exam may reveal distention and a succession splash.

Standard laboratory studies are usually normal. Hemoglobin (Hb)A_{1c} levels vary. Thyroid-stimulating hormone (TSH) levels and fasting cortisol should be measured to screen for Addison's disease and hypothyroidism. Vitamin D levels are frequently low.

The symptoms of GP display periods of quiescence interrupted by periods of severe nausea and vomiting; the intensity of the latter is frequently a reason to visit emergency rooms or be interned in hospital. Patients may lose large amounts of fluid, which leads to dehydration, hypovolemia, and alterations in serum electrolytes as well as to pH imbalance because of loss of hydrogen chloride (HCl), and volume contraction sometimes combined with full-blown diabetic ketoacidosis (DKA).

TESTS FOR GASTROPARESIS

The clinical standard test to confirm GP is nuclear medicine gastric scintigraphy following a standardized solid meal followed by 1-min sampling at each hour for a total of 4 h.[22] An upper endoscopy to rule out esophagitis, peptic ulcer disease, or mechanical obstruction may be indicated. Before ordering a gastric emptying test, it is important to stop medications that can induce a delay in gastric emptying for at least 48 h. Those include narcotics, anticholinergic agents, glucagon-like peptide 1 (GLP-1) analogs, and amylin analogs. Also controlling hyperglycemia before and during testing is important as markedly elevated blood glucose levels may delay gastric emptying further. Thus, the preferred gastric emptying test, which consists of a 257 kcal Eggbeaters® sandwich, usually is not tolerated while the patient is the hospital. The gastric emptying and electrogastrography tests are better tolerated after discharge or when the patient is able to comfortably ingest Step 3 of the GP diet described in Table 20.1. An emerging technology is the Wireless Capsule Motility Test, which measures intraluminal pH. The capsule is swallowed during ingestion of a nutrient bar; no further food intake is allowed for 5 h. A sudden change from a low pH (acid) to a neutral or alkaline pH indicates exit of the capsule from stomach into duodenum. If the capsule does not empty from the stomach into the duodenum in 5 h, then delayed gastric emptying is confirmed.

Consulting a gastroenterologist to assist in the diagnosis and hospital management of suspected or confirmed GP should be considered. For instance, GP can be associated with gastroesophageal reflux disease in many patients. Also, an increased risk of bacterial overgrowth of the small intestine has been reported, which requires a targeted therapy.[23]

TREATMENT OF THE PATIENT WITH DIABETES AND GASTROPARESIS IN A HOSPITAL SETTING

The main reasons for patients with DM and GP to be hospitalized are as follows:

1. Acute exacerbations of GP symptoms (nausea, vomiting, pain) leading into dehydration, hypovolemia, and rarely into vascular collapse.
2. Hyperglycemic crisis, usually ketoacidosis, the symptoms of which resemble closely those of acute exacerbation of GP.
3. Severe hypoglycemia.
4. More commonly, a combination of 1 and 2 or 1 and 3.

Table 20.1—Diet for Nausea and Vomiting in Patients with Diabetic Gastroparesis

Diet	Goal	Avoid
Step 1: Sports drinks and bouillon		
For severe nausea and vomiting: Small volumes of salty liquids, with some caloric content to avoid volume depletion Chewable multiple vitamin each day	1000–1500 mL/day in multiple servings (e.g., twelve 120-mL servings over 12–14 h) Patient can sip 30–60 mL at a time to reach approximately 120 mL/h	Citrus drinks of all kinds; highly sweetened drinks
Step 2: Soups and smoothies		
If Step 1 is tolerated: Soup with noodles or rice and crackers Smoothies with low-fat dairy Peanut butter, cheese, and crackers in small amounts Caramels or other chewy confections Ingest above foods in at least six small-volume meals/day Chewable multiple vitamin each day	Approximately 1500 calories/day to avoid volume depletion and maintain weight (often more realistic than weight gain)	Creamy, milk-based liquids
Step 3: Starches, chicken, and fish		
If Step 2 is tolerated: Noodles, pastas, potatoes (mashed or baked), rice, baked chicken breast, fish (all easily mixed and emptied by the stomach) Ingest solids in at least six small-volume meals/day Chewable multiple vitamin each day	Common foods that patient finds interesting and satisfying and that provoke minimal nausea/vomiting symptoms	Fatty foods that delay gastric emptying; red meats and fresh vegetables that require considerable trituration; pulpy fibrous foods that promote formation of bezoars

There has been no clinical trial to define the best treatment approaches for inpatient treatment of patients with diabetes and GP. The recommendations that follow derive from the experience of the authors of this chapter and impute a great amount from the model that has been generated in the GLUMIT (Glucose Monitoring and Insulin Pump Therapy) study, which was mainly an outpatient program.[24]

The initial treatment must focus on restoration of volume status, correction of electrolyte imbalances, and stabilization of glucose with IV insulin drip (in the presence of hyperglycemia or DKA) or dextrose infusion (in the presence of hypoglycemia). Approaches for all of these abnormalities are presented in other chapters of this book. This chapter will focus on the transition from the acute management to management in the general medicine ward, assuming that there is no etiology for these alterations other than the combination of diabetes and GP.

ACUTE NUTRITION MANAGEMENT OF EXACERBATION OF SYMPTOMS ASSOCIATED WITH GASTROPARESIS

After hemodynamic stabilization, patients are transitioned to PO intake using a three-step diet. Step 1 (Table 20.1) is aimed at maintaining hydration with oral fluids. Patients are encouraged to sip small volumes (e.g., 2 ounces every 30–60 min) of liquids containing electrolytes (may be accomplished with commercially available sports drinks) and bouillon-like soup broths throughout the day. The purpose is to restore hydration with salt and water. Nausea and vomiting often improve substantially with hydration, and the patient may then advance to steps 2 and 3 as outlined in Table 20.1.[9]

One of the keys in the American Diabetes Association's recommended medical nutrition therapy for patients with diabetes is an increase in consumption of nutrient-rich food items, such as salads, fresh raw fruits, and fresh raw vegetables.[25] These foods, however, are some of the most difficult foods for the gastroparetic stomach to triturate and empty.

Therefore, nutritious liquids, such as soups or smoothies that require much less gastric neuromuscular work to empty, are advised for patients with GP. Solid foods such as potatoes and pastas require less trituration and are emptied with less gastric neuromuscular work compared with red meats and fibrous foods. Highly fibrous foods, such as fresh oranges, celery, prunes, leeks, and sunflower-seed shells may contribute to the formation of bezoars. Carbohydrates may be limited for the patient with diabetes, but often, it is the soft, starchy carbohydrate foods that are most well tolerated by patients with GP. In addition, meals should be of low fat content because both fat and fiber tend to delay gastric emptying. The three-step diet for patients with GP is a guide to help patients select foods that both limit postprandial gastrointestinal symptoms and maintain hydration and nutrition (Table 20.1).

These nutrition changes require reeducation of the patient with diabetes and GP and their physicians. Consultation by a registered dietitian nutritionist who is knowledgeable in GP is invaluable. The goal is good nutrition and minimal postprandial symptoms while selecting appropriate foods for the severity of GP. Unfortunately, less than 40% of patients with diabetes with GP have had a dietary or nutrition consultation.[25]

GLUCOSE CONTROL IN THE PATIENT WITH DIABETES AND GASTROPARESIS

Glucose control in the patient with diabetic GP can be extremely difficult both in the outpatient and inpatient environments. This difficulty is dictated to a great extent by a bidirectional relationship between glycemia and gastric emptying,[26] whereby hyperglycemia slows further gastric emptying and GP imposes unpredictable swings in glucose excursions.

The rate of gastric emptying of ingested nutrients is influenced by the severity of GP; on a day-to-day basis, gastric emptying is not predictable and eating is compromised by nausea and vomiting. Vomiting reduces absorption of anticipated calories. Liquid nutrients and solid foods may be retained in the stomach much longer than expected by the patient or by the treating physician. Thus, both postprandial hypoglycemia or hyperglycemia are distinctive feature of patients with diabetes and GP resulting from the mismatch of insulin absorption and the slow and frequently erratic entry of food-derived nutrients (Figure 20.3).

Pharmacological Glucose Management

Patients with T1D require insulin replacement as do most (if not all) patients with T2D and GP. We do not recommend use of oral agents or noninsulin injectable medications (pramlintide, GLP analogues) for management of glycemia in patients with T2D and GP. First, because of GP, oral medications[27] may not empty from the stomach for hours, resulting in erratic pharmacokinetics and pharmocodynamics. The sulfonylureas are associated with protracted hypoglycemia in these patients. The GLP-1 incretin mimetics slow stomach peristalsis and are associated with nausea and vomiting themselves and hence are not recommended.[28] Although dipeptidyl peptidase-4 (DPP-4) inhibitors do not have much effect on slowing gastric emptying,[29] their efficacy depends on good insulin reserve, and most patients with T2D and GP have a longer duration of diabetes and likely have severely decreased capacity to secrete insulin. In addition to the latter, no clinical trials have been published on the possible safety or efficacy of the use of these agents in patients with GP. The use of the peroxisome proliferator–activated-receptor (PPAR) agonists in diabetes (without GP) is controversial, and other agents (sodium-glucose linked transporter [SGLT2] inhibitors) have not been tested in these patients or may cause diarrhea and abdominal distension (i.e., disacharidase inhibitors) aggravating gastrointestinal symptoms. Thus, we strongly favor the use of insulin in the patient with T2D and GP.

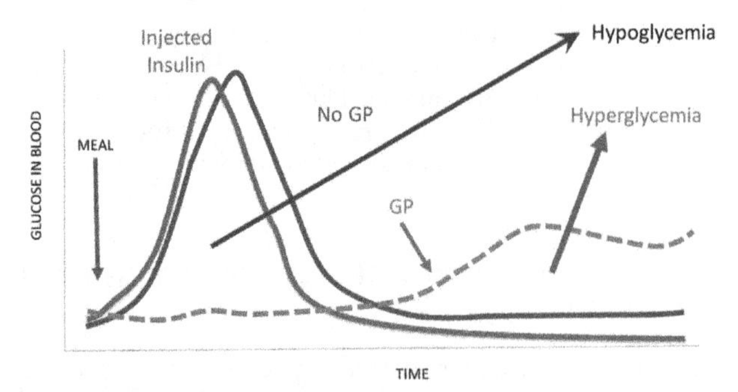

Figure 20.3—Mismatch of insulin pharmacokinetics and food absorption in patients with diabetes and GP. The current paradigm of meal insulin administration is not appropriate for patients with DM and GP because peaks of insulin concentration in the blood occurs much earlier than the peak of food absorption. Thus, hypoglycemia and hyperglycemia occur if the classical model of insulin administration is applied in this setting.

The current paradigm of insulin administration in T1D and insulin-using T2D is based on the basal-bolus model, which is often easier to achieve with use of insulin pumps rather than multiple insulin injections of rapid and long-acting insulins.[30] A basic assumption of the mealtime bolus is that gastric emptying of the ingested meal is completed within 4 h and intestinal absorption of nutrients is completed within 4–6 h. The administration of mealtime insulin is timed to match anticipated nutrient absorption. This is problematic for patients with GP because the onset and duration of the small intestinal absorption phase is critically dependent on the rate of gastric emptying. Besides the slow emptying of the stomach, the day-to-day variability in gastric emptying of common foods is unknown.

INSULIN ADMINISTRATION FOR THE PATIENT WITH GASTROPARESIS

Whenever possible, we recommend use of continuous insulin infusion (insulin pump) to manage glycemia in patients with diabetes and GP. A published study[31] and our own data support this modality of insulin administration. If insurance coverage and costs present an unsurmountable obstacle, then multiple daily injections are the next best option. We do not favor the use of premixed insulin preparations. Monitoring glycemia for insulin adjustment is preferably established with a system based on fingerstick testing augmented with a continuous glucose monitoring system (CGMS).

BASAL INSULIN ADMINISTRATION

The estimated initial dose of basal insulin can be calculated using a formula of 0.3 units/kg/day for a T2D patient and 0.15 units/kg/day for someone with T1D. In the inpatient setting, for the patient receiving an intravenous (IV) drip of insulin, the basal dose can be estimated from the hourly rate of infusion, extrapolated to 24 h and reduced by 25%, provided that the infusion has lasted for more than 12 h and has been stable in the past 4–6 h of administration (<10% variance in the hourly rate). For patients with diabetic GP, we recommend an overlap of at least 4 h (we prefer 6–8 h) between initiation of the basal insulin and cessation of the IV drip. Our preferred basal insulin is insulin glargine. If the patient routinely uses an insulin pump, we restart the pump.

Traditional adjustment of the basal insulin is based on the blood glucose level measured before breakfast, which assumes postabsorptive state (some 11–14 h after last meal). In patients with diabetic GP, however, the postabsorptive state is not so easy to define because gastric emptying may be delayed all day and an unknown amount of food (accumulated breakfast, lunch, or dinner from the previous day) is emptied during the night. Thus, the prebreakfast glycemia may not reflect real basal glycemia but rather ongoing postprandial glycemic excursions.

There are several approaches to attempt to better estimate the postabsorptive glycemia in these patients. First, the patient may skip breakfast for 2 to 3 days in a row and measure capillary glycemia every 1 to 2 h after waking up until lunch time to determine whether glycemia remains stable or falls slightly, reflecting the postabsorptive state. Second, the patient may skip dinner and measure capillary glycemia frequently through the night. Third, a better approach is to use CGMS to detect trends. Patients and physicians need to examine in detail overnight trends. An overnight surge of glucose starting near or at midnight may suggest late gastric emptying from the last supper or even from combined supper and lunch, as opposed to a steady and gradual increase that may indicate a need to adjust the basal insulin. The identification of these trends is demanding, but it is useful to avoid hypoglycemia and severe hyperglycemia.

BOLUS INSULIN ADMINISTRATION FOR MEALS

The challenges in determining meal bolus are much more complex than for the basal insulin. Instead of discrete postprandial "peaks" of increase and decrease of glycemia, most of the patients with diabetes and GP in whom we examined profiles of glycemia using CGMS, display almost-constant hyperglycemia interrupted by unpredictable dips into the normal or low glucose ranges.[32] This persistent hyperglycemia is probably the result of efforts of patients and doctors to avoid hypoglycemia in a setting in which tools to deliver insulin for these patients have not been tested in robust clinical trials. In spite of the noted caveats, some general recommendations can be made regarding the insulin mealtime bolus for patients with GP to reduce the risk of hypoglycemia and attempt to minimize hyperglycemia. If using injections, we suggest the following alternatives:

- Use regular insulin (rather than rapid-acting insulin analogues) in some patients because it has longer duration effect
- Administer insulin after the meal (not before)
- Give dose-fractionated insulin in two to three "mini-shots" spaced within 4–6 h after meal ingestion

If using pumps, we suggest the following:

- Start mealtime bolus ~15–30 min after meal ingestion
- Use the dual-wave bolus delivery feature and program a small initial first wave (i.e., 10 to 20%) and program the second wave to last for 4–6 h

MONITORING BLOOD GLUCOSE FOR MEALTIME BOLUSES

We recommend that whenever feasible CGMS be used. The patterns of the 24-h readings of pre- and postprandial glycemia in the individual patient should be examined carefully. We recently finished GLUMIT, a trial that tested the safety and efficacy of using continuous subcutaneous insulin infusion (CSII) and CGMS in 45 patients with GP and diabetes (Figure 20.4; Table 20.2). In this study we used some the previously noted principles and found that this approach reduced HbA_{1c} by 1.1% and was associated with a reduction in the time that patients spent in the hypoglycemic and hyperglycemic range. Patients also reported improvement in gastric symptoms.[32] Pending further testing in hospital settings, these guidelines may be used in the inpatient setting.

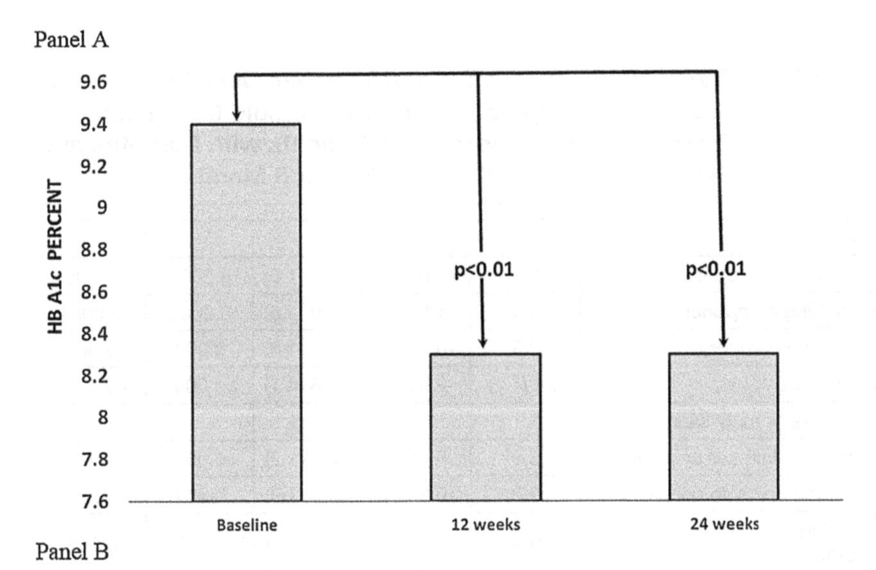

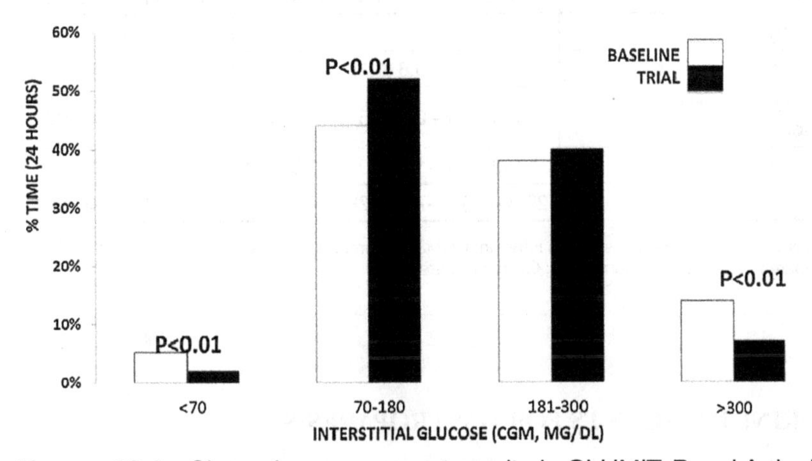

Figures 20.4—Glycemia management results in GLUMIT. Panel A depicts the HbA_{1c} levels and panel B the time spent in hypoglycemia, euglycemia, and hyperglycemia (using CGMS) in patients with diabetes and GP treated with CSII and GCMS.

Table 20.2—The GLUMIT Study: Effects of Improved Diabetes Glycemic Control on Gastric Symptoms and Liquid Mixed Meal (Ensure) Volume Tolerance in Patients with Diabetes and GP Treated with CSII and CGMS for 6 Months

Nausea					
Nausea component	3.5	−1.0 (1.5)	−1.0 (1.5)	0.0001	<0.0001
Retching component	2.4	−1.0 (1.6)	−1.0 (1.6)	0.0002	0.0001
Vomiting component	2.3	−0.8 (1.7)	−0.9 (1.8)	0.003	0.003
Subscore	8.1 (4.2)	−2.9 (4.0)	−2.8 (4.1)	<0.0001	<0.0001
Fullness or early satiety					
Stomach fullness component	3.9	−0.9 (1.0)	−0.7 (1.2)	<0.0001	0.0006
Not able to finish component	3.3	−0.8 (1.7)	−0.6 (1.9)	0.004	0.05
Feeling excessively full component	3.9	−0.7 (1.4)	−0.7 (1.4)	0.003	0.001
Loss of appetite component	3.0	−0.6 (1.5)	−0.6 (1.4)	0.01	0.01
Subscore	14.1 (3.6)	−3.1 (4.5)	−2.4 (4.5)	<0.0001	0.002
Bloating					
Bloating component	3.7	−0.8 (1.1)	−0.8 (1.2)	<0.0001	<0.0001
Stomach visibly larger component	3.4	−0.5 (1.5)	−0.7 (1.5)	0.04	0.003
Subscore	7.1 (2.3)	−1.3 (2.9)	−1.5 (2.5)	0.0009	0.0007
Total GCSI	29.3 (7.1)	−7.2 (8.2)	−6.6 (8.8)	<0.0001	<0.0001

CSII, continuous subcutaneous insulin infusion; CGMS, continuous glucose monitoring system; GCSI, gastroparesis cardinal symptom index; GP, gastroparesis.

PHARMACOLOGICAL AND OTHER TREATMENTS FOR THE SYMPTOMS OF GASTROPARESIS IN THE HOSPITAL

PROKINETIC AGENTS FOR GASTROPARESIS

Drugs that increase the rate of gastric emptying (prokinetic agents) have been used to treat diabetic GP for many years.[33] Unfortunately, many drugs designed to improve the rate of gastric emptying have not improved the symptoms associated with GP. Studies of prokinetics and gastric stimulation have shown that the rate of gastric emptying does not correlate with the symptoms associated with GP.[34] The only prokinetic drugs currently available to treat GP are metoclopramide (Reglan) and erythromycin (Table 20.3). Metoclopramide is a drug with effects on several receptors: dopamine$_2$ receptors, 5HT$_3$ receptor antagonist, and acetylcholinesterase inhibitor.[34] Gastric emptying is increased by metoclopramide, but the drug also crosses the blood-brain barrier and causes a variety of central nervous system

Table 20.3—Drug Therapies Used to Treat Upper Gastrointestinal Symptoms in Patients with Diabetic GP

Therapy	Mechanisms and sites of action	Dosage	Adverse effects
Prokinetic therapy			
Macrolides			
Erythyromycin	Motilin receptor agonist	125–250 mg four times daily	Nausea, diarrhea abdominal cramps, rash
Substituted benzamides			
Metoclopramide	Dopamine (D_2) receptor antagonist; 5-HT_3 receptor antagonist; 5-HT_4 receptor agonist	5–20 mg before meals and at bedtime	Extrapyramidal symptoms, dystonic reactions, anxiety, depression, hyperprolactinemia, tardive dyskinesia
Domperidone	D_2-receptor antagonist (peripheral)	10–20 mg before meals and at bedtime	Hyperprolactinemia, breast tenderness, galactorrhea
Antinauseant therapy			
Serotonin antagonists			
Ondansetron	5-HT_3 receptor antagonist	4–8 mg twice daily, either orally or intravenously	Headache, increased liver enzymes
Granisetron	5-HT_3 receptor antagonist	2 mg once daily or 3.1 mg patch	Headache, increased liver enzymes
Phenothiazines			
Prochlorperazine	Central nervous system (CNS) sites	5–10 mg three times daily	Hypotension, extrapyramidal symptoms
Antihistamines			
Promethazine	CNS, H_1 receptor antagonist	25 mg twice daily	Drowsiness
Dimenhydrinate	H_1 receptor antagonist	50 mg four times daily	Drowsiness
Cyclizine	H_1 receptor antagonist	50 mg four times daily	Drowsiness
Butyrophenones			
Droperidol	Central dopamine receptor antagonist	2.5–5 mg intravenously every 2 h	Sedation, hypotension

continued

Table 20.3—Drug Therapies Used to Treat Upper Gastrointestinal Symptoms in Patients with Diabetic GP *(continued)*

Therapy	Mechanisms and sites of action	Dosage	Adverse effects
Antidepressants			
Mirtazapine	CNS sites	15 mg at bedtime	Weight gain
Benzodiazepines			
Lorazepam	CNS sites	0.5–1 mg four times daily	Drowsiness, lightheadedness
Alprazolam	CNS sites	0.25–0.5 mg three times daily	Drowsiness, lightheadedness
Dronabinol	CNS	5–10 mg two times daily	Sedation

symptoms, ranging from nervousness to Parkinson's disease and irreversible tardive dyskinesia. Erythromycin is a macrolide antibiotic that stimulates motilin receptors and contractions in the corpus and antrum, which increases the rate of gastric emptying.[35] Domperidone is a dopamine$_2$ agonist that does not cross the blood-brain barrier, improves nausea and gastric dysrhythmias, and may improve the rate of gastric emptying in some patients with diabetic GP.[36] Domperidone, however, is not available in the U.S. except through a special U.S. Food and Drug Administration program.

ANTINAUSEA DRUGS

The quality of life for patients with GP is extremely poor because of constant nausea and episodic vomiting. These symptoms may lead to dehydration, which requires frequent emergency room visits or hospitalizations. In unremitting nausea and vomiting, normal weight cannot be maintained. Total parenteral nutrition may be needed in a minority of patients to support nutrition. Table 20.3 lists a number of drugs that are used empirically to treat nausea for patients with GP. At the present time, there is no way to predict which medication will decrease nausea in an individual patient. Each drug may be tried to see whether nausea and vomiting improve. These drugs have not been specifically approved for use in patients who have symptoms associated with diabetic GP.

PYLORIC THERAPIES (BOTULINUM TOXIN INJECTION, SURGICAL MYOTOMY) AND GASTRIC ELECTRICAL STIMULATION

Several modalities of treatment are being used in the outpatient setting. A small subset of patients with GP has pyloric dysfunction, which traditionally has been diagnosed with manometry. Promising diagnostic tools for diagnosis of pyloric dysfunction include the use of wireless capsule motility and impedance planimetry. Treatment of suspected pylorospasm with injections of botulinum toxin into the pylorus has resulted in no better symptom improvement than placebo in patients with GP.[37] Patients with idiopathic GP and normal 3 cpm myoelectrical activity (obstructive GP) who underwent pyloroplasty had improvement in symptoms and gastric emptying rates, but the patients with diabetic GP did not have improvement in gastric emptying.[38] Gastric electrical stimulation is provided to relieve nausea and vomiting, possibly working via vagal afferents. In controlled trials, this treatment relieves nausea and vomiting in patients with diabetes with GP.[39] Severe GP with malnutrition requires jejunostomy for enteral feeding tubes or venting gastrostomy. Placement of stimulators or any gastric operations are not suited for the acute management of GP in the hospital, with the exception of jejunostomy for the placement of feeding tubes.[40]

CONCLUSION

GP is a complication of long-standing T1D and T2D. Symptoms associated with GP include early satiety, prolonged postprandial fullness, bloating, nausea, vomiting, and abdominal pain. Mortality is increased in patients with diabetic GP. ICCs are depleted and gastric enteric neurons are abnormal, suggesting the disease is a neuropathy affecting control of gastric smooth muscle relaxation and contraction, and a Cajalopathy affecting gastric electrical rhythm. A subset of patients with diabetic GP has pylorospasm that results in obstructive GP.

GP delays gastric emptying of food and hence also retards entry of nutrients from the small intestine into the bloodstream. As a consequence of the latter, there is a mismatch of exogenous prandial insulin peak activity and postprandial glycemia. Thus, GP increases substantially the risk of hypo- and hyperglycemia. Patients with diabetic GP frequently require emergency department services and hospital admission for treatment of severe hypoglycemia, ketoacidosis, and dehydration secondary to vomiting or a combination of all of these issues.

Current treatment goals for patients with GP in the hospital are to restore volume and correct electrolyte imbalances with IV fluids, correct and avoid hypoglycemia and severe hyperglycemia with judicious doses of insulin, and attempt to minimize symptoms with use of antinauseant and prokinetic drugs. Diet should be reintroduced slowly following the three-step GP diet. Selected diagnostic tests, such as endoscopy or abdominal ultrasound or computed tomography, should be selected to exclude other diseases that mimic the nonspecific symptoms that are associated with GP. Transition from the hospital to the outpatient clinic requires education and close follow-up to avoid readmissions.

REFERENCES

1. Camilleri M, Parkman H, Shafi M, et al. Clinical guideline: Management of gastroparesis. *Am J Gastroenterol* 2013;108:18–37

2. Koch KL. Diabetic gastropathy: Gastric neuromuscular dysfunction in diabetes mellitus. A review of symptoms, pathophysiology, and treatment. *Dig Dis Sci* 1999;44:1061–1075
3. Hasler WL, Soudah HC, Dulai G, Owyang C. Mediation of hyperglycemia-evoked gastric slow-wave dysrhythmias by endogenous prostaglandins. *Gastroenterology* 1995;108:726–736
4. Fraser R, Horowitz M, Maddox A, et al. Hyperglycemia slows gastric emptying in type 1 diabetes mellitus. *Diabetologia* 1990;33:675–680
5. Bharucha A. Epidemiology and natural history of gastroparesis. In *Gastroparesis, Gastroenterology Clinics of North America.* Parkman H, Pasricha P, Eds., Philadelphia, Elsevier, 2015, p. 9–19
6. Syed A, Calles-Escandon J, Wolfe M. Epidemiology of gastroparesis with and without diabetes in a large cohort from 340 USA hospitals. *Gastroenterology* 2015;148(Suppl. 1):S505–S506
7. The Diabetes Control and Complications Trial Research Group. The effect of intensive diabetes therapy on measures of autonomic nervous system function in the Diabetes Control and Complications Trial (DCCT). *Diabetologia* 1998;4:416–4238
8. Koch KL, Hasler WL, et al. for the Gastroparesis Clinical Research Consortium. Contrasting gastroparesis in type 1 (T1DM) vs. type 2 (T2DM) diabetes: Clinical course after 48 weeks of follow-up and relation to comorbidities and health resource utilization. *Gastroenterology* 2013;144(5 Suppl.):S926–S927
9. Dickman R, Kislov J, Boaz M, et al. Prevalence of symptoms suggestive of gastroparesis in a cohort of patients with diabetes mellitus. *J Diab Comp* 2013;27:376–379
10. Koch KL. Gastric neuromuscular function and neuromuscular disorders. In *Sleisenger and Fordtran's Gastrointestinal and Liver Disease: Pathophysiology/Diagnosis/Management.* Feldman M, Friedman LS, Brandt LJ, Eds. Philadelphia, Elsevier, 2015, p. 811–838
11. Moran TH, Wirth JB, Schwartz GJ, et al. Interactions between gastric volume and duodenal nutrients in the control of liquid gastric emptying. *Am J Physiol* 1999; 276:R997–1002
12. Camilleri M. Integrated upper gastrointestinal response to food intake. *Gastroenterology* 2006;131:640–658
13. Ordog T. Interstitial cells of Cajal in diabetic gastroenteropathy. *Neurogastroenterol Motil* 2008;20:8–18
14. Rayner CK, Verhagen MA, Hebbard GG, et al. Proximal gastric compliance and perception of distension in type 1 diabetes mellitus: Effects of hyperglycemia. *Am J Gastroenterology* 2000;95:1175–1183

15. Won KJ, Sanders KM, Ward SM. Interstitial cells of Cajal mediate mechanosensitive responses in the stomach. *Proc Natl Acad Sci USA* 2005;102:14913–14918

16. He C-L, Soffer EE, Ferris CD, et al. Loss of interstitial cells of Cajal and inhibitory innervation in insulin-dependent diabetes. *Gastroenterology* 2001;121:427–434

17. Lin Z, Sarosiek I, Forster J, et al. Association of the status of interstitial cells of Cajal and electrogastrogram parameters, gastric emptying, and symptoms in patients with gastroparesis. *Neurogastroenterol Motil* 2010;22(1):56–61

18. Mearin F, Camilleri M, Malagelada JR. Pyloric dysfunction in diabetics with recurrent nausea and vomiting. *Gastroenterology* 1986;90:1919–1925

19. Brzana RJ, Bingaman S, Koch KL. Gastric myoelectrical activity in patients with gastric outlet obstruction and idiopathic gastroparesis. *Am J Gastroenterol* 1998;93:1083–1089

20. Parkman HP, Yates K, Hasler WL, et al. Similarities and differences between diabetic and idiopathic gastroparesis. *Clin Gastroenterol Hepatol* 2011;9:1056–1064

21. Tougas G, Eaker EY, Abell TL, et al. Assessment of gastric emptying using a low fat meal: Establishment of international control values. *Am J Gastroenterol* 2000;95:1456–1462

22. George NS, et al. Small intestinal overgrowth in gastroparesis. *Dig Dis Sci* 2014;59:645–652

23. American Diabetes Association. Clinical practice guidelines 2014. *Diabetes Care* 2014;37(Suppl. 1):S28–S30

24. Calles-Escandon J, Van Natta M, Koch KL, Hasler W, et al. (on behalf of the NIH Gastroparesis Consortium). Pilot study of the safety, feasibility, and efficacy of continuous glucose monitoring (CGM) and insulin pump therapy in diabetic gastroparesis (GLUMIT-DG): A multicenter, longitudinal trial by the NIDDK gastroparesis clinical research consortium (GPCRC). *Gastroenterology* 2015;146(Suppl.):S295

25. Parkman HP, et al. Dietary intake and nutritional deficiencies in patients with diabetic or idiopathic gastroparesis. *Gastroenterology* 2011;141:486–498

26. Marahe C, et al. Relationship between gastric emptying, postprandial glycemia and incretin homones. *Diabetes Care* 2013;36:1396–1405

27. Bolen S, Feldman L, Vassy J, et al., Systematic review: Comparative effectiveness and safety of oral medications for type 2 diabetes mellitus. *Ann Intern Med* 2007;147:386–399

28. Amori RE, Lau J, Pittas AG. Efficacy and safety of incretin therapy in type 2 diabetes: Systematic review and meta-analysis. *JAMA* 2007;298(2):194–206

29. Stevens J, et al. The effect of sitagliptin on gastric emptying in healthy humans—a randomized controlled study. *Aliment Pharmacol Ther* 2012;36:379–390

30. Jeitler K, Horvath K, Berghold A, et al. Continuous SQ insulin infusion versus multiple daily insulin injections in patients with diabetes mellitus: systematic review and meta-analysis. *Diabetologia* 2008;51:941–951

31. Sharma D, Morrison G, Joseph F, et al. The role of continuous SQ insulin infusion therapy in patients with diabetic gastroparesis. *Diabetologia* 2011;54:2768–2770

32. Calles-Escandón J, Hasler WL, Koch KL, et al. Continuous blood glucose patterns in patients with diabetes with gastroparesis: Baseline findings from the GpCRC GLUMIT-DG study. *Gastroenterology* 2014;146(Suppl. 1):S616

33. Lata PF, Pigarelli DL. Chronic metoclopramide therapy for diabetic gastroparesis. *Ann Pharmacother* 2003;37:122–126

34. Janssen P, Harris MS, Jones M, Masaoka T, et al. The relation between symptom improvement and gastric emptying in the treatment of diabetic and idiopathic gastroparesis. *Am J Gastroenterology* 2013;108(9):1382–1391

35. Rayner CK, Su YC, Doran SM, et al. The stimulation of antral motility by erythromycin is attenuated by hyperglycemia. *Am J Gastroenterol* 2000;95:2233–2241

36. Koch KL, Stern RM, Stewart WR, Vasey MW. Gastric emptying and gastric myoelectrical activity in patients with symptomatic diabetic gastroparesis: Effects of long-term domperidone treatment. *Am J Gastroenterol* 1989;84:1069–1075

37. Friedenberg FK, Palit A, Parkman HP, et al. Botulinum toxin A for the treatment of delayed gastric emptying. *Am J Gastroenterol* 2008;103:416–423

38. Scott BK, Koch KL, Westcott, CJ. Pyloroplasty for patients with medically-refractory functional obstructive gastroparesis. *Gastroenterology* 2014;146 (1 Suppl.):S615.39

39. McCallum RW, Snape W, Brody F, et al. Gastric electrical stimulation with Enterra improves symptoms from diabetic gastroparesis in a prospective study. *Clin Gastroenterol Hepatol* 2010;8:947–954

40. Sarosiek I, Davis B, Eichler E, McCallum R. Surgical approaches to treatment of gastroparesis: Gastric stimulation, pyloroplasty, total gastrectomy and enteral feeding tubes. In *Gastroparesis, Gastroenterology Clinics of North America*, Parkman H, Pasricha P, Eds., Philadelphia, Elsevier, 2015, pp. 151–167

Chapter 21

Inpatient Management of the Pregnant Woman with Diabetes

Elizabeth O. Buschur, MD,[1] Marie E. McDonnell, MD,[2]
M. Kathleen Figaro, MD,[3] and Emma M. Eggleston, MD,[2,4]

INTRODUCTION

The inpatient management of diabetes in pregnancy poses unique challenges because of the need for tight antepartum and peripartum glycemic control, the inherent ketosis-prone nature of pregnancy, and pregnancy-specific conditions that may complicate management. The prevalence of the three primary types of diabetes in pregnancy—type 1 diabetes (T1D), type 2 diabetes (T2D), and gestational diabetes (GDM)—are each on the rise, with increases in GDM and T2D being the most prominent.[1,2] The rise of diabetes in pregnancy has significant individual and public health implications in light of the well-described linear relationship between hyperglycemia and adverse maternal and fetal outcomes.[3,4] In the inpatient setting, evidence-based interdisciplinary care is critical to minimize complications and address the unique needs of women with diabetes. This chapter will review the antepartum and peripartum inpatient management of diabetes in pregnancy and highlight pregnancy-specific complications that may influence care.

ANTEPARTUM CARE

Historically, pregnant women with pregestational diabetes were universally admitted to the hospital for glycemic management. Today, pregnant women with diabetes are primarily managed in the outpatient setting and inpatient admission is reserved for acute conditions. These may be diabetes-related (intensive glucose management and titration of insulin as needed for erratic glycemic control, recurrent hypoglycemia, diabetic ketoacidosis [DKA], gastroparesis) or may be due to other complications of pregnancy for which women with diabetes are at higher risk (e.g., preeclampsia, preterm labor, infection). The goal of diabetes care during

[1]Division of Endocrinology, Diabetes and Metabolism, The Ohio State University Wexner Medical Center, Columbus, OH. [2]Division of Endocrinology, Diabetes and Hypertension, Section of Diabetes, Brigham and Women's Hospital, Boston, MA. [3]Genesis Diabetes Care Center, Bettendorf, IA. [4]Department of Population Medicine, Harvard Pilgrim Health Care Institute and Harvard Medical School, Boston, MA.

DOI: 10.2337/9781580406086.21

pregnancy is to achieve glycemia in the normal range to the extent possible without significant hypoglycemia and to manage diabetes-associated complications and comorbidities.

GLYCEMIC TARGETS

Glycemic control goals vary among endocrine organizations and type of diabetes (Table 21.1). The American Diabetes Association (ADA) recommends the following glycemic targets for women with preexisting diabetes during pregnancy: preprandial, bedtime, and overnight glucose 60–99 mg/dL; 1- or 2-h postprandial glucose 100–129 mg/dL; and hemoglobin A_{1c} <6%. For women with GDM, the ADA recommends fasting values of ≤95 mg/dL, 1-h postprandial ≤140 mg/dL, and 2-h postprandial ≤120 mg/dL glucose targets. The Endocrine Society recommends fasting ≤95 mg/dL, 1-h postprandial ≤140 mg/dL, and 2-h postprandial ≤120 mg/d[5] glucose targets for women with pregestational diabetes or GDM. The American College of Obstetrics and Gynecology has similar glycemic goals for women with GDM or pregestational diabetes.

Maturity onset diabetes of the young (MODY) also can complicate pregnancy, but prevalence rates are unclear. Mutations in the glucokinase (GCK) gene (MODY 2) and hepatocyte nuclear factor-1α (HNF1α) gene (MODY 3) represent the majority of cases.[6,7] With the exception of MODY 2, in which excessively tight control may contribute to intrauterine growth retardation (IUGR), management of MODY in pregnancy is similar to that of other forms of diabetes in pregnancy.

Table 21.1—American Diabetes Association glycemic targets in the anterpartum, peripartum, and postpartum periods.

Time period	Glycemic goals (mg/dL)	
	PDM	GDM
Antepartum	60-99 overnight and fasting 100-129 postprandial (1h or 2h)	Fasting ≤95, 1h postprandial ≤140, and 2h postprandial ≤120
Peripartum	70-110	70-110
Postpartum	<120-140 overnight and preprandial <150-170 postprandial 140-180 inpatient	<100

The Endocrine Society has similar recommendations for antepartum glycemic goals: fasting ≤95 mg/dL, 1h postprandial ≤140, and 2h postprandial ≤140 mg/dL and peripartum glycemic goals of 72-126 mg/dL. [Endocrine Society Clinical Practice Guidelines for Diabetes during Pregnancy, 2013].
The American College of Obstetrics and Gynecology has similar recommendations for preexisting diabetes: fasting ≤95 mg/dL, premeal ≤100 mg/dL, 1h postprandial ≤140, and 2h postprandial ≤120 mg/dL and the same intrapartum glycemic goals of 70-110 mg/dL.[ACOG Practice Bulletin for GDM, 2013].
PDM = preexisting diabetes
GDM = gestational diabetes
Data extracted from Kitzmiller, et al.[9]

INSULIN

There are several detailed reviews of insulin use in pregnancy.[8,9] In the following sections, we provide a basic overview to inform inpatient management. Insulins approved by the U.S. Food and Drug Administration (FDA) for use in pregnancy include NPH, insulin detemir, regular insulin, regular U-500, lispro, and aspart. Each of these is pregnancy category B. Glargine and glulisine insulin are currently pregnancy category C.

NPH and insulin detemir insulins are both given twice daily as basal regimens; however, either can be administered as a bedtime or morning dose alone in patients with GDM or T2D, depending on glycemic patterns. NPH has been used in pregnancy for decades and is the basal insulin for which there is the most post-marketing safety data. The peak of NPH can be used to an advantage with morning dosing as it can help cover carbohydrate intake at lunch. It also can lead to hypoglycemia in the late morning to late afternoon, and the nocturnal peak can be problematic in some women. Midmorning, midafternoon, and pre-bed snacks are particularly important in women using insulin, and these snacks can help prevent hypoglycemia associated with NPH peaks. If continued hypoglycemia occurs, a trial of insulin detemir, which has a less pronounced peak, may be of benefit. Although glargine currently is not recommended as a first-line insulin in pregnancy, several recent studies have suggested it is safe during pregnancy.[10–12] Glargine typically is dosed once daily at bedtime or in the morning. In some women with T2D, or women with T1D for whom the duration of action is <24 h, glargine can be dosed twice daily with care to avoid insulin stacking and hypoglycemia. In women with pregestational diabetes, it is our practice to use NPH or insulin detemir twice daily as first-line basal insulin. However, in women with excellent control on glargine for whom changing the regimen could cause unstable glycemia or those for whom once-daily dosing is strongly preferable and the risk of hyperglycemia or DKA is high (e.g., women with difficult social circumstances, work constraints, or developmental delays), glargine may be the best option.

Regular U-500 is a concentrated insulin (five times the concentration of U-100 regular insulin) used for women with extreme insulin resistance. Typically, U-500 is started if a woman injects more than 100 units at a time or if the total daily insulin dose exceeds 300 units. It tends to have a longer duration and a longer absorption period than regular insulin and may be used as basal insulin in pregnancy, with a prandial rapid-acting insulin analog as needed. No randomized trials of U-500 use in pregnancy are available, but several case reports describe no adverse maternal or neonatal outcomes.[13–15] U-500 has also been used in continuous infusion pumps for pregnant women with high insulin resistance.[13] Because of the risk of dosing confusion and profound hypoglycemia, the inpatient use of U-500 insulin requires standardized pharmacy protocols, detailed instructions for the patient, and targeted training for nursing and the inpatient care team.

Prandial insulins that are FDA approved for use in pregnancy include aspart, lispro, and regular insulin. All are pregnancy category B. In women with pregestational diabetes, the preferred method for dosing of prandial insulin is based on an insulin-to-carbohydrate ratio with a correction (or sensitivity) factor to address acute blood glucose levels outside the target range. For those women with preexisting diabetes who are not familiar or comfortable with carbohydrate counting, a standing dose of prandial insulin can be used at meals in addition to a scale for premeal correction. Regardless of approach, flexibility in dosing is important and allowing the patient to play a role in determining her prandial doses may be an important part of achieving glycemic controls. Women with longstanding diabetes are generally familiar with their glycemic response to specific foods or circumstances and are practiced in adjusting their regimen to a variety of variable factors. Rigid approaches to dosing may lead to erratic control, particularly in the inpatient setting in which patient self-management is often secondary to standardized protocols. Although the latter are important for consistency of care and safety, a more patient-centered approach that integrates patient knowledge, when communicated across the care team and documented clearly, may achieve better glycemic control.

In women with low appetite, nausea, or vomiting, dosing with lispro or aspart right after meals, when actual intake is known, may be helpful in avoiding hypoglycemia. If this approach is used, tight timing of insulin administration, ideally upon immediate completion of the meal but no longer than 15 min postmeal, is recommended. Dosing for snacks in the inpatient setting is not generally instituted because of concern for insulin stacking and hypoglycemia. For some women, however, correction for snacks at a looser carbohydrate ratio than for standard meals, is needed to avoid hyperglycemia. Because of their flexibility and lower potential for hypoglycemia, rapid-acting insulin analogs are preferred by many providers, but regular insulin may be used as an alternative if needed, with attention to later onset and longer duration of action.

CONTINUOUS SUBCUTANEOUS INSULIN INFUSION

Continuous subcutaneous insulin infusion (CSII) via an insulin pump offers pregnant women with pregestational diabetes a convenient way to deliver insulin. CSII is an excellent alternative to multiple daily injections of insulin, with no apparent differences in glycemic control, maternal outcome, or neonatal outcome.[16] Some studies suggest that pregnant women using CSII have similar rates of severe hypoglycemia and DKA as those on multiple daily injections,[17] but pump malfunction or infusion site problems can increase the risk of DKA and awareness of this risk by the patient and inpatient management team is of critical importance. Unless necessary for glycemic control, initiation of pump therapy in pregnancy is not recommended. In the absence of significant acute illness, many patients on CSII can continue wearing their pumps during an antepartum hospital admission if the patient has the mental and physical capacity to adjust the pump. It is important to train nursing staff regarding the basic principles of pump therapy and to document accurately basal rates and bolus doses taken during the inpatient stay. Backup pump supplies, including battery, reservoirs, and infusion sites, are also needed and can be provided either by the patient or the hospital pharmacy. Continuous glucose monitors (CGM) can be used in conjunction with CSII or separately with multiple daily injections to provide glucose trend data that can be helpful for pregnant women with diabetes who are trying to achieve recommended tight glycemic control and avoidance of hypoglycemia. As with pump therapy, education of the inpatient care team and nursing staff on CGM is central to successful integration into the care plan.

ORAL AGENTS

Although insulin is the first-line agent recommended by the ADA and the Endocrine Society for management of hyperglycemia in pregnancy, the oral antiglycemics glyburide and metformin are used in some women with GDM or T2D. Both of these agents are approved by the FDA and are classified as category B and B/C depending on manufacturer, respectively, during pregnancy. Randomized data, however, suggest they are safe for use in pregnancy.[18,19] Unless a patient is stable and admitted for observation alone, discontinuation of metformin and glyburide and use of insulin is recommended during inpatient admissions because of the potential for metabolic and glycemic instability with acute illness.

MEDICAL NUTRITION THERAPY

Careful attention to nutrition is a central component of managing diabetes during pregnancy, and this is as true in the inpatient setting as it is in the outpatient setting. The inpatient setting may provide an excellent opportunity for a patient and her family to meet with a registered dietitian nutritionist (RD or RDN) or dietitian and certified diabetes educator (CDE) as part of her diabetes care team. Adjustments to the patient's insulin regimen while inpatient should be made with consideration of a patient's meal patterns at home. A pregnant woman's diet in the hospital may be different than her diet at home. To the extent possible, flexibility in the timing of meals, snacks, and sleep should mimic her home situation. Similarly, women with specific food needs (vegetarian, allergies, celiac disease) should have tailored diets as needed, and if not possible with a hospital menu, patients should be allowed to have food brought in from home. This requires flexibility and communication among the patient, care team, and family, but it is worthwhile in reducing the occurrence of hypo- and hyperglycemia.

In sum, the inpatient setting can present several advantages (ostensibly controlled timing, type, and amounts of nutrient intake and regulated insulin administration) and challenges (different meal content and timing compared with the patient's home regimen, less patient control over the self-care regimen, erratic sleep and other interruptions, and delayed insulin administration pending other competing clinical factors). Care must be taken to achieve glycemic goals while avoiding hypoglycemia. We recommend adjusting a patient's insulin regimen on a daily basis with the help of an inpatient team, including an RD or RDN, CDE, endocrinologist, maternal fetal medicine specialist, and social worker, as needed. Although there are no randomized data on outcomes when a multidisciplinary team provides care, our experience supports the importance of flexibility and clear communication among the patient, family, and health-care team.

CONDITIONS COMPLICATING INPATIENT MANAGEMENT

In addition to the practical parameters that influence inpatient glycemic control, multiple clinical situations can exacerbate control, resulting in hyperglycemia or hypoglycemia.

DIABETIC KETOACIDOSIS

Pregnancy is a ketosis-prone state because of increased insulin resistance, increased lipolysis, and physiologically compensated respiratory alkalosis with decreased ability to buffer ketoacids. DKA is more common, occurs at lower levels of glycemia, and carries a higher risk of mortality in pregnant women with diabetes as compared with nonpregnant women with diabetes. DKA has been reported in 1–10% of pregnant women with T1D and can occur at glucose values ≤200 mg/dL (13.9 mmol/L). There are also multiple case reports of euglycemic DKA in pregnant women.[20–23] The risk of fetal demise is substantial, with rates of 9–35% reported in the literature; however, these rates have been declining over time with improvements in care.[24] Other complications include fetal hypoxia and acidosis, preterm delivery, and maternal or neonatal intensive care unit admission.[25] Although uncommon, inpatient care teams should be alert to the possibility that DKA can occur in individuals with ketosis-prone T2D and GDM.[24]

Triggers of DKA include gastroparesis, vomiting, preeclampsia, insulin pump malfunction, infection, and use of steroids and β-sympathomimetics. As women with diabetes may be admitted for management of acute stressors or are given therapies that may exacerbate risk of DKA (e.g., corticosteroids for preterm labor or β-sympathomimetics for tocolysis), a low index of suspicion is required and a general approach of ensuring adequate insulinization for physiologic demands is critical. This may require transition from subcutaneously (SQ) delivered insulin to an intravenous (IV) insulin infusion to ensure glycemic stability until the acute process is resolved. In labor, the majority of women with pregestational T1D require IV insulin with simultaneous dextrose-containing fluids to avoid DKA. Particular attention is needed during the transition to *and* from IV insulin and prior SQ or CSII regimens because DKA can occur if the overlap in insulin action between the two modes of insulin delivery is inadequate.

Management of DKA in pregnancy is similar to management in the nonpregnant state, with a DKA protocol that incorporates IV insulin, aggressive hydration with intravenous fluids, and electrolyte repletion. There are several excellent reviews of management of DKA during pregnancy.[8,26] If not already in place, women admitted with DKA in pregnancy should receive inpatient education on prevention and instruction regarding how and when to contact the care team. They also should be instructed regarding purpose and use and should be discharged with urine ketone strips. If using CSII, a backup supply of insulin syringes and basal insulin to be used in case of pump failure or other pump-related problems should be provided.

GASTROPARESIS

Pregnant women with autonomic neuropathy are at increased risk of gastroparesis, hypoglycemia unawareness, and orthostatic hypotension. Gastroparesis poses particular risks and, when severe, is one of the few relative contraindications to pregnancy in women with pregestational diabetes as it can lead to extreme hypo- and hyperglycemia, increased risk of DKA, weight loss, and malnutrition.[9] Women with significant gastroparesis often experience frequent hospitalizations and may require prokinetic therapy and parenteral nutrition. Initial management of gastroparesis consists of dietary modification, optimization of glycemic control, and hydration, but therapy with antiemetics, metoclopramide (pregnancy class B) or erythromycin (pregnancy class B), and intravenous fluids may be needed. In severe cases, parenteral nutrition may be required. Patients with gastroparesis may need to administer prandial insulin following completion of their meal to ensure that they were able to tolerate the anticipated carbohydrate intake. A more frequent, but lower dose, prandial dosing may be required if eating five to six small meals per day. Attention should be paid to avoid potential insulin stacking. Careful inpatient team management that includes an RD or RDN and adjustment of traditional inpatient meal times and sizes is needed to optimize nutritional status and glycemic control with attention to timing of insulin injections. As vomiting associated with gastroparesis can trigger DKA, a low threshold should be held for transition to IV insulin administration until symptoms are controlled.

NEPHROPATHY

Women with normal albumin excretion or microalbuminuria are at low risk for development of kidney disease in pregnancy. In contrast, women with poorly controlled hypertension or reduced glomerular filtration rate (GFR), serum creatinine level >1.5 mg/dL, or proteinuria >3 g in 24 h at the onset of pregnancy are at risk of worsening of renal disease. A recent study showed the increased prevalence of hypertension, preeclampsia, preterm birth, cesarean section rates, and neonatal intensive care unit admissions among pregnant women with diabetic nephropathy.[27] In the inpatient setting, women with significant renal disease require particular attention to blood pressure control and fluid management and a nephrology consultation may be needed. Angiotensin-converting enzyme (ACE) inhibitors and angiotensin receptor blockers are contraindicated during pregnancy because of teratogenic effects. As insulin is renally cleared, insulin dosing adjustments often are required when changes in renal status occur and avoidance of hypoglycemia can be challenging.

RETINOPATHY

The large majority of women with diabetic retinopathy will not experience worsening of retinopathy during or following pregnancy. For some, however, particularly those with proliferative retinopathy, retinopathy may worsen transiently during pregnancy, and in a small subset with severe pregestational retinopathy, visual changes may persist postdelivery. Retinopathy may worsen rapidly and result in permanent loss of vision. The likelihood of retinopathy progression is related to maternal duration of diabetes, severity of existing retinopathy, and degree of glycemic control before and during pregnancy.[28] Hypertension, smoking, hyperlipidemia, and hypoglycemia also have been associated with acceleration of retinopathy during pregnancy.[29] As in nonpregnant individuals, rapid tightening of glycemic control has been associated with early worsening of retinopathy in women with diabetes. In the inpatient setting, attention to vision changes and glycemic control, in consultation with the obstetrics and ophthalmology teams, is needed if acute inpatient vision changes develop.

CARDIAC DISEASE

Pregnant women with longstanding diabetes are at increased risk of macrovascular cardiac disease (coronary artery disease, heart failure, stroke) and microvascular cardiovascular disease (microvascular angiopathy, cardiac autonomic neuropathy). The risk is related both to diabetes and to the frequent presence of other cardiovascular and renal risk factors, such as hypertension and nephropathy.[9] The volume expansion and physiologic stressors of pregnancy may reveal previously subclinical disease or worsen existing disease, and preemptive awareness of the potential for cardiac dysfunction, particularly under the stress of labor or other acute conditions that may have precipitated inpatient admission are important. Cardiac monitoring, appropriate management of fluids, and specialty cardiology care may be needed for women with longstanding diabetes and known or recently diagnosed cardiovascular disease.

BETAMETHASONE THERAPY

Betamethasone therapy typically is prescribed (two doses of 12 mg given intramuscularly every 24 h for 48 h) for preterm labor to assist with fetal lung maturity. Hyperglycemia can be significant and typically ensues by the third day after receiving betamethasone and lasts for up to 5 days following administration. Inpatient titration of the insulin regimen is commonly needed for maintenance of glycemic control during this time. Insulin doses during treatment with betamethasone typically need to be increased by the first day after the first betamethasone dose (day 2 of betamethasone therapy) by 10, 40, 40, 20, and 20%, respectively, on days 2–6 after the first betamethasone dose.[30]

PRETERM BIRTH AND PROGESTERONE

Progesterone typically is given from 16 to 36 weeks of gestation in women with a history of preterm birth at doses of 250 mg intramuscularly weekly or intravaginal suppository daily. This may cause increased insulin resistance and hyperglycemia, and insulin should be adjusted accordingly; however, the glycemic rise is typically less than that observed with betamethasone therapy.

CELIAC DISEASE

Women with diabetes and celiac disease may require hospitalization for abdominal symptomatology during pregnancy. Women with celiac disease are at increased risk for miscarriage, preterm labor, and fetal growth restriction, which are all independently associated with diabetes. There is a lack of data on management of coexisting celiac disease and diabetes during pregnancy. Celiac disease can make the medical management of diabetes difficult because of the constraints of the diet and high glycemic index which is found in some gluten-free foods. For women with concurrent celiac disease and diabetes, we recommend inpatient nutrition consultation by the RD or RDN.

PERIPARTUM MANAGEMENT

During the peripartum period, clinical care goals include preventing maternal hyperglycemia and other hyperglycemia-related adverse outcomes. Maternal glycemic control during labor is associated with neonatal hypoglycemia, independent of antepartum glycemic control.[31,32] Reduced neonatal hypoglycemia among offspring of mothers with preexisting and gestational diabetes has been associated with maternal euglycemia achieved through insulin and dextrose infusion protocols.[31,33,34] Both the American College of Obstetrics and Gynecology and the American College of Endocrinology recommend the goal glucose range of 70–110 mg/dL during labor and delivery for both gestational and pregestational diabetes.[35,36] Similarly, the Endocrine Society recommends a target blood glucose range of 72–126 mg/dL during labor and delivery for women with preexisting and gestational diabetes.[5] Several studies have shown that maternal glycemia during labor is inversely related to neonatal hypoglycemia (Table 21.2). Some studies have suggested that higher levels of maternal glycemia (15–30 mg/dL higher than the 110 mg/dL upper range recommended) may be permissible during labor and delivery without increased risk of neonatal hypoglycemia.[37–39]

In one study of women with GDM, neonatal hypoglycemia occurred despite maternal glycemia falling within the recommended goals, suggesting that other factors may be affecting the risk of neonatal hypoglycemia.[40] Two large randomized controlled trials in patients with GDM also showed a nonsignificant trend toward lowering of neonatal hypoglycemia with targeted treatment of gestational diabetes compared with placebo care (no treatment of GDM).[41,42]

For most pregnant women with pregestational diabetes, glycemic management at induction of labor includes an IV infusion of regular insulin carefully titrated with low-dose dextrose infusion. Women with well-controlled T2D on SQ insulin may remain on this regimen during labor, unless glycemic targets are not met, in which case an IV infusion of regular insulin should be started. Similarly, in women with T1D of more recent onset who are well controlled and without signs of brittle diabetes or a recent history of DKA (e.g., glycemic patterns suggestive of residual β-cell function), consideration of remaining on a subcutaneous regimen during labor is an option. In light of the ketosis-prone state of pregnancy and the increased potential for delivery complications, however, careful consideration and review of pros and cons with the patient are recommended. Regardless of the type of diabetes, transition to IV insulin is recommended if glycemic control has not been achieved with the SQ regimen (glucose >70–110 mg/dL range × 2). There are several published protocols for IV insulin and dextrose infusion for the treatment of preexisting diabetes during

Table 21.2—Peripartum maternal glucose targets and frequency of neonatal hypoglycemia

Article	Patients (n), type of diabetes	HbA1c at delivery (%)	Glucose targets (mg/dL) (mmol/L)	Maternal hypoglycemia (n)/severe hypoglycemia (n)	Neonatal hypoglycemia, n (%)	Insulin protocol	Findings
Taylor et al.[34]	107, T1DM	7.2 mean HbA1c during pregnancy	72-144 mg/dL (4-8)	13/0	50 (46.7%) (<2.5 mmol/L or 45 mg/dL)	500 ml 10% dextrose to contain 16 units Actrapid insulin and 10 mmol KCl per bag. This was given over 8 h (i.e. 1 ml/min) via an infusion pump	Neonatal hypoglycemia is associated with maternal glucoses during labor more so than HbA1c during pregnancy
Barrett et al.[37]	137 23 PDM (18 T1DM, 5 T2DM), 114 GDM (52 diet-controlled, 62 on insulin)	Not provided	72-144 mg/dL (4-8) (met by 129 patients)	11	30 (21.9%) (<2.6 mmol/L or 47 mg/dL)	Intravenous dextrose and insulin infusion (details not provided)	Mostly women with GDM, neonatal hypoglycemia occurred despite maternal glucoses <144 mg/dL
Lepercq et al.[39]	174 patients, T1DM 229 pregnancies	6.0 +/- 0.8 in group 1 (induced labor) and 6.0 +/- 0.9 in group 2 (spontaneous labor)	61-141 mg/dL (3.4–7.8)	16/0	30 (13%)	10% dextrose (80 ml/h) intravenous was given along with short-acting insulin, starting at 1 IU/h intravenous	With slightly broader glucose range during labor, there were not higher rates of neonatal hypoglycemia
Rosenberg et al.[40]	36, 28 insulin requiring GDM, 8 PDM	Not provided	100 mg/dL	0	5 (13.9%)	5% dextrose in normal saline at 125 mL/hr and a continuous insulin drip vs glucose containing intravenous fluids alternating with non-glucose containing fluids depending on glucose	In patients with insulin-requiring GDM with glycemic goals at target during labor, neonatal hypoglycemia still occurred

PDM = preexisting diabetes
GDM = gestational diabetes
T1DM = type 1 diabetes mellitus
T2DM = type 2 diabetes mellitus

pregnancy.[26,35,39] For planned inductions or cesarean sections, the usual dose of intermediate or long-acting insulin is given at bedtime and the morning dose is held. The patient is typically kept without eating, and IV insulin and normal saline infusion are begun. Once active labor begins or glucose is <70 mg/dL, the normal saline infusion is changed to 5% dextrose, infused at a rate of 100–150 cc/h (2.5 mg/kg/min) with a goal of achieving glucose near 100 mg/dL. Glucose levels are checked hourly with a bedside glucose meter and insulin and dextrose infusion rates are adjusted according to blood glucose with a goal range of 70–110 mg/dL. A bolus of insulin typically is not given before starting the insulin infusion. In women with T1D, a dextrose infusion is needed during active and prolonged labor to prevent ketosis. In women with GDM, euglycemia can be maintained without insulin infusion in most cases.[43]

For pregnant women on CSII, there are two options for peripartum glucose management: discontinuation of CSII and beginning IV insulin infusion versus continuing insulin pump therapy.[8] Typically, pregnant women transition to an IV insulin infusion for optimal glycemic control and safety during labor and delivery. Some women who are in excellent control on insulin pumps and in whom an uncomplicated delivery is anticipated, can remain on their pumps during labor and delivery with careful attention to changing insulin requirements during labor and in the immediate postpartum period. A small retrospective observational study suggests that maintenance of insulin pump therapy with a reduction of basal rates during active labor may be safe in both vaginal deliveries and cesarean sections.[44] Of note, in this study, glycemic goals were broader than the goals recommended in the U.S. (70–140 mg/dL vs. 70–110 mg/dL, respectively). Care should be taken to reduce the risk of DKA during labor in women with T1D using CSII because of the possible occlusion of infusion sites during labor and kinking of tubing. Furthermore, unexpected changes may arise that prevent a woman from managing her insulin pump during labor, such as anesthesia, sedation, and clinical deterioration. It generally is not considered safe to have a third party (medical staff or family) manage a patient's insulin pump if the patient is not able to do so. If continuation of an insulin pump is chosen for a particular patient, pump settings need to be adjusted during labor and the postpartum period. If CSII is maintained, consent should be obtained and documented. Basal rates typically need to be reduced by 50% during the second stage of labor and postpartum. In the peripartum period, reasons for discontinuing the pump and starting an IV insulin infusion include hyperglycemia (glucose above the recommended 70–110 mg/dL range × 2), preeclampsia, chorioamnionitis, and placental abruption or urgent cesarean section, among others.

Once oral feeding resumes postdelivery, SQ injection of rapid-acting insulin (such as aspart or lispro) is needed for carbohydrate intake despite the continuation of the IV insulin infusion to avoid hypoglycemia associated with uptitration of the drip.

Women with Gestational Diabetes

Labor's effect to lower glucose is often likened to prolonged exercise, and in most women with GDM, labor has a glucose regulatory effect. On the basis of observational studies, the majority (86%) of women with GDM do not require insulin therapy during labor to achieve glycemic targets. Women who do require insulin therapy during labor are generally suboptimally controlled in the antepartum period or did not have standard perinatal care.[42] In such women, the GDM diagnosis may be misleading and poor control could indicate pregestational T2D or T1D, in which case careful transitional insulin and insulin therapy in the early postpartum period may be indicated.

KEY POINTS FOR INPATIENT GLYCEMIC MANAGEMENT DURING THE PERIPARTUM PERIOD:

- Recognize and treat DKA early
- During labor, glycemic goals are 70–110 mg/dL
- Insulin infusion and low-dose dextrose protocols should be used in most patients with preexisting diabetes during labor and delivery
- Use of insulin pumps may be continued in select patients who achieve glycemic goals during labor
- SQ insulin injection regimen may be continued in select patients with mild well-controlled T2D
- Most patients with GDM can achieve euglycemia during labor without IV insulin
- U-500 may be used for severe insulin resistance with careful patient and staff education
- Flexibility of insulin and dietary regimen, and engagement of patient and family in care plan, is important
- Education of care team, including nursing staff, on parameters specific to diabetes in pregnancy (e.g., risk of DKA, use of insulin drip, CSII, and CGM) is paramount

THE POSTPARTUM PERIOD

The period of time between early labor, peak labor and parturition, and placental delivery is a time of dramatic metabolic flux. Following the delivery of the placenta, the physiological insulin requirement generally falls sharply in women with both T1D and T2D. This is presumed to be due to withdrawal of human placental lactogen (HPL) and other hormones produced by the placenta at increasing concentrations with advancing gestation.[45] Other factors are likely at play however, such as a fall in the elevated levels of cytokines and plasma lipid concentrations identified to be present during later pregnancy.[46,47] The potentially prominent role of cytokines may explain why some women with diabetes who have peripartum complications may not have dramatically improved insulin sensitivity and may require careful monitoring and uninterrupted insulin therapy. As discussed in the following section, breast-feeding is another factor that may improve insulin sensitivity in the later postpartum period, and hence lower insulin requirements after delivery.[48]

GLYCEMIC GOALS IN THE POSTPARTUM PERIOD

In the postpartum period, glycemic goals are altered to reflect those considered reasonable and standard for the adult inpatient population. Although data are lacking to support specific postpartum glycemic targets, the ADA and the American College of Endocrinology have suggested a glucose goal of 100–139 mg/dL before meals and <180 mg/dL at all times during a typical hospital stay, with monitoring of glucose before meals in noncritically ill adult medical and surgical inpatients. In patients who are critically ill, the glycemic goals during therapy with an IV insulin protocol may vary, but the recommended goal ranges generally approximate the range from 140 to 180 mg/dl. These goals, however, should be individualized to the specific patient and clinical scenario.[49] For example, if chorioamnionitis or wound infection is present, tighter glycemic goals may be indicated.

WOMEN WITH PREGESTATIONAL DIABETES

Although there are no randomized studies or other rigorous data to support a specific insulin reduction protocol for the postpartum period, insulin doses should be reduced proactively by 25–50%,[8,35] depending on peripartum glucose control to prevent maternal hypoglycemia. For example, if glucose control prepartum was suboptimal and insulin was continued during labor, the planned insulin reduction may be 25%. If glycemic control was optimal, and the woman plans to breast-feed, a 50% reduction may be more appropriate. Eating should be encouraged after delivery, regardless of the route of delivery, to avoid hypoglycemia. For the majority of women who are stable and able to eat on the general postpartum ward, SQ insulin should be proactively dosed and divided to support estimated basal, nutritional, and supplemental insulin needs per standard guidelines and practice in adults.[49] Insulin-requiring women who are not expected to take in calories in the next 8 h should have frequent glucose monitoring and may require IV dextrose therapy to maintain optimal glycemia. Women requiring intensive monitoring because of postpartum complications should be considered for variable-rate continuous IV insulin therapy per standardized protocol. Moreover, special considerations apply to women with T1D as compared with T2D or other subtypes.

TYPE 1 DIABETES

Patients with T1DM are expected to require basal insulin throughout labor and the postpartum period. Although many women experience mild hypoglycemia and extremely low insulin needs during labor and immediately after delivery, it is difficult to predict which women are more likely to experience ketoacidosis because of a gap in basal insulin therapy. For this reason, it is best to formally transition all women with known or suspected T1D to an insulin regimen that (1) includes and prioritizes a long or intermediate acting basal insulin such as NPH or glargine and (2) is dosed to overlap with the insulin infusion by at least 2 h. Once food intake resumes, the antepartum insulin-to-carbohydrate ratios may be decreased by half to a third, and correction factors are increased by a similar percentage to accommodate higher insulin sensitivity in the postpartum state. Women with brittle diabetes, severe gastroparesis, preeclampsia, or delivery complications (blood loss, infection, thrombosis) may require a longer duration on IV insulin, and timing the transition to SQ regimen should be tailored to their clinical status.

Women who were using CSII antepartum may restart with a reduction of predelivery basal rates by 30–50%. The basal dose is typically reduced by 50% of a patient's peripartum basal needs and slightly lower than the prepregnancy basal insulin requirement. In many cases, there is basal insulin "onboard," which should be considered in determining the appropriate timing and dosage of the basal insulin dose. To avoid hypoglycemia after the transition to SQ insulin while ensuring adequate insulin overlap, it is reasonable to continue the IV dextrose infusion for several hours. Glucose should be monitored during sleep on the first night after delivery to prevent hypoglycemia. Insulin-to-carbohydrate ratios and correction doses (insulin sensitivity) should both be loosened (i.e., less insulin given for meals and for correction of hyperglycemia). If breast-feeding is planned, a slight further reduction in insulin doses, especially basal insulin, and frequent snacking are recommended.

TYPE 2 DIABETES

Depending on pregestational glucose control and medication requirement, a percentage of women with T2D may not require medication therapy in the immediate postpartum period. Metformin, glyburide, and most insulins are considered safe to use when breast-feeding.[50]

TRANSITIONING TO HOME

Although most women with true GDM will no longer have glucose intolerance after delivery, it is important to engage them in self-care and monitoring, and arrange for postpartum testing before discharge given the implication of their diagnosis on future health risks. Not only are women at risk of GDM in subsequent pregnancies,[48] the risk of developing overt T2D accumulates over time and is sevenfold higher than in women without gestational diabetes.[48,51] One relatively recent investigation reported subsequent diabetes rates of >90% in German women who required insulin during pregnancy.[52] A postgestational 75g oral glucose tolerance test is recommended per ADA guidelines in the outpatient setting at 6–12 weeks postpartum after the effects of pregnancy have resolved.[53,54] If negative, women with GDM should be screened every 1–3 years with any standard diabetes screening test.[53]

Women with pregestational diabetes should continue self-monitoring of blood glucose (SMBG) according to a schedule that is personalized for them and considers their early postpartum glucose control, their medications, and expected change over time. For women who required insulin before pregnancy, SMBG is recommended fasting, premeal, and postmeal. SMBG in the fasting state and 2 h postmeal is indicated both to determine insulin requirements and ensure safety. Prompt follow-up with an endocrinologist or internist is encouraged.

For women with T2D who appear to require oral agents only (e.g., metformin), daily SMBG is a minimal requirement until outpatient follow-up occurs. Women who are discharged on sulfonylurea therapy should be advised of the risk of hypoglycemia and SMBG is recommended at least twice daily.

A preponderance of evidence also supports encouraging women with GDM or overt diabetes to breast-feed their babies and for >3 months whenever possible.[5] Breast-feeding lowers fasting plasma glucose and insulin levels and is associated with reduced prevalence of subsequent diabetes both at the postpartum screen and after a decade.[48,52,55]

TEAM-BASED CARE

Management of a pregnant woman with diabetes admitted either for acute antepartum conditions or for delivery of her infant is complex. Therefore, teams of physicians, midlevel providers and nurses as well as RDs or RDNs, CDEs, pharmacists, and social workers are needed to deliver the best care. Multiple studies have shown that a patient-centered care plan with multiple specialists integrated to provide detailed, specific care is the best model for caring for diabetes during pregnancy.[9] An integrated approach to health care of diabetes during pregnancy yields the best perinatal maternal and neonatal outcomes and lowers total health-care costs.[5,9] The ADA recommends shared responsibility for health care during pregnancy between a pregnant woman and her medical providers and family.[9] The diabetes self-management education team consists of multiple clinicians that coordinate care for the pregnant woman with diabetes. Members of the team include endocrinologists, obstetricians, perinatologists, maternal fetal medicine specialists, nurses, RDs or RDNs, social workers, CDEs, ophthalmologists, and other health-care professionals specifically trained in the care of women with diabetes during pregnancy.[9] At times other specialists are needed, including cardiologists, podiatrists, nephrologists, and mental health providers. A team approach to care has shown lasting changes in self-management behaviors both during pregnancy and following delivery, which helps prepare the woman with diabetes for her next desired pregnancy.[56]

In the hospital, effective communication between the nursing team and other members of any interdisciplinary team is key. Communication focuses on consulting, collaborating, and therapeutic interactions to build morale and accomplish goals. Mutual respect and trust among members of the team lead to better care and patient outcomes. Communication between the endocrinologist or other diabetes specialist who cared for the patient before admission, the inpatient on-call obstetrician, and nurses of various shifts is crucial to ensure that the sudden changes in insulin requirements postpartum do not lead to lapses in care that could either cause significant hyper- or hypoglycemia during the postpartum period or after discharge. Consistent and data-filled provider transitions or hand-offs minimize safety gaps both throughout the admission and following discharge into the community.

REFERENCES

1. Albrecht SS, et al. Diabetes trends among delivery hospitalizations in the U.S., 1994–2004. *Diabetes Care* 2010;33(4):768–773

2. Temple RC, et al. Glycaemic control throughout pregnancy and risk of pre-eclampsia in women with type I diabetes. *BJOG* 2006;113(11):1329–1332

3. Evers IM, de Valk HW, Visser GH. Risk of complications of pregnancy in women with type 1 diabetes: nationwide prospective study in the Netherlands. *BMJ* 2004;328(7445):915

4. Persson M, Norman M, Hanson U. Obstetric and perinatal outcomes in type 1 diabetic pregnancies: A large, population-based study. *Diabetes Care* 2009;32(11): 2005–2009

5. Blumer I, et al. Diabetes and pregnancy: an Endocrine Society clinical practice guideline. *J Clin Endocrinol Metab* 2013;98(11):4227–4249

6. Colom C, Corcoy R. Maturity onset diabetes of the young and pregnancy. *Best Pract Res Clin Endocrinol Metab* 2010;24(4):605–615

7. Misra S, Dornhorst A. Gestational diabetes mellitus: primum non nocere. *Diabetes Care* 2012;35(9):1811–1813

8. Gabbe SG, Carpenter LB, Garrison AE. New strategies for glucose control in patients with type 1 and type 2 diabetes mellitus in pregnancy. *Clin Obstet Gynecol* 2007;50(4):1014–1024

9. Kitzmiller JL, et al. Managing preexisting diabetes for pregnancy: summary of evidence and consensus recommendations for care. *Diabetes Care* 2008;31(5):1060–1079

10. Bruttomesso D, et al. Type 1 diabetes control and pregnancy outcomes in women treated with continuous subcutaneous insulin infusion (CSII) or with insulin glargine and multiple daily injections of rapid-acting insulin analogues (glargine-MDI). *Diabetes Metab* 2011;37(5):426–431

11. Negrato CA, et al. Glargine vs. NPH insulin therapy in pregnancies complicated by diabetes: an observational cohort study. *Diabetes Res Clin Pract* 2010;89(1):46–51

12. Price N, Bartlett C, Gillmer M. Use of insulin glargine during pregnancy: a case-control pilot study. *BJOG* 2007;114(4):453–457

13. Hatipoglu B, Soni S, Espinosa V. Glycemic control with continuous subcutaneous insulin infusion with use of U-500 insulin in a pregnant patient. *Endocr Pract* 2006;12(5):542–544

14. Okeigwe I, et al. U-500R and aspart insulin for the treatment of severe insulin resistance in pregnancy associated with pregestational diabetes. *J Perinatol* 2013;33(3):235–238

15. Zuckerwise LC, et al. Pregestational diabetes with extreme insulin resistance: use of U-500 insulin in pregnancy. *Obstet Gynecol* 2012;120(2 Pt. 2):439–442.

16. Mello G, et al. Continuous subcutaneous insulin infusion (CSII) versus multiple daily injections (MDI) of rapid-acting insulin analogues and detemir in type 1 diabetic (T1D) pregnant women. *J Matern Fetal Neonatal Med* 2015;28(3):276–280

17. Kallas-Koeman MM, et al. Insulin pump use in pregnancy is associated with lower HbA1c without increasing the rate of severe hypoglycaemia or diabetic ketoacidosis in women with type 1 diabetes. *Diabetologia* 2014;57(4):681–689
18. Langer O, et al. A comparison of glyburide and insulin in women with gestational diabetes mellitus. *N Engl J Med* 2000;343(16):1134–1138
19. Rowan JA, et al. Metformin versus insulin for the treatment of gestational diabetes. *N Engl J Med* 2008;358(19):2003–2015
20. Guo RX, et al. Diabetic ketoacidosis in pregnancy tends to occur at lower blood glucose levels: case-control study and a case report of euglycemic diabetic ketoacidosis in pregnancy. *J Obstet Gynaecol Res* 2008;34(3):324–330
21. Madaan M, et al. Diabetic ketoacidosis occurring with lower blood glucose levels in pregnancy: a report of two cases. *J Reprod Med* 2012;57(9–10):452–455
22. Tarif N, Al Badr W. Euglycemic diabetic ketoacidosis in pregnancy. *Saudi J Kidney Dis Transpl* 2007;18(4):590–593
23. Tarif N, Al Badr W. Euglycemic diabetic ketoacidosis in pregnancy. *Saudi J Kidney Dis Transpl* 2007;18(4):590–593
24. Sibai BM, Viteri OA. Diabetic ketoacidosis in pregnancy. *Obstet Gynecol* 2014; 123(1):167–178
25. Parker JA, Conway DL. Diabetic ketoacidosis in pregnancy. *Obstet Gynecol Clin North Am* 2007;34(3):533–543, xii
26. Garrison EA, Jagasia S. Inpatient management of women with gestational and pregestational diabetes in pregnancy. *Curr Diab Rep* 2014;14(2):457
27. Klemetti MM, et al. Obstetric and perinatal outcome in type 1 diabetes patients with diabetic nephropathy during 1988–2011. *Diabetologia*, 2015;58(4): 678–686
28. Arun CS, Taylor R. Influence of pregnancy on long-term progression of retinopathy in patients with type 1 diabetes. *Diabetologia* 2008;51(6):1041–1045
29. Rasmussen KL, et al. Progression of diabetic retinopathy during pregnancy in women with type 2 diabetes. *Diabetologia* 2010;53(6):1076–1083
30. Mathiesen ER, et al. Insulin dose during glucocorticoid treatment for fetal lung maturation in diabetic pregnancy: test of an algorithm [correction of analgoritm]. *Acta Obstet Gynecol Scand* 2002;81(9):835–839
31. Andersen O, et al. Influence of the maternal plasma glucose concentration at delivery on the risk of hypoglycaemia in infants of insulin-dependent diabetic mothers. *Acta Paediatr Scand* 1985;74(2):268–273
32. Nold JL, Georgieff MK. Infants of diabetic mothers. *Pediatr Clin North Am* 2004;51(3):619–637, viii
33. Balsells M, et al. Gestational diabetes mellitus: metabolic control during labour. *Diabetes Nutr Metab* 2000;13(5):257–262

34. Taylor R, et al. Clinical outcomes of pregnancy in women with type 1 diabetes. *Obstet Gynecol* 2002;99(4):537–541
35. ACOG Committee on Practice Bulletins. ACOG Practice Bulletin. Clinical management guidelines for obstetrician-gynecologists. Number 60, March 2005. Pregestational diabetes mellitus. *Obstet Gynecol* 2005;105(3):675–685
36. Garber AJ, et al. American College of Endocrinology position statement on inpatient diabetes and metabolic control. *Endocr Pract* 2004;10(Suppl. 2):4–9
37. Barrett HL, Morris J, McElduff A. Watchful waiting: a management protocol for maternal glycaemia in the peripartum period. *Aust N Z J Obstet Gynaecol* 2009;49(2):162–167
38. Carron Brown S, et al. Effect of management policy upon 120 Type 1 diabetic pregnancies: policy decisions in practice. *Diabet Med* 1999;16(7):573–578
39. Lepercq J, et al. A standardized protocol to achieve normoglycaemia during labour and delivery in women with type 1 diabetes. *Diabetes Metab* 2008; 34(1):33–37
40. Rosenberg VA, et al. Intrapartum maternal glycemic control in women with insulin requiring diabetes: a randomized clinical trial of rotating fluids versus insulin drip. *Am J Obstet Gynecol* 2006;195(4):1095–1099
41. Crowther CA, et al. Effect of treatment of gestational diabetes mellitus on pregnancy outcomes. *N Engl J Med* 2005;352(24):2477–2486
42. Landon MB, et al. A multicenter, randomized trial of treatment for mild gestational diabetes. *N Engl J Med* 2009;361(14):1339–1348
43. Flores-Le Roux JA, et al. Peripartum metabolic control in gestational diabetes. *Am J Obstet Gynecol* 2010;202(6):568, e1–6
44. Fresa R, et al. Experiences of continuous subcutaneous insulin infusion in pregnant women with type 1 diabetes during delivery from four Italian centers: a retrospective observational study. *Diabetes Technol Ther* 2013;15(4):328–334
45. Ryan EA, Enns L. Role of gestational hormones in the induction of insulin resistance. *J Clin Endocrinol Metab* 1988;67(2):341–347
46. Kirwan JP, et al. TNF-alpha is a predictor of insulin resistance in human pregnancy. *Diabetes* 2002;51(7):2207–2213
47. Xiang AH, et al. Multiple metabolic defects during late pregnancy in women at high risk for type 2 diabetes. *Diabetes* 1999;48(4):848–854
48. Gunderson EP, et al. Lactation intensity and postpartum maternal glucose tolerance and insulin resistance in women with recent GDM: the SWIFT cohort. *Diabetes Care* 2012;35(1):50–56
49. Moghissi ES, et al. American Association of Clinical Endocrinologists and American Diabetes Association consensus statement on inpatient glycemic control. *Diabetes Care* 2009;32(6):1119–1131

50. Kjos SL. After pregnancy complicated by diabetes: postpartum care and education. *Obstet Gynecol Clin North Am* 2007;34(2):335–349, x
51. Bellamy L, et al. Type 2 diabetes mellitus after gestational diabetes: a systematic review and meta-analysis. *Lancet* 2009;373(9677):1773–1779
52. Ziegler AG, et al. Long-term protective effect of lactation on the development of type 2 diabetes in women with recent gestational diabetes mellitus. *Diabetes* 2012;61(12):3167–3171
53. American Diabetes Association. Standards of medical care in diabetes—2015: summary of revisions. *Diabetes Care* 2015;38(Suppl.):S4
54. Committee on Practice Bulletins—Obstetrics. Practice Bulletin No. 137: Gestational diabetes mellitus. *Obstet Gynecol* 2013;122(2 Pt. 1):406–416
55. O'Reilly MW, et al. Atlantic DIP: high prevalence of abnormal glucose tolerance post partum is reduced by breast-feeding in women with prior gestational diabetes mellitus. *Eur J Endocrinol* 2011;165(6):953–959
56. Feig DS, Cleave B, Tomlinson G. Long-term effects of a diabetes and pregnancy program: does the education last? *Diabetes Care* 2006;29(3):526–530

Chapter 22

Diabetic Ketoacidosis and Hyperglycemic Hyperosmolar State

J. Sonya Haw, MD,[1] Robert Rushakoff, MD,[2] and Guillermo E. Umpierrez, MD[1]

EPIDEMIOLOGY

Diabetic ketoacidosis (DKA) and hyperglycemic hyperosmolar state (HHS) are serious acute metabolic complications of diabetes. Recent data indicate there are more than 144,000 hospital admissions per year for DKA and HHS in the U.S. and an overall upward trend, with a 30% increase in the annual number of cases between 1995 and 2009 (Figure 22.1).[1] The incidence of HHS is lower than DKA and accounts for <1% of all primary diabetic admissions. Mortality rate from DKA or HHS has significantly decreased during the past 2 decades (Figure 22.1*B*). In children and young adults, the overall DKA mortality is less than 1%, but a rate >5% is reported in the elderly and in patients with concomitant life-threatening illnesses.[2] Mortality in patients with HHS is higher than in DKA and is between 5 and 16% of patients.[3] The prognosis of both conditions is substantially worse at the extremes of age in the presence of coma, hypotension, and severe comorbidities.[4,5] In adult patients, mortality of patients with hyperglycemic crises increases with aging, with mortality rates for those >65–75 years reaching 20–40%.[1] In the older age-groups, the major cause of death relates to the underlying medical illness (i.e., trauma, infection) that precipitated ketoacidosis,[6] but in the younger patient, mortality is more likely to be due to the metabolic disarray.[7]

Both DKA and HHS are characterized by insulinopenia, dehydration, and severe hyperglycemia. Clinically, they differ only by the degree of dehydration and the severity of metabolic acidosis.[3] DKA has long been considered a key clinical feature of type 1 diabetes (T1D), but in recent years, DKA has been increasingly reported in adult patients with type 2 diabetes (T2D).[8] In community-based studies, >40% of patients with DKA are >40 years and >20% are >55 years.[8] In children, T2D now accounts for up to one-half of all newly diagnosed diabetes between the ages of 10 and 21 years.[7,9] The SEARCH for Diabetes in Youth Study reported that 31.1% of participants <20 years of age with T1D presented with DKA as compared with 5.7% of youth with T2D.[10] Patients with T2D may develop DKA under stressful conditions, such as trauma, surgery, or infections,[8] but some children and adult patients present with DKA without an apparent precipitating cause.[11] HHS occurs most commonly in older patients with T2D, but also occurs in children and young adults.[6]

[1]Department of Medicine, Emory University, Atlanta, GA. [2]Department of Medicine, University of California San Francisco (UCSF), San Francisco, CA.

 DOI: 10.2337/9781580406086.22

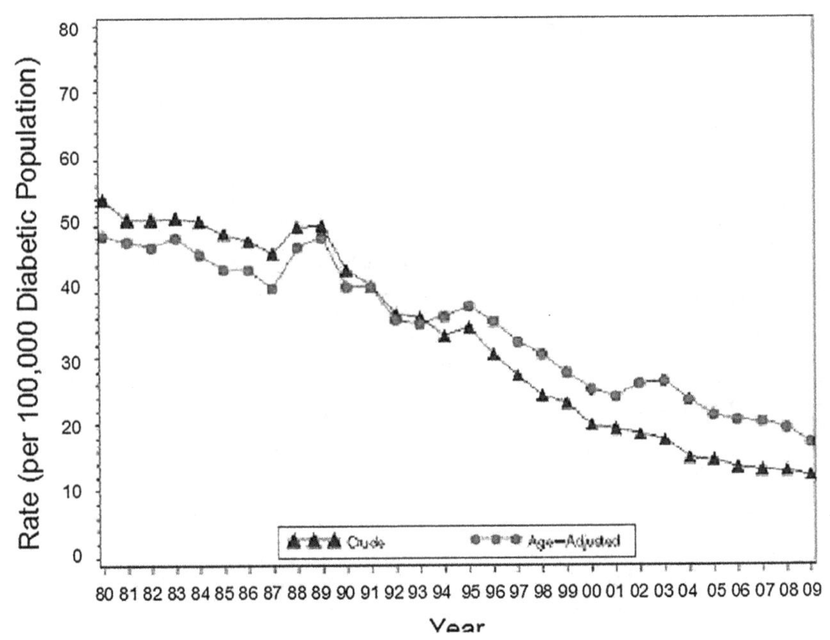

Figure 22.1—Epidemiology of hyperglycemic crisis in the U.S. *A*: Number (in thousands) of hospital discharges with diabetic ketoacidosis (DKA) as first-listed diagnosis, U.S., 1988–2009. *B*: Crude and age-adjusted death rates for hyperglycemic crises as underlying cause per 100,000 diabetic population, U.S., 1980–2009. The age-adjusted rate decreased 64% from 48.4 per 100,000 diabetic population in 1980 to 17.3 per 100,000 diabetic population in 2009.

Source: Adapted from Centers for Disease Control and Prevention, National Center for Chronic Disease Prevention and Health Promotion, Division of Diabetes Translation (www.cdc.gov/diabetes/data/national.html).

PATHOGENESIS

The basic underlying mechanism for DKA and HHS is the reduction in the net effective concentration of circulating insulin coupled with a concomitant elevation of counterregulatory hormones (glucagon, catecholamines, cortisol, and growth hormone).[3,12] Hyperglycemia results from increased hepatic and renal glucose production (gluconeogenesis and glycogenolysis) and impaired glucose utilization in peripheral tissues (Figure 22.2). From a quantitative standpoint, increased hepatic glucose production represents the major pathogenic disturbance responsible for hyperglycemia in patients with DKA.[3] Increased gluconeogenesis results from the high availability of noncarbohydrate substrates (alanine, lactate,

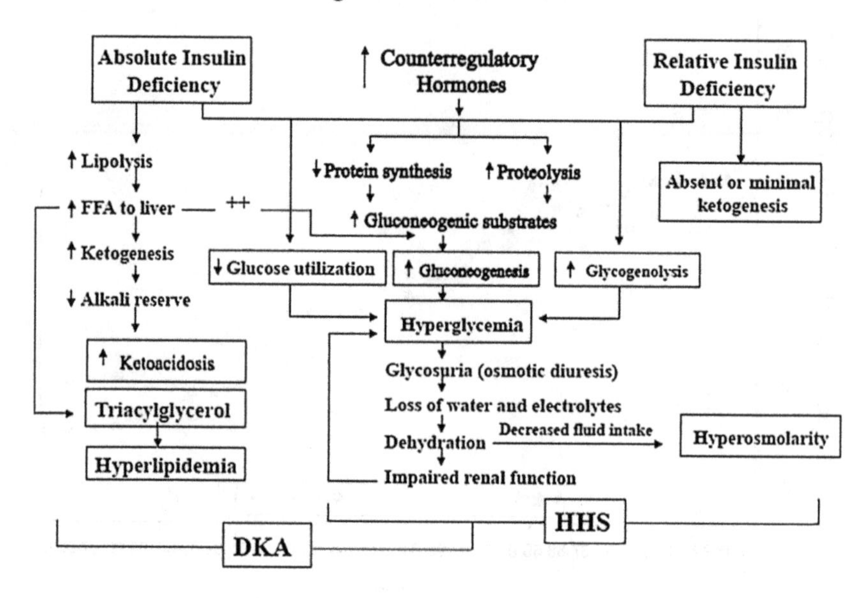

Figure 22.2—Pathogenesis of diabetic ketoacidosis (DKA) and hyperglycemic hyperosmolar state (HHS). Hyperglycemia results from increased hepatic glucose production and impaired glucose utilization in peripheral tissues (primarily muscle). From a quantitative standpoint, increased hepatic glucose production represents the major pathogenic disturbance responsible for hyperglycemia. Ketogenesis results from increased release of free fatty acids from adipose tissue. In the liver, free fatty acids are oxidized to ketone bodies. The two major ketone bodies are β-hydroxybutyrate and acetoacetic acid.

and glycerol in the liver and glutamine in the kidney) and from the increased activity of gluconeogenic enzymes.[12,13] In addition, hyperglycemia causes both an osmotic diuresis and decreased glomerular filtration rate, which further aggravate hyperglycemia.[3]

The mechanisms that underlie the increased production of ketones recently have been discussed in a number of reviews on DKA.[12,14] The combination of insulin deficiency and increased concentration of counterregulatory hormones causes the activation of hormone-sensitive lipase in adipose tissue. The increased activity of tissue lipase causes a breakdown of triglyceride into glycerol and free fatty acids (FFAs). In the liver, FFAs are oxidized to ketone bodies, a process predominantly stimulated by glucagon.[15] Increased concentration of glucagon lowers the hepatic levels of malonyl coenzyme A (CoA) by blocking the conversion of pyruvate to acetyl CoA through inhibition of acetyl CoA carboxylase,[15] the first rate-limiting enzyme in de novo fatty acid synthesis. Malonyl CoA inhibits carnitine palmitoyl-transferase I (CPT I), the rate-limiting enzyme for transesterification of fatty acyl CoA to fatty acyl carnitine, allowing oxidation of fatty acid to ketone bodies.[15] The increased fatty acyl CoA in DKA leads to increased ketogenesis in DKA.[15] Increased production of ketone bodies (acetoacetate and β-hydroxybutyrate) leads to ketonemia and metabolic acidosis.

Studies in animals and humans with diabetes have shown that lower insulin levels are needed for antilipolysis than for peripheral glucose uptake.[16] In HHS, there is not enough insulin secretion to maintain normoglycemia, but there is sufficient insulin to prevent exaggerated lipolysis and ketogenesis.[17] Patients with HHS have been shown to have higher insulin concentration and reduced concentration of FFA, cortisol, growth hormone, and glucagon compared with patients with DKA.[17]

A strong body of evidence indicates that DKA and HHS are associated with systemic inflammation and oxidative stress. Several studies have reported significant elevation of interleukin (IL)-6, -1B, and -8 and tumor necrosis factor-α (TNF-α) and increased counterregulatory hormones in patients with uncontrolled diabetes and ketoacidosis.[18] These elevations of circulating proinflammatory cytokines are reduced to normal levels promptly in response to insulin therapy and normalization of blood glucose concentration. Of interest, similar high levels of inflammation and oxidation markers are present in patients with DKA and HHS, indicating that hyperglycemia, independent of the presence of ketoacidosis, is the cause of the increase in proinflammatory cytokines.[18] The increased cytokine release during DKA and HHS results in capillary perturbation and endothelial dysfunction, which could explain why hyperglycemia is associated with poor outcomes in patients with acute myocardial infarction, stroke, and cardiac surgery.[19]

PRECIPITATING FACTORS

DKA is the initial manifestation of diabetes in 20% of adult patients and in up to 40% of children with T1D.[7,16] The most common precipitating factors for DKA include infections, coexisting illnesses, psychological stress, and poor compliance with therapy.[20,21] Infection accounts for 30–50% of cases, with urinary tract infections and pneumonia representing the majority of infections. Noncompliance and psychological factors account for a significant number of recurrent cases of DKA in inner-city populations.[20,22] Other less common precipitating causes are pancreatitis, cerebrovascular accident, alcohol abuse, myocardial infarction, and trauma.[8] Certain drugs that affect carbohydrate metabolism, including corticosteroids, thiazides, sympathomimetic agents, antipsychotics, and pentamidine, also may precipitate the development of DKA.[8,23] Recently, the sodium glucose cotransporter 2 (SGLT2) inhibitors, a new class of oral antidiabetic agents that decrease concentrations of plasma glucose by inhibiting proximal tubular reabsorption of glucose in the kidney, have been reported to be associated with the development of euglycemic DKA in patients with T1D and T2D.[24,25]

HHS commonly occurs in older adults with T2D, especially in residents of nursing homes who may not be aware of the need for hydration. Infection is the major precipitating factor occurring in 30–60% of HHS patients, with urinary tract infections and pneumonia being the most common infections.[6,26] Newly diagnosed diabetes is reported between 7 and 17% of patients admitted with HHS.[21] Other common precipitating causes of HHS include cerebrovascular and cardiac events, pancreatitis and use of certain drugs, including glucocorticoids, diazoxide, and β-blockers.[8,23]

PRESENTATION AND DIAGNOSIS

The typical clinical presentation of DKA and HHS includes a history of polyuria, polydipsia, weight loss, dehydration, weakness, clouded sensorium, altered respiratory status (Kussmaul breathing), and possibly coma. The clinical presentation of DKA usually develops rapidly, over a time span of <24–48 hours; in contrast, HHS usually evolves over several days to weeks. Nausea, vomiting, and abdominal pain are reported in 40–75% of cases of DKA[27] and are associated with a severe metabolic acidosis and with a history of alcohol or cocaine abuse. In a group of 200 consecutive patients with DKA, abdominal pain was present in 86% of patients with serum bicarbonate <5 mmol/L, in 66% of patients with levels between 5 and <10 mmol/L, in 36% of patients with levels between 10 and <15 mmol/L, and in 13% of patients with bicarbonate levels 15–18 mmol/L.[28] In the majority of patients, abdominal pain spontaneously resolves after correction of the metabolic disturbance.[27]

Physical findings may include poor skin turgor, Kussmaul respirations (if acidotic), tachycardia, hypotension, alteration in mental status, shock, and, ultimately, coma, which is more frequent in HHS. In some patients, focal neurologic signs and seizures may be the dominant clinical features, resulting in a common misdiagnosis of stroke.[29,30] Despite the focal nature of neurological findings, the neurologic manifestations often reverse completely after correction of the metabolic disorder.[30] The degree of mental obtundation has been shown to correlate with serum osmolarity in DKA and HHS.[26] A recent retrospective analysis, however, showed that the degree of acidosis predicted altered mental status better than osmolarity.[31]

LABORATORY FINDINGS

The syndrome of DKA is defined by a triad of hyperglycemia, ketosis, and metabolic acidosis. As indicated in Table 22.1, DKA can be classified as mild, moderate, or severe, depending on the extent of metabolic acidosis and level of sensorium.[2] The diagnostic criteria for HHS includes a plasma glucose concentration >600 mg/dL, a serum osmolality >320 mOsm/kg of water, and the absence of significant metabolic acidosis (Table 22.1). Approximately 30% of the patients with hyperglycemic crises have mixed features of DKA and HHS, presenting with severe hyperglycemia, high anion gap metabolic acidosis, positive ketones, and hyperosmolality.[32]

Table 22.1—Diagnostic Criteria for Diabetic Ketoacidosis (DKA) and Hyperglycemic Hyperosmolar State (HHS)

	DKS			**HHS**
	Mild	**Moderate**	**Severe**	
Plasma glucose (mg/dL)	>250	>250	>250	>600
Arterial pH	7.25–7.30	7.00–<7.24	<7.00	>7.30
Serum bicarbonate (mEq/L)	15–18	10–<15	< 10	>15
Urine ketone	Positive	Positive	Positive	Small
Serum ketone	Positive	Positive	Positive	Small
Effective Serum Osmolality	Variable	Variable	Variable	>320 mOsm/kg
Anion Gap	>10	>12	>12	<12
Alteration in sensorium	Alert	Alert/Drowsy	Stupor/Coma	Stupor/Coma

The presence of augmented ketosis is the key diagnostic feature of ketoacidosis. This can be assessed by increased acetoacetic acid, by the nitroprusside reaction, or by direct measurement of β-hydroxybutyrate, the main ketoacid in DKA.[33] The nitroprusside reaction has been shown to underestimate the level of ketosis. Direct measurement of β-hydroxybutyrate is available by fingerstick method, which is a more accurate indicator of ketoacidosis and response to medical treatment.[33]

Electrolyte abnormalities are common in patients with DKA and HHS on admission. The serum sodium is usually low because of the osmotic flux of water from the intracellular to the extracellular space in the presence of hyperglycemia. To assess the severity of sodium and water deficit, serum sodium may be corrected by adding 1.6 mg/dL to the measured serum sodium for each 100 mg/dL of glucose >100 mg/dL.[3] The admission serum potassium concentration usually is elevated in patients with DKA and HHS. Hyperkalemia is caused by a shift of potassium from the intracellular to the extracellular space because of acidemia, insulin deficiency, and hypertonicity. Similarly, the admission serum phosphate level may be normal or elevated because of metabolic acidosis.[3] In addition, leukocytosis in the absence of infection is common as well as an increased level of amylase, which is reported in 21 to 79% of patients with DKA.[34] Of note, there is little correlation between hyperamylasemia and the presence of symptoms or pancreatic imaging studies consistent with acute pancreatitis.[34]

TREATMENT

Several reviews and clinical guidelines have reported on the management of DKA and HHS.[2,3] The goals of therapy are to *1*) correct dehydration and circulatory volume deficit; *2*) correct hyperglycemia, ketosis, and hyperosmolality; *3*) correct electrolyte imbalances; and *4*) identify and treat precipitating events. During treatment, frequent monitoring of vital signs, mental status, blood glucose concentration, and acid-base status are needed to assess response to medical treatment. Patients should be admitted to an area with adequate nursing supervision and capability to monitor status and administer intravenous (IV) or frequent subcutaneous (SQ) insulin injections. The majority of patients with mild to moderate DKA can be safely managed in the emergency department or in stepdown units, and only patients with severe DKA or those with a critical illness as the precipitating cause (i.e., myocardial infarction, gastrointestinal bleeding, sepsis) should be treated in the intensive care unit.

FLUID THERAPY

IV hydration is a mainstay of management; it serves to decrease counter regulatory hormone concentrations, improve metabolic acidosis, and decrease serum glucose and ketones through urinary clearance. Patients with DKA and HHS are invariably volume depleted with an estimated water deficit of ~100 mL/kg of body weight.[3] The initial fluid replacement is most often isotonic saline to restore perfusion and expand intravascular volume. Subsequent fluid replacement choice and infusion rate are determined by hydration status, serum electrolytes, and urine output. Isotonic saline is usually continued in patients with low serum sodium, whereas patients with normal or elevated sodium or hyperosmolality often receive 0.45% NaCl. IV dextrose is added when the glucose is 200–250 mg/dL to avoid hypoglycemia and allow insulin therapy to continue. The choice and rate of subsequent fluid will be based on the patient's sodium concentration and hydration status. The water deficit can be estimated (Table 22.2), based on corrected serum sodium concentration, using the following

Table 22.2—Useful Formulas for the Evaluation of DKA and HHS

1. Calculation of anion gap (AG):

   $$AG = [Na+] - [Cl- + HCO3-]$$

2. Total and effective serum osmolality:

   $$\text{Total} = 2[Na+] + \frac{\text{glucose (mg/dL)}}{18} + \frac{\text{BUN (mg/dL)}}{2.8}$$

   $$\text{Effective} = 2[Na+] + \frac{\text{glucose (mg/dL)}}{18}$$

3. Corrected serum sodium:

   $$\text{Corrected } [Na+] = \frac{1.6 \times \text{glucose (mg/dl)} - 100}{100} + [\text{measured Na+}]$$

4. Total body water (TBW) deficit:

   $$\text{TBW deficit} = \frac{[\text{wt (kg)} \times 0.6] - [1 - (\text{corrected Na+})]}{140}$$

equation: water deficit = 0.6 × (body weight in kilograms) × (1 – [corrected sodium / 140]).[6] The goal is to replace half the estimated water deficit over a period of 24 h. Iatrogenic fluid overload can be avoided by frequent patient monitoring.

INSULIN THERAPY

The common practice of priming with an IV bolus of regular insulin has been shown to be unnecessary as long as a continuous infusion of IV regular insulin is initiated at a dose of 0.1 units/kg/h (Table 22.3).[35,36] The goal is to achieve a rate of decline of 50–100 mg/dL/h. Once the serum glucose has declined to ~250 mg/dL, an infusion of glucose (D5% 0.45 normal saline) should be started at 150–200 mL/h, and the insulin infusion rate should be reduced to 0.05 units/kg/h. Thereafter, the rate of insulin administration may need to be adjusted to maintain glucose levels at ~200 mg/dL, and this rate may need to be continued until ketoacidosis is resolved.

Patients with DKA also can be treated with SQ rapid-acting insulin analogs either every 1 or 2 h. If hourly, patients should receive an initial "priming" dose of rapid-acting insulin of 0.2 to 0.3 units/kg of body weight, followed by 0.1 unit/kg/h until blood glucose of 250 mg/dL is reached (Table 22.2). At that time, insulin

Table 22.3 —Treatment Protocol

1. IV Fluids

- 0.9% saline at 500–1,000 mL/hour for 2 h, then
- 0.45% saline at 250–500 mL/h until blood glucose <250 mg/dL, then
- Dextrose 5% in 0.45% saline at 150–250 ml/h until resolution of DKA

2. Insulin Therapy

IV regular insulin:

a) Give IV bolus of regular insulin of 0.1 U/kg
b) Start continuous insulin infusion at 0.1 U/kg/h
c) When blood glucose <250 mg/dL (13.8 mmol/L), change IV fluids to D5%–0.45% saline and reduce insulin infusion rate to 0.05 unit/kg/h to keep glucose ~200 mg/dL (11.1 mmol/l) until resolution of DKA

SQ rapid-acting insulin every 1 h (SQ-1 h):

a) Initial dose SQ: 0.2 U/kg of body weight, followed by 0.1 unit/kg/h
b) When blood glucose <250 mg/dL (13.8 mmol/L), change IV fluids to D5%–0.45% saline and reduce SQ rapid-acting insulin to 0.05 unit/kg/h to keep glucose ~200 mg/dL (11.1 mmol/l) until resolution of DKA

SQ rapid-acting insulin every 2 h (SQ-2 h):

a) Initial dose SQ: 0.3 U/kg of body weight, followed by 0.2 U/kg 1 h later, then
b) SQ rapid-acting insulin at 0.2 U/kg every 2 h
c) When blood glucose <250 mg/dL (13.8 mmol/L), change IV fluids to D5%–0.45% saline and reduce SQ rapid-acting insulin to 0.1 U/kg every 2 h to keep glucose ~200 mg/dL (11.1 mmol/l) until resolution of DKA

(continued)

Table 22.3 —Treatment Protocol *(continued)*

3. Potassium Replacement

a) Initially, if serum K^+ >5.5 mmol/L, do not give K^+ but check serum K^+ every 2 h
b) Add K^+ as needed based on subsequent values:

- K^+ = 4–5.5 mmol/L, add 20 mmol of KCl to each liter of IV fluid
- K^+ = 3–<4 mmol/L, add 40 mmol of KCl to each liter of IV fluid
- K^+ = <3 mmol/L, give 10–20 mmol of KCl per hour until serum K^+ >3 mmol/L, then add 40 mmol of KCl to each liter of IV fluid

4. Bicarbonate

- Arterial pH <6.9, administer 44.6 mEq of sodium bicarbonate in 200 ml 0.45% saline over 1 h until pH increases to 6.9–7.0
- Do not give bicarbonate if pH >7.0

5. Laboratory Assessment

Admission: Cell blood count with differential, complete metabolic profile, venous pH, and serum β-hydroxybutyrate.

During treatment: Basic metabolic profile (glucose, bicarbonate, sodium, potassium, chloride, urea, and creatinine), venous pH, phosphorus, and β-hydroxybutyrate at 2 h, 4 h, and every 4 h until resolution of DKA.

Glucose monitoring: During therapy, capillary blood glucose should be determined every 1–2 h at the bedside using a glucose oxidase reagent strip.

6. Transition to Subcutaneous (SQ) Insulin Therapy

- Continue insulin infusion until resolution of ketoacidosis (glucose <200 mg/dL, bicarbonate ≥18 mEq/L, pH ≥7.30, anion gap ≥14 mEq/L)
- Once resolved, begin SQ insulin regimen
- In patients with known diabetes who were receiving insulin before admission, restart previous insulin regimen if they had adequate glycemic control before admission
- In patients with newly diagnosed diabetes, start insulin at 0.6 units/kg/day
- Consider basal-bolus regimen with basal insulin (glargine once daily or detemir once or twice daily) and rapid-acting insulin analogs (lispro, aspart, glulisine) before meals
- To prevent recurrence of DKA during the transition period to SQ insulin, IV insulin should be continued for 2–4 h after SQ insulin is given

dose is reduced to 0.05 unit/kg/h, and the IV fluids changed to D5% 0.45 normal saline to maintain blood glucose ~200 mg/dL until resolution of DKA. Patients treated with SQ rapid-acting insulin analogs every 2 h should receive an initial dose of 0.3 unit/kg followed by 0.2 unit/kg 1 h later and subsequently every 2 h until blood glucose of 250 mg/dL is reached. At that time, insulin dose is reduced to 0.1 unit/kg every 2 h, and the IV fluids changed to D5% 0.45 normal saline to keep blood glucose ~200 mg/dL until resolution of DKA.

Low-dose insulin infusion protocols have been shown to be effective in patients with HHS with resolution of hyperglycemia in ~9±2 hours and improvement in mental status and hyperosmolality in 11±1 hours.[2,6,21] Despite the lack of prospective randomized studies in patients with HHS, the most recent ADA position statement on the management of hyperglycemic crises in adult patients proposed a single-treatment algorithm for the management of DKA and HHS.[2]

During therapy, capillary blood glucose should be determined every 1–2 h at the bedside and laboratory should be drawn every 4 h during therapy for determination of serum electrolytes, glucose, blood urea nitrogen, creatinine, phosphorus, and venous pH. Measurement of β-hydroxybutyrate levels correlates with resolution of ketoacidosis.[2]

POTASSIUM

Total body potassium depletion is present in patients with DKA and HHS, although initial serum potassium levels may be normal or even high. Initiation of fluids and insulin will lower serum potassium concentrations and as a result, hypokalemic cardiac arrest may ensue without appropriate attention to this critical concept. Consequently, most patients with hyperglycemic crises require early IV potassium therapy. Potassium should be initiated when the serum level is below the upper limit of normal, generally 5–5.5 mmol/L with the goal level of 4–5 mmol/L during therapy.[2,3] The exception to this is the patient with low urine output or severely decreased renal function; in this case, potassium should be repleted if it is low, and the patient should be monitored carefully.

The total body potassium deficit in patients with DKA and HHS has been estimated to be ~ 3–5 mmol/kg of body weight.[37] Despite this deficit, most patients with DKA have a serum potassium level at or above the upper limits of normal on presentation.[37,38] These high levels occur because of a shift of potassium from the intracellular to the extracellular space because of acidosis, insulin deficiency, and hypertonicity. Both insulin therapy and correction of acidosis decrease serum potassium levels by stimulating cellular potassium uptake in peripheral tissues. In patients with serum potassium levels <3.3 mmol/L, aggressive potassium replacement should begin immediately by an infusion of potassium chloride at a rate of 20 mmol/h, and insulin therapy should be delayed for 1 or 2 h until sufficient potassium is given.[3] In addition, for patients with severe renal failure, end-stage renal disease, or with low urine output, frequent monitoring and cautious potassium replacement is needed to avoid hyperkalemia.

BICARBONATE

Bicarbonate therapy in DKA is seldom indicated and generally limited to patients with severe metabolic acidosis (pH <6.9 mmHg). Although severe metabolic acidosis can lead to impaired myocardial contractility, cerebral vasodilatation, coma, and several gastrointestinal complications,[39] the administration of bicarbonate offers no advantage in improving outcomes or in the rate of recovery from ketoacidosis in patients with arterial pH >7.0.[40,41] Several studies have pointed to potential deleterious effects of bicarbonate therapy, including increased risk of hypokalemia, decreased tissue oxygen uptake, and cerebral edema.[40] In patients with severe metabolic acidosis (pH <6.9), however, clinical guidelines recommend that 50–100 mmol of sodium bicarbonate be given as an isotonic solution (in 200 ml of water) every 2 h until pH rises to ~6.9–7.0.[2,3]

COMPLICATIONS OF THERAPY

The two most common acute complications associated with the treatment of DKA in adult subjects are hypoglycemia and hypokalemia. Hypoglycemia is reported in 10–25% of patients during insulin therapy.[21] Hypoglycemic events most commonly occur after several hours of insulin infusion (between 8 and 16 h) or during the transition phase. The failure to reduce the insulin infusion rate or to use dextrose-containing solutions when glucose levels reach 250 mg/dL are the most common causes of hypoglycemia during insulin therapy.[21] Frequent blood glucose monitoring (every 1–2 h) is mandatory to recognize hypoglycemia because many patients with DKA who develop hypoglycemia during treatment do not experience adrenergic manifestations of sweating, nervousness, fatigue, hunger, and tachycardia. Both insulin therapy and correction of acidosis decrease serum potassium levels by stimulating intracellular potassium uptake in peripheral tissues and may lead to hypokalemia. Aggressive potassium replacement early in management has been shown to minimize the risk of hypokalemia.

IMMEDIATE FOLLOW-UP CARE AFTER HYPERGLYCEMIC CRISIS

IV insulin therapy should continue until the hyperglycemic crisis has resolved. Criteria for resolution of DKA include glucose <200 mg/dL, serum bicarbonate level ≥18 mEq/L, venous pH >7.3, and calculated anion gap ≤14 mEq/L.[2] Criteria for resolution of HHS include total serum osmolarity <320 mOsm/kg and blood glucose ≤250 mg/dL, with a gradual recovery to mental alertness.

A basal-bolus insulin regimen with the combination of a long-acting basal insulin (glargine or detemir) once daily and rapid-acting insulin analogues (aspart, lispro, glulisine) before meals is recommended after discontinuation of IV insulin infusion. The use of insulin analogs has been shown to improve glucose control with a significantly lower rate of hypoglycemia compared with human insulin formulations with NPH and regular insulin.[42]

The best time to transition from IV to SQ insulin is when the patient is alert and able to take food by mouth. Because the half-life of IV regular insulin is less than 10 min, the first dose of SQ insulin should be given 2–4 h before stopping the insulin infusion. The administration of SQ basal insulin early in the course of treatment may facilitate treatment and prevent rebound hyperglycemia after discontinuation of IV insulin therapy.[43] In patients with previously known diabetes, resuming the outpatient insulin regimen is recommended if they had adequate glycemic control before admission. Insulin-naïve patients can be started on a total dose of SQ insulin of 0.5–0.8 unit/kg of body weight.[21,42]

REFERENCES

1. Department of Health and Human Services, National Center for Chronic Disease Prevention and Health Promotion. Diabetes Data & Trends. Crude and age-adjusted hospital discharge rates for diabetic ketoacidosis as first-listed diagnosis per 1,000 diabetic population, United States, 1988–2009
2. Kitabchi AE, Umpierrez GE, Miles JM, Fisher JN. Hyperglycemic crises in adult patients with diabetes. *Diabetes Care* 2009;32:1335–1343
3. Kitabchi AE, Umpierrez GE, Murphy MB, Barrett EJ, Kreisberg RA, Malone JI, Wall BM. Management of hyperglycemic crises in patients with diabetes. *Diabetes Care* 2001;24:131–153

4. Fadini GP, de Kreutzenberg SV, Rigato M, Brocco S, Marchesan M, Tiengo A, Avogaro A. Characteristics and outcomes of the hyperglycemic hyperosmolar non-ketotic syndrome in a cohort of 51 consecutive cases at a single center. *Diabetes Res Clin Pract* 2011;94:172–179
5. Bhowmick SK, Levens KL, Rettig KR. Hyperosmolar hyperglycemic crisis: an acute life-threatening event in children and adolescents with type 2 diabetes mellitus. *Endocr Pract* 2005;11:23–29
6. Pasquel FJ, Umpierrez GE. Hyperosmolar hyperglycemic state: a historic review of the clinical presentation, diagnosis, and treatment. *Diabetes Care* 2014;37:3124–3131
7. Wolfsdorf J, Craig ME, Daneman D, Dunger D, Edge J, Lee W, Rosenbloom A, Sperling M, Hanas R. Diabetic ketoacidosis in children and adolescents with diabetes. *Pediatric Diabetes* 2009;10(Suppl. 12):118–133
8. Davis SN, Umpierrez GE. Diabetic ketoacidosis in type 2 diabetes mellitus—pathophysiology and clinical presentation. *Endorincol Metab* 2007;3:730–731
9. Wolfsdorf J, Glaser N, Sperling MA, American Diabetes Association. Diabetic ketoacidosis in infants, children, and adolescents: A consensus statement from the American Diabetes Association. *Diabetes Care* 2006;29:1150–1159
10. Dabelea D, Rewers A, Stafford JM, Standiford DA, Lawrence JM, Saydah S, Imperatore G, D'Agostino RB, Jr., Mayer-Davis EJ, Pihoker C, Group SfDiYS. Trends in the prevalence of ketoacidosis at diabetes diagnosis: the SEARCH for diabetes in youth study. *Pediatrics* 2014;133:e938–e945
11. Umpierrez GE, Smiley D, Kitabchi AE. Narrative review: ketosis-prone type 2 diabetes mellitus. *Ann Intern Med* 2006;144:350–357
12. Foster DW, McGarry JD. The metabolic derangements and treatment of diabetic ketoacidosis. *New Engl J Med* 1983;309:159–169
13. van de Werve G, Jeanrenaud B. Liver glycogen metabolism: an overview. *Diabetes Metab Rev* 1987;3:47–78
14. Maletkovic J, Drexler A. Diabetic ketoacidosis and hyperglycemic hyperosmolar state. *Endrocinol Metab Clin N Am* 2013;42:677–695
15. McGarry JD, Foster DW. Regulation of hepatic fatty acid oxidation and ketone body production. *Ann Rev Biochem* 1980;49:395–420
16. Rewers A, Klingensmith G, Davis C, Petitti DB, Pihoker C, Rodriguez B, Schwartz ID, Imperatore G, Williams D, Dolan LM, Dabelea D. Presence of diabetic ketoacidosis at diagnosis of diabetes mellitus in youth: the Search for Diabetes in Youth Study. *Pediatrics* 2008;121:e1258–1266
17. Gerich JE, Martin MM, Recant L. Clinical and metabolic characteristics of hyperosmolar nonketotic coma. *Diabetes* 1971;20:228–238
18. Stentz FB, Umpierrez GE, Cuervo R, Kitabchi AE. Proinflammatory cytokines, markers of cardiovascular risks, oxidative stress, and lipid peroxidation in patients with hyperglycemic crises. *Diabetes* 2004;53:2079–2086

19. Chaudhuri A, Umpierrez GE. Oxidative stress and inflammation in hyperglycemic crises and resolution with insulin: implications for the acute and chronic complications of hyperglycemia. *J Diabetes Complications* 2012;26: 257–258

20. Randall L, Begovic J, Hudson M, Smiley D, Peng L, Pitre N, Umpierrez D, Umpierrez G. Recurrent diabetic ketoacidosis in inner-city minority patients: behavioral, socioeconomic, and psychosocial factors. *Diabetes Care* 2011;34:1891–1896

21. Umpierrez GE, Kelly JP, Navarrete JE, Casals MM, Kitabchi AE. Hyperglycemic crises in urban blacks. *Arch Intern Med* 1997;157:669–675

22. Lohiya S, Kreisberg R, Lohiya V. Recurrent diabetic ketoacidosis in two community teaching hospitals. *Endrocr Pract* 2013;19:829–833

23. Jin H, Meyer JM, Jeste DV. Atypical antipsychotics and glucose dysregulation: a systematic review. *Schizophrenia Res* 2004;71:195–212

24. Taylor SI, Blau JE, Rother KI. SGLT2 inhibitors may predispose to ketoacidosis. *J Clin Endocrinol Metab* 2015;100:2849–2852

25. Peters AL, Buschur EO, Buse JB, Cohan P, Diner JC, Hirsch IB. Euglycemic diabetic ketoacidosis: a potential complication of treatment with sodium-glucose cotransporter 2 inhibition. *Diabetes Care* 2015;38:1687–1693

26. Wachtel TJ. The diabetic hyperosmolar state. *Clin Geriatic Med* 1990;6:797–806

27. Pant N, Kadaria D, Murillo LC, Yataco JC, Headley AS, Freire AX. Abdominal pathology in patients with diabetes ketoacidosis. *Am J Med Sci* 2012;344: 341–344

28. Umpierrez G, Freire AX. Abdominal pain in patients with hyperglycemic crises. *J Crit Care* 2002;17:63–67

29. Harden CL, Rosenbaum DH, Daras M. Hyperglycemia presenting with occipital seizures. *Epilepsia* 1991;32:215–220

30. Guisado R, Arieff AI. Neurologic manifestations of diabetic comas: correlation with biochemical alterations in the brain. *Metab Clin Experiment* 1975;24:665–679

31. Nyenwe EA, Razavi LN, Kitabchi AE, Khan AN, Wan JY. Acidosis: the prime determinant of depressed sensorium in diabetic ketoacidosis. *Diabetes Care* 2010;33:1837–1839

32. Kitabchi AE, Wall BM. Diabetic ketoacidosis. *Med Clin N Am* 1995;79:9–37

33. Sheikh-Ali M, Karon BS, Basu A, Kudva YC, Muller LA, Xu J, Schwenk WF, Miles JM. Can serum beta-hydroxybutyrate be used to diagnose diabetic ketoacidosis? *Diabetes Care* 2008;31:643–647

34. Vantyghem MC, Haye S, Balduyck M, Hober C, Degand PM, Lefebvre J. Changes in serum amylase, lipase and leukocyte elastase during diabetic ketoacidosis and poorly controlled diabetes. *Acta Diabetologica* 1999;36:39–44

35. Kitabchi AE, Murphy MB, Spencer J, Matteri R, Karas J. Is a priming dose of insulin necessary in a low-dose insulin protocol for the treatment of diabetic ketoacidosis? *Diabetes Care* 2008;31:2081–2085

36. Goyal N, Miller JB, Sankey SS, Mossallam U. Utility of initial bolus insulin in the treatment of diabetic ketoacidosis. *J Emer Med* 2010;38:422–427

37. Adrogue HJ, Wilson H, Boyd AE, 3rd, Suki WN, Eknoyan G. Plasma acid-base patterns in diabetic ketoacidosis. *New Engl J Med* 1982;307:1603–1610

38. Arora S, Cheng D, Wyler B, Menchine M. Prevalence of hypokalemia in ED patients with diabetic ketoacidosis. *Am J Emer Med* 2012;30:481–484

39. Mitchell JH, Wildenthal K, Johnson RL, Jr. The effects of acid-base disturbances on cardiovascular and pulmonary function. *Kidney Intl* 1972;1:375–389

40. Morris LR, Murphy MB, Kitabchi AE. Bicarbonate therapy in severe diabetic ketoacidosis. *Ann Intern Med* 1986;105:836–840

41. Soler NG, Bennett MA, Dixon K, FitzGerald MG, Malins JM. Potassium balance during treatment of diabetic ketoacidosis with special reference to the use of bicarbonate. *Lancet* 1972;2:665–667

42. Umpierrez GE, Jones S, Smiley D, Mulligan P, Keyler T, Temponi A, Semakula C, Umpierrez D, Peng L, Ceron M, Robalino G. Insulin analogs versus human insulin in the treatment of patients with diabetic ketoacidosis: a randomized controlled trial. *Diabetes Care* 2009;32:1164–1169

43. Hsia E, Seggelke S, Gibbs J, Hawkins RM, Cohlmia E, Rasouli N, Wang C, Kam I, Draznin B. Subcutaneous administration of glargine to diabetic patients receiving insulin infusion prevents rebound hyperglycemia. *J Clin Endocrinol Metab* 2012;97:3132–3137

Chapter 23

Hypoglycemia Prevention and Treatment

Janice L. Gilden, MS, MD, FCP, FACE,[1] Daniel J. Rubin, MD, MSc, FACE,[2] Kristen Kulasa, MD,[3] and Greg Maynard MD, MSc, SFHM[4]

INTRODUCTION

Hypoglycemia is a common problem for hospitalized patients and is a prominent limiting factor for inpatient glycemic control efforts. Symptomatic hypoglycemia is unpleasant, and severe hypoglycemia may result in serious adverse events, including seizure, coma, and even death. Hypoglycemia has been associated with mortality, although whether it serves as a marker of illness or a causal agent per se at the population level remains to be established. As such, prevention and management of hypoglycemia are important goals for managing hospitalized patients with diabetes that every medical center needs to address as part of comprehensive glycemic control efforts. Overtreatment of hypoglycemia and fear of hypoglycemia, which often leads to clinical inertia, can lead to hyperglycemia and increased glucose variability. In addition, overuse of sliding-scale insulin (SSI) also is associated with adverse outcomes. Judicious, protocol-based treatment of hypoglycemia is therefore another important goal for the management of inpatients with diabetes.

INCIDENCE AND COSTS

Patients with diabetes who experience hypoglycemia during hospitalization have longer lengths of stay, higher costs (including more venipunctures, point-of-care [POC] glucose testing, administration of intravenous dextrose solutions, and nursing time), and greater odds of being discharged to a skilled nursing facility than their counterparts without hypoglycemia.[1–3] Patients with impaired cognition

[1]Chief of Endocrinology and Professor of Medicine, Endocrine Fellowship Program Director, Rosalind Franklin University of Medicine and Science/Chicago Medical School, Captain James A. Lovell Federal Health Care Center, Presence Saints Mary and Elizabeth Medical Center, Chicago, IL. [2]Assistant Professor of Medicine, Temple University School of Medicine, Section of Endocrinology, Diabetes, and Metabolism, Philadelphia, PA. [3]Assistant Clinical Professor of Medicine, Director, Inpatient Glycemic Control, Division of Endocrinology, Diabetes, and Metabolism, University of California, San Diego, San Diego, CA. [4]Clinical Professor of Medicine, Department of Medicine, Chief Quality Officer, University of California Davis Medical Center, Sacramento, CA.

DOI: 10.2337/9781580406086.23

or communication skills, common conditions in the elderly, are at highest risk for unrecognized hypoglycemia or delayed responses from the health-care team.[4–7] The Institute for Safe Medication Practices (ISMP) identifies insulin as a high-alert medication in the inpatient setting.[8] Approximately one-quarter of all patient safety incidents involving insulin result in patient harm, and insulin has been implicated in one-third of all medication-related deaths.[3,8–11]

Iatrogenic hypoglycemia is a top source of inpatient adverse drug events (ADEs). The Office of the Inspector General (OIG) recently released a study of ADEs in hospitals.[12] ADEs represent one-third of all hospital-acquired conditions in the hospital, affect 1.9 million stays annually, and cost $4.2 billion per year; additionally, 57% of these ADEs were associated with the use of hypoglycemic agents. To qualify as an ADE, a hypoglycemic event must be induced by an anti-hyperglycemic agent and have documented signs or symptoms of hypoglycemia or require therapy. On the basis of 25,145 hospital visits in the Medicare Patient Safety Monitoring System sample, an estimated 10.2% of inpatients exposed to insulin or hypoglycemic agents experienced an ADE, representing 930,000 ADEs per year nationally.[7]

The true incidence of inpatient hypoglycemia, however, is underestimated because of the lack of standardized definitions and varying methods of data collection and reporting among hospital systems.[13,14] Furthermore, hospital costs can result from morbidities associated with insulin-induced hypoglycemia and endothelial injury, abnormal coagulation, and increases in counterregulatory hormones, which are all associated with increased risks for cardiovascular events and sudden death.[15–18]

SIGNS, SYMPTOMS, AND DEFINITIONS

Blood glucose values <70 mg/dL (3.9 mmol/L) have been defined as hypoglycemia and correspond to the threshold for increases in counterregulatory hormones.[13,14] In hospitalized patients, severe hypoglycemia has been variably defined as <40 mg/dL (2.2 mmol/L) or <50 mg/dL (2.8 mmol/L), when cognitive decline normally begins.[13,14,19] Early recognition and treatment of mild to moderate hypoglycemia (40–69 mg/dL [2.2–3.8 mmol/L]) can prevent deterioration to a more severe episode.[13,14]

The acute effects of hypoglycemia can range from asymptomatic to severe. Signs and symptoms are divided into adrenergic and neuroglycopenic disturbances. Adrenergic symptoms generally are associated with mild hypoglycemia and generally are the first to occur with decreasing blood glucose levels.[20] These symptoms include diaphoresis, anxiety, palpitations, hunger, tremors, tachycardia, pallor, headache, and even visual disturbances. As hypoglycemia progresses and becomes more severe, neuroglycopenic effects become more likely. These include headache, confusion, personality changes (aggressive or passive behavior) mental status changes, confusion, lack of responsiveness, seizures, hemiplegia or other neurologic changes that can mimic a cerebrovascular accident or transient ischemic event, or even coma.[21] Although not commonly occurring, a blood glucose level of about 10 mg/dL (0.6 mmol/L) may even be associated with pupillary dilation, shallow breathing, bradycardia, hypotonicity, and death.[22] Therefore, treatment of neuroglycopenic effects requires more aggressive and rapid interventions.

HYPOGLYCEMIA UNAWARENESS AND OTHER CHANGES IN SYMPTOMATOLOGY

Hypoglycemia unawareness is defined by the absence of symptoms with blood glucose levels <70 mg/dL (3.9 mmol/L).[23] Patients at risk for hypoglycemia unawareness include those with absent or impaired counterregulatory responses; long-standing duration of diabetes; recurrent low blood glucose events with the development of hypoglycemia-associated autonomic failure (HAAF); extremely tight glycemic control with normal blood glucose and HbA_{1c} levels (which increases risks for hypoglycemia); type 1 diabetes (T1D) and severely insulin-deficient type 2 diabetes (T2D); pharmacologic therapy with medications that blunt adrenergic response, such as β-blockers; deficient glucagon stores as in alcoholism or in the malnourished; or advanced age.[24] Hypoglycemia unawareness can severely limit achievement of stringent diabetes control. People with hypoglycemia unawareness are also less likely to be awakened from sleep if nocturnal low blood glucose episodes occur. Several weeks of avoiding hypoglycemia can improve counterregulatory mechanisms and improve hypoglycemic awareness.[25]

In addition, patients with previously poor glycemic control can experience symptoms of hypoglycemia at or near normal levels of blood glucose. Symptoms of hypoglycemia also may occur as blood glucose levels fall or may even mimic those of other conditions, such as hypotensive episodes or infection.

RISK FACTORS FOR INPATIENT HYPOGLYCEMIA

Although hypoglycemia in hospitalized patients with diabetes is often due to overtreatment of hyperglycemia, some conditions predispose patients to hypoglycemia that are not related to antidiabetic medications. In addition, studies by Kosiborod et al.[26] and Boucai et al.[4] suggest that inpatient hypoglycemia may be a marker of illness severity, rather than a cause of an adverse event.

Other risk factors that predispose to hypoglycemia involve changes in clinical status, diet, and medication regimens, as well as a breakdown of hospital processes. Thus, risk factors for inpatient hypoglycemia in patients with diabetes can be divided into patient factors, nutrition factors, and system issues (Table 23.1).

PATIENT FACTORS

Patient-specific risk factors for hypoglycemia include long duration of diabetes, low BMI, malnutrition, HbA_{1c} <7 %, history of previous cardiovascular events, insulin treatment on admission, older age, and a higher albumin-to-creatinine ratio.[27] Patients with T2D generally have less risk for hypoglycemia than those with T1D. Insulin sensitivity can be affected by underlying illness, such as acute renal failure, sepsis, and changes in medications, such as quinolone antibiotics, vasopressors, and corticosteroids. The counterregulatory hormonal responses to

Table 23.1—Risk Factors for Inpatient Hypoglycemia

Patient Factors

- Underlying illness: renal insufficiency, liver disorder, sepsis
- Changes in medications: β-blockers, antibiotics, vasopressors, corticosteroids
- Characteristics of diabetes: type of diabetes (more commonly T1D); long duration of disease; complications, such as cardiovascular risks, renal function, and increased insulin sensitivity; prior glycemic control with history of recurrent asymptomatic or severe hypoglycemia; resolution of glucotoxicity
- Other: older age, lower BMI, malnutrition

Nutrition Factors

- Inadequate insulin adjustment for prandial intake because of erratic oral intake or missed meals
- Interruption of enteral or parenteral nutrition with inadequate glucose replacement
- Inadequate adjustment of insulin for feedings being held before procedures
- Elevated gastric residuals
- Loss of intravenous or enteral access

System Factors

- Lack of hospital and hospital-system protocols regarding patient safety and quality control
- Lack of knowledge and training of staff, nursing errors, and communication errors
- Lack of communication between multidisciplinary teams writing orders
- Lack of hospital and hospital-system protocols regarding bedside glucose monitoring, standardized insulin treatment, transitions of care from inpatient to outpatient
- Use of sliding-scale insulin as sole treatment of hyperglycemia or overly aggressive insulin correction factor or supplements
- Lack of hospital and hospital-system hypoglycemic prevention and treatment protocols

hypoglycemia may be impaired by angiotensin-converting enzyme inhibitors and β-blockers. It is important to assess the current level of glycemic control, which may need to be relaxed in patients with previously aggressive tight control, to avoid hypoglycemia while in the hospital.

Elderly adults with diabetes mellitus are at increased risk for hypoglycemia because of multiple factors: *1*) impaired renal function and increased time for drug clearance; *2*) polypharmacy, which makes them more susceptible to hypoglycemia resulting from drug interactions or other therapies that can affect glucose control; and *3*) age- or comorbid disease-related cognitive deficiencies, which impair recognition of hypoglycemic symptoms.

NUTRITION FACTORS

A number of factors related to the content and timing of nutrition can predispose patients to hypoglycemia. The diet should be carefully designed to provide adequate calories and to meet the patient's needs for growth, activity, and tissue repair. The carbohydrate amount of the diet needs to be determined with the patient and individualized to consider the pharmacologic regimen and patient preferences.

This is best done by registered dietitian nutritionists (RDs or RDNs), knowledgeable in diabetes management and skilled in evaluating the patient's clinical condition, meal planning, and lifestyle preferences. Carbohydrate amount may be used to calculate prandial insulin dosing with timing of meal content matched to prandial insulin. Nursing staff should calculate the prandial insulin based on the amount of the meal that is consumed—for example, less insulin when less of the meal is eaten. In patients receiving enteral or parenteral nutrition, glucose monitoring should be performed to guide control of hyperglycemia during feedings and avoid hypoglycemia if feedings are interrupted.[28,29] Hypoglycemia may occur when a fixed dose of mealtime (prandial) insulin is administered without accounting for erratic oral intake, missed meals, the timing of meal delivery, and blood glucose monitoring. Similarly, interruption of enteral or parenteral nutrition with inadequate glucose replacement, and inadequate adjustment of insulin when nutrition is held may lead to low blood glucose levels.

SYSTEM ISSUES

Inpatient management systems should be designed around patient safety and quality control with a well-coordinated and trained multidisciplinary team (consisting of primary care physicians, endocrinologists, intensive care specialists, hospitalists, nurse practitioners, physician assistants, nursing personnel, and RDs or RDNs). System-wide approaches and protocols to prevent hypoglycemia, as well as root cause analyses, have proven to be useful.[11,30] In addition, hypoglycemia unawareness and inadequate frequency of glucose monitoring in the inpatient setting can lead to underestimation of the true rates of hypoglycemia. Additional system failures that can account for increased rates of hypoglycemia include the following: *1*) lack of evaluation of patient-specific trends in blood glucose values; *2*) lack of recognition for individual insulin sensitivities; *3*) delays in making appropriate changes in glycemic management; *4*) use of SSI as the sole treatment for hyperglycemia; *5*) lack of administration of sufficient glucose with insulin for the acute treatment of hyperkalemia; *6*) administration of enteral tube feeds or parenteral nutrition, when different teams give nutrition orders that are not coordinated or communicated with those for insulin administration; *7*) lack of down-titrating insulin in conjunction with decreasing corticosteroid doses; and *8*) others, such as nursing errors, communication errors, and lack of hospital policies.[11,13,28] Other contributions to the occurrence of hypoglycemia include poor communication among various teams with conflicting glycemic orders, lack of standardized protocols or order sets, and lack of planning for transitions of care between different phases of hospital stay and from the inpatient to the outpatient setting.

BEDSIDE BLOOD GLUCOSE MONITORING

During hospitalization, bedside POC blood glucose monitoring or laboratory glucose values should be used to monitor glycemic control and guide insulin dosing. Any glucose value that does not correlate with the patient's clinical status should be confirmed with a laboratory plasma glucose measurement. The frequency of glucose monitoring should be designed to match the patient's medication regimen and nutritional intake, as well as monitor for hypoglycemia. Hypoglycemia also can suggest clinical deterioration.[28,29] In the patient receiving enteral or parenteral nutrition, the timing of glucose monitoring should match carbohydrate intake. For patients who are eating, blood glucose monitoring should be performed at least before meals and at bedtime. In the patient not receiving nutrition (NPO), glucose monitoring is performed every 4–6 h.[28] For patients receiving intravenous insulin infusions, blood glucose should be monitored every 30 min to 2 h.

HYPOGLYCEMIA TREATMENT

Rapid treatment of hypoglycemia requires a well-coordinated team approach. Early recognition of the signs and symptoms is crucial (Table 23.2). Although bedside blood glucose monitoring usually is performed on a scheduled basis, signs and symptoms may occur at any time during the day or night, requiring more frequent measurement as needed. In addition, blood glucose evaluation for nocturnal hypoglycemia, frequently under-recognized, also should be done. Protocols need to be established on a hospital- or system-wide basis. The first step is education of nursing staff and patients on the recognition of the causes as well as signs and symptoms of hypoglycemia. Bedside monitoring must be available at all times with rapid assessment of the patient's level of consciousness, respiratory status, and other parameters.

Hypoglycemia treatment requires ingestion of glucose or other carbohydrate-containing foods and can be administered using the 15-15 rule (15 g of rapid-acting or simple carbohydrate, wait 15 min, and if the blood glucose if still low, then administering another 15 g of carbohydrate with repetition of these steps until the blood glucose level is normalized).[28] The oral route is preferred for patients able to swallow, and easily digestible carbohydrates (glucose tablets, gel, or liquid) should be administered. Adding fat may delay and prolong the acute glycemic response. If the patient is NPO or has impaired mental status, however, then administration of intravenous dextrose of 50% by bolus or 1 mg glucagon intramuscularly are the preferred treatments. Overtreatment (such as 1 quart of orange juice with 5 packets of sugar) should be avoided. This can result in hyperglycemia, which can trigger the need for more insulin and can lead to a vicious cycle of low and high blood glucose levels. Frequent bedside glucose monitoring should then be done until the patient's glucose levels are stable. Insulin activity may be ongoing from previously administered insulin, which may lead to recurrent hypoglycemia; therefore, this situation requires vigilance. Following any hypoglycemic episode, an evaluation should be done for cause with correction of the problem, which may include appropriate medication adjustments, changes in nutrient intake, or system changes.

INSULIN PROTOCOLS

The American Diabetes Association (ADA) currently recommends that all patients should be assessed for a history of diabetes, and, if previously known, the type of diabetes and an assessment for adequacy of their home insulin regimen when admitted to the hospital.[28] Although insulin therapy is the current standard of care for achieving glycemic control in hospitalized patients, it is also the drug

Table 23.2—Hypoglycemia Protocol

A. Education of Nursing Staff and Patients Regarding Recognition of Signs and Symptoms, Bedside Glucose Monitoring, and Treatment of Hypoglycemia

Symptoms: may include any or any combination of the following—shakiness, nervousness or anxiety, sweating, chills and clamminess, irritability or impatience, confusion, including delirium, rapid/fast heartbeat, lightheadedness or dizziness, hunger or nausea, sleepiness, blurred/impaired vision, tingling or numbness in the lips or tongue, headaches, weakness or fatigue, anger, stubbornness, sadness, lack of coordination, nightmares or crying out during sleep, seizures, unconsciousness.

B. Determine Blood Glucose Level and Consciousness of Patient and Ability to Comply with Oral Intake

If able to consume fast-acting carbohydrates, treat using 15-15 Rule:

1. Administer 15–20 g of glucose or readily digestible rapid-acting carbohydrates.
2. Recheck blood glucose after 15 min.
3. If hypoglycemia continues, repeat above steps until blood glucose >70 mg/dL (3.9 mmol/L).
4. Once blood glucose returns to normal, administer a small snack if next planned meal or snack is more than 1–2 h away.

Examples of 15 g of readily digestible carbohydrates:

- 3–4 glucose tablets
- gel tube
- 4 ounces (1/2 cup) of juice or regular (not diet) soda
- 1 tablespoon sugar
- 8 ounces of nonfat or 1% milk

If confused, unconscious, or NPO, treat as follows:

- If IV access and blood glucose level is 50–70 mg/dL (2.8–3.9 mmol/L), administer 25 ml of 50% dextrose over 5 min. If IV access and blood glucose level is <50 mg/dL (2.8 mmol/L), administer 50 ml of 50% dextrose over 5 min.
- If no IV access, inject 1 mg glucagon intramuscularly or subcutaneously into patient's buttock, arm, or thigh.
- When the individual regains consciousness (usually in 5–15 min), give a carbohydrate and protein snack. Be aware of potential for nausea and vomiting.
- Notify provider.

Notify provider of hypoglycemic episode.

C. Assess possible cause of hypoglycemia to avoid recurrence. Common causes of hypoglycemia include an interruption of food, tube feedings, or IV dextrose and decreased steroids. Does the treatment regimen need to be revised or are other patient and system factors contributing to the hypoglycemia?

associated with the greatest number of medication errors in hospitals.[30,31] Therefore, insulin treatment in hospital settings requires careful planning and monitoring. In general, glucose levels should be maintained <180 mg/dL (11.2 mmol/L). This decreases the risk for acute hyperglycemic symptoms, as well as minimizes fluid and electrolyte abnormalities, reduces risk for infection resulting from changes in immune function, and minimizes hypoglycemia. Clinical guidelines for most non–intensive care unit patients recommend targeting a glucose level of <140 mg/dL (7.8 mmol/L) before meals and a random glucose level of

<180 mg/dL (10.0 mmol/L). For critically ill patients, standardized protocol-driven intravenous insulin infusions should be used to control hyperglycemia, with a starting threshold of no higher than 180 mg/dL (10.0 mmol/L). Blood glucose levels with use of an intravenous insulin infusion should be maintained between 140 and 180 mg/dL (7.8–10.0 mmol/L), provided that these targets can be achieved safely (i.e., minimizing hypoglycemia).[28] If blood glucose levels fall <100 mg/dL (5.6 mmol/L), then insulin orders should be reviewed and adjustments made for levels <70 mg/dL (3.9 mmol/L), unless the event can be explained easily by other factors. Less stringent glycemic targets may be appropriate for some patients who are older, have multiple comorbidities, are at high risk for hypoglycemia, and have reduced life expectancy.

Structured insulin order sets and management algorithms not only improve rates of hyperglycemia but also decrease the rates of hypoglycemia.[28,31] Standardized protocols should be utilized but must be individualized in the following situations: *1*) use of continuous intravenous insulin infusions, *2*) use of subcutaneous (SQ) insulin (basal, prandial, and correction insulins), *3*) when transitioning from intravenous to SQ insulin, and *4*) for nurse-driven hypoglycemia treatment. Caution is advised when administering supplemental (also termed correction factor) insulin to correct hyperglycemia at night to avoid nocturnal hypoglycemia. The use of SSI alone is nonphysiologic and should not be used as the sole treatment of hyperglycemia.[32]

Insulin doses should be readjusted based on the previous day's blood glucose responses and should be reduced by ~20% for unexplained blood glucose results <70 md/dL (3.9 mmol/L). Insulin doses should also be reduced if blood glucose levels are between 70 (3.9 mmol/L) and 100 mg/dL (5.6 mmol/L), because these values may increase risk for subsequent hypoglycemia.[28] Patients receiving insulin therapy may need to have doses adjusted as their medical status and diet improve. Studies such as RABBIT 2 (Randomized Study of Basal Bolus Insulin Therapy in the Inpatient Management of Patients with Type 2 Diabetes Undergoing General Surgery), the DEAN TRIAL (Insulin Detemir versus NPH Insulin in Hospitalized Patients with Diabetes), and the BASAL PLUS TRIAL have confirmed the benefits and feasibility of the use of basal with meat-related bolus insulin, while avoiding significant hypoglycemia.[33–35] In addition, Rubin et al.[36] showed that the odds of hypoglycemia increase with starting insulin doses >0.6 units/kg/day compared with doses <0.2 units/kg/day, whereas the odds do not increase with 0.2–0.6 units/kg/day.[36]

Other types of insulin, such as neutral protamine Hagedorn (NPH) and premixed 70/30 are not recommended for use in the hospital setting because of their high rates of hypoglycemia. NPH is an intermediate-acting preparation with variable and suboptimal onset of action, variable absorption, and varying peaks of activity and increased risks for hypoglycemia. The pharmacologic properties of basal insulin analogs (such as detemir or glargine) provide relatively peakless 20- to 24-h coverage with less associated hypoglycemia. Premixed insulins, such as 70/30 or 75/25, generally do not have adequate prandial flexibility and often fall short of achieving desired glycemic control. There are also higher rates of hypoglycemia associated with these insulin preparations.[35] Therefore, these insulin preparations generally should not be used in the inpatient setting.

SPECIAL SITUATIONS FOR INSULIN MANAGEMENT

Hypoglycemia may occur if enteral tube feedings are interrupted and insulin is not adjusted appropriately, or the glucose content from feedings is not replaced. This happens most frequently when feedings are held before procedures, for elevated gastric residuals, or if intravenous or enteral access is lost. Dextrose infusion may be required in cases of interrupted tube feedings to avoid hypoglycemia.[37] Other special situations that warrant careful insulin adjustment because of increased risks for hypoglycemia include *1*) patients with increased sensitivity (e.g., those with T1D); *2*) patients with inadequate oral intake or who will be kept NPO; *3*) patients on tapering glucocorticoid doses (most commonly used in conjunction with chemotherapy or solid organ and bone marrow transplants or immunologic disorders); *4*) patients experiencing renal failure (estimated glomerular filtration rate [eGFR] <60 mL/min); or *5*) patients with peritoneal dialysis.

Glucose monitoring should be designed to match the patient's medication regimen and nutritional intake and should monitor for hypoglycemia. Hypoglycemia also can suggest clinical deterioration.[28,29] In the majority of patients who are eating, blood glucose monitoring should be performed before meals and at bedtime. Patients who are NPO should have their glucose monitored every 4–6 h.[28,29] Any glucose value that does not correlate with the patient's clinical status should be confirmed with a laboratory plasma glucose measurement. For patients receiving intravenous insulin infusions, blood glucose should be monitored every 30 min to 2 hours.

OTHER ANTIHYPERGLYCEMIC PHARMACOLOGIC AGENTS

In general, oral diabetes medications and noninsulin injectables are not used in the inpatient setting because of the inability to quickly titrate to achieve desired blood glucose effect and the associated side effects that limit their use in the hospital setting. Sulfonylureas, especially glibencamide, are a low-cost option for home use but are associated with an increased risk of hypoglycemia because of a long duration of action and decreased clearance. Although metformin often is considered a first-line treatment for T2D in the outpatient setting because of its low risk of hypoglycemia, lactic acidosis may occur during situations of changing renal function, when GFR is <30 mL/min, and during various surgical and radiology procedures. Therefore, these antihyperglycemic agents are not recommended to be administered in the acute hospital setting.

Recently, incretin-based therapy, such as dipeptidyl peptidase-4 (DDP-4) inhibitors and glucagon-like peptide-1 (GLP-1) agonists, have been reported to decrease postprandial hyperglycemia with less hypoglycemia in the acute hospital setting, especially when glucocorticoids are used.[38] Additional randomized studies are needed to further evaluate the safety and efficacy of incretin therapy in the management in hospital settings.

CONCLUSION

Patients with or without diabetes may experience hypoglycemia while in the hospital setting because of changes in nutritional state (inadequate or erratic caloric intake, emesis, new NPO status, reduced infusion rate of intravenous dextrose, or unexpected interruption of enteral feedings or parenteral nutrition), heart failure, renal or liver disease, malignancy, infection, or sepsis. Other factors that may increase the risk of hypoglycemia include sudden decreases in corticosteroid dose, altered cognition affecting the patient's ability to recognize and report hypoglycemic symptoms, and inappropriate timing of short- or rapid-acting insulin relative to caloric intake. Prevention of hypoglycemia involves proper coordination of inpatient diabetic management with appropriate treatment options depending on the type of diabetes and individual patient circumstances. Furthermore, use of SSI in the inpatient hospital setting as the sole agent for insulin management is inadequate for the treatment of hyperglycemia and is strongly discouraged to avoid unanticipated hypoglycemic episodes.

A hypoglycemia management protocol or plan for prevention and treatment of hypoglycemia is essential for each hospital or hospital system (Table 23.3). The management plan should include a nurse-driven protocol for timely recognition and treatment of hypoglycemic events methods to record and track hypoglycemic events and should use root-cause analysis principles by an inpatient diabetes management safety committee to drive continuous improvement.[11,31,39] Finally, as recommended by the PRIDE Group (Planning Research in Inpatient Diabetes Group),[31] well-controlled randomized studies are needed to answer questions regarding acceptable rates of hypoglycemia as well as determine best practices for glycemic control with avoidance of hypoglycemia in the inpatient setting.

Table 23.3—Summary of Principles for Hypoglycemia Prevention

System Approaches

- Develop and implement hypoglycemia protocols
- Assess for ongoing factors that increase risks of hypoglycemia
- Adopt system protocols for prevention of hypoglycemia
- Apply preventive measures to minimize hypoglycemia risks in the inpatient setting on a system-wide basis
- Monitor hypoglycemic episodes on a hospital- or system-wide basis
- Adopt a hypoglycemia risk assessment plan utilizing the root cause analysis principles

Patient Care Approaches

- Avoid sole use of sliding-scale for treatment
- Avoid overaggressive insulin supplementation to correct hyperglycemia
- Assess for ongoing factors that increase risks of hypoglycemia
- Assess all patients for symptomatic and asymptomatic hypoglycemia
- Assess all patients for cognitive function and acute changes in cognitive function
- Increase monitoring for hypoglycemia by the entire health-care team as well as the patient
- Reevaluate patients for hypoglycemia unawareness or nocturnal hypoglycemia, or patients with a history of one or more episodes of severe hypoglycemia for changes in treatment regimen (unexplained by inadequate caloric intake)

REFERENCES

1. Curkendall SM, Natoli JL, Alexander CM, Nathanson BH, Haidar T, Dubois RW. Economic and clinical impact of inpatient diabetic hypoglycemia. *Endocr Pract* 2009;15(4):302–312
2. Farrokhi F, Smiley D, Umpierrez GE. Glycemic control in non-diabetic critically ill patients. *Best Pract Res Clin Endorcinol Metab* 2011;25(5): 813–824
3. Cobaugh DJ, Maynard G, Cooper L, et al. Enhancing insulin-use safety in hospitals: Practical recommendations from an ASHP Foundation expert consensus panel. *Am J Health Syst Pharm* 2013;70(16):1404–1413
4. Boucai L, Southern WN, Zonszein J. Hypoglycemia-associated mortality is not drug-associated but linked to comorbidities. *Am J Med* 2011;124:1028–1035
5. Kagansky N, Levy S, Rimon E, et al. Hypoglycemia as a predictor of mortality in hospitalized elderly patients. *Arch Int Med* 2003;163(15):1825–1829
6. Amori RE, Pittas AG, Siegel RD, et al. Inpatient medical errors involving glucose-lowering medications and their impact on patients: review of 2,598 incidents from a voluntary electronic error-reporting database. *Endocr Pract* 2008;14(5):535–542
7. Classen DC, Jaser L, Budnitz DS. Adverse drug events among hospitalized Medicare patients: epidemiology and national estimates from a new approach to surveillance. *Jt Comm J Qual Patient Saf* 2010;36(1):12–21
8. Institute for Safe Medication Practices. ISMP's list of high-alert medications. Available from http://www.ismp.org/tools/highalertmedicationLists.asp. Accessed 5 December 2014
9. Cousins D, Rosario C, Scarpello J. Insulin, hospitals and harm: a review of patient safety incidents reported to the National Patient Safety Agency. *Clin Med* 2011;11:28–30
10. Deal EN, Liu A, Wise LL et al. Inpatient insulin orders: are patients getting what is prescribed? *J Hosp Med* 2011;6:526–529
11. Hellman R. A systems approach to reducing errors in insulin therapy in the inpatient setting. *Endocr Pract* 2004;10(Suppl. 2):100–108
12. Office of the Inspector General. Adverse events in hospitals: national incidence among Medicare beneficiaries. Washington, DC, 2010
13. Seaquist ER, Anderson J, Childs B, et al. Hypoglycemia and diabetes: a report of a workgroup of the American Diabetes Association and the Endocrine Society. *Diabetes Care* 2013;36:1384–1395
14. Moghissi ES, Korytkowski MT, DiNardo M, Einhorn D, Hellman R, Hirsch IB, et al. American Association of Clinical Endocrinologists and American Diabetes Association consensus statement on inpatient glycemic control. *Endocr Pract* 2009;15:353–369. doi:10.4158/EP09102.RA

15. Razavi Nematollahi L, Kitabchi AE, Stentz FB, Wan JY, Larijani BA, Tehrani MM, et al. Proinflammatory cytokines in response to insulin-induced hypoglycemic stress in healthy subjects. *Metabolism* 2009;58:443–448. doi:10.1016/j.metabol.2008.10.018

16. Fisher BM, Hepburn DA, Smith JG, Frier BM. Responses of peripheral blood cells to acute insulin-induced hypoglycaemia in humans: effect of alpha-adrenergic blockade. *Horm Metab Res* 1992;26(Suppl.):109–110

17. Chow E, Bernjak A, Williams S, Fawdry RA, Hibbert S, Freeman J, Sheridan PJ, Heller SR. Risk of cardiac arrhythmias during hypoglycemia in patients with type 2 diabetes and cardiovascular risk. *Diabetes* 2014;63(5):1738–1747. doi: 10.2337/db13-0468

18. Goto A, Arah OA, Goto M, et al. Severe hypoglycaemia and cardiovascular disease: systemic review and meta-analysis with bias analysis. *BMJ* 2013;347:f4533

19. Cryer PE. Hypoglycaemia: the limiting factor in the glycaemic management of type I and type II diabetes. *Diabetologia* 2002;45:937–948

20. Hepburn DA, Deary IJ, Frier BM, Patrick AW, Quinn JD, Fisher BM. Symptoms of acute insulin-induced hypoglycemia in humans with and without IDDM. Factor-analysis approach. *Diabetes Care* 1991;14(11):949–957. doi:10.2337/diacare.14.11.949

21. Towler DA, Havlin CE, Craft S, Cryer P. Mechanism of awareness of hypoglycemia. Perception of neurogenic (predominantly cholinergic) rather than neuroglycopenic symptoms. *Diabetes* 1993;42:1791–1798. doi:10.2337/diab.42.12.1791

22. Cryer PE. Hypoglycemia, functional brain failure and brain death. *J. Clin Invest* 2007;117(4):868–870

23. Gerich JE, Mokan M, Veneman T, Korytkowski M, Mitrakou A. Hypoglycemia Unawareness. *Endocrine Rev* 1991;12(4):356–371. doi:http://dx.doi.org/10.1210/edrv-12-4-356

24. Cryer PE. Diverse causes of hypoglycemia-associated autonomic failure in diabetes. *N Engl J Med* 2004;350:2272–2279

25. Fanelli CG, Epifano L, Rambotti AM, et al. Meticulous prevention of hypoglycemia normalizes the glycemic thresholds and magnitude of most of neuroendocrine responses to, symptoms of, and cognitive function during hypoglycemia in intensively treated patients with short-term IDDM. *Diabetes* 1993;42:1683–1689

26. Kosiborod M, Inzucchi SE, Goyal A, Krumholz HM, Masoudi FA, Xiao L, et al. Relationship between spontaneous and iatrogenic hypoglycemia and mortality in patients hospitalized with acute myocardial infarction. *JAMA* 2009;301:1556–1564 doi:10.1001/jama.2009.496

27. Farrokhi F, Klindukhova O, Chandra P, Peng L, Smiley D, Newton C, et al. Risk factors for inpatient hypoglycemia during subcutaneous insulin therapy

in non-critically ill patients with type 2 diabetes. *J Diabetes Sci Technol* 2012;6:1022–1029

28. ADA. Diabetes care in the hospital, nursing home, and skilled nursing facility. American Diabetes Association standards of medical care in diabetes. *Diabetes Care* 2015;38(Suppl. 1):580–585. doi:10.2337/dc15-S016

29. Maynard G, Wesorick DH, O'Malley C, Inzucchi SE, Society of Hospital Medicine, Glycemic Control Task Force. Subcutaneous insulin order sets and protocols: effective design and implementation strategies. *J Hosp Med* 2008;3:29–41. doi:10.1002/jhm.354

30. Rashidee A, Hart J, Chen J, Kumar S. High-alert medications: error prevalence and severity. *Pat Safe Qual Health Care*. July August 2009. Available from http://www.psqh.com/julyaugust-2009/164-data-trends.html. Accessed 12 December 2015

31. Draznin B, Gilden J, Golden SH, Inzucchi SE, for the PRIDE Investigators. Pathways to quality inpatient management: a call to action. *Diabetes Care* 2013;36:1807–1814. doi:10.2337/dc12-2508

32. Hirsch IB. Sliding scale insulin: time to stop sliding. *JAMA* 2009;301:213–214

33. Umpierrez GE, Smiley D, Jacobs S, et al. Randomized study of basal-bolus insulin therapy in the inpatient management of patients with type 2 diabetes undergoing general surgery (RABBIT 2 surgery). *Diabetes Care* 2011;34:256–261

34. Umpierrez GE, Hor T, Smiley D, Temponi A, Umpierrez D, Ceron M, Munoz C, Newton C, Peng L, Baldwin D. Comparison of inpatient insulin regimens with detemir plus aspart versus neutral protamine Hagedorn plus regular in medical patients with type 2 diabetes. *J Clin Endocrinol Metab* 2009;94:564–569

35. Riddle MC, Rosenstock J, Vlajnic A, Gao L. Randomized, 1-year comparison of three ways to initiate and advance insulin for type 2 diabetes: twice-daily premixed insulin versus basal insulin with either basal-plus one prandial insulin or basal-bolus up to three prandial injections. *Diabetes Obes Metab* 2014;16(5):396–402. doi:10.1111/dom.12225

36. Rubin DJ, Rybin D, Doros G, McDonnell ME. Weight-based, insulin dose-related hypoglycemia in hospitalized patients with diabetes. *Diabetes Care* 2011;34(8):1723–1728

37. Baldwin D, Kinnare K, Draznin B, et al. Insulin treatment of hyperglycemia in hospitalized patients receiving total parenteral nutrition (TPN). *Diabetes* 2012;61(Suppl. 1):A1070

38. Umpierrez GE, Schwartz S. Use of incretin-based therapy in hospitalized patients with hyperglycemia. *Endocr Pract* 2014;20(9):933–944. doi:10.4158/EPI 13471.RA

39. Korytkowski M, Dinardo M, Donihi AC, Bigi L, Devita M. Evolution of a diabetes inpatient safety committee. *Endocr Pract*. 2006;12(Suppl. 3):91–99

Chapter 24

Use of Continuous Subcutaneous Insulin Infusions in the Inpatient Setting: A Guide to Management

Eileen Faulds, CNP, CDE,[1] Robert Rushakoff, MD,[2] Umesh Masharani, MD,[3] and Kathleen Dungan, MD, MPH[4]

INTRODUCTION

Continuous subcutaneous insulin infusions (CSII), commonly referred to as insulin pumps, are being used with increasing frequency, such that many users likely will require hospitalization over time.[1] Many insulin pump patients would prefer to continue pump therapy during their hospitalization.[2] Patient knowledge varies, however, and most physicians and nurses in the inpatient setting have little understanding of CSII. Professional guidelines recommend the continuation of CSII in the hospital in conjunction with a pump expert, if the patients mentally and physically equipped to operate their pump.[3–5] This chapter will focus on evidence for continued use of CSII in the hospital, potential advantages and disadvantages, identifying patients best suited to continue, use and management strategies for use of CSII in this setting.

EVIDENCE FOR USE OF CSII IN THE HOSPITAL

In the ambulatory setting, studies have demonstrated modest but inconsistent HbA_{1c} reductions, lower insulin requirements, and better patient satisfaction with CSII compared with multiple dose injection (MDI).[6-9] Most studies, however, do not demonstrate a reduced risk of hypoglycemia.

Limited studies have addressed the inpatient use of CSII. Most of the studies are small and retrospective or address policy development and patient selection and many were performed at centers with expertise and resources for managing insulin pumps. Cook et al.[10] published guidelines for management of CSII in the inpatient setting, including a discussion on patient selection and the development of a standardized order set.[10] The most recent retrospective analysis by Cook et al. spanned 5 years and examined 136 patient records, totaling 253 hospitalizations.[11] CSII was continued through the entire admission in 65% of hospitalizations and

[1]Division of Endocrinology, Diabetes & Metabolism, Wexner Medical Center Inpatient Diabetes Consults, The Ohio State University, Columbus, OH. [2]Medical Director, Inpatient Diabetes, Professor of Medicine, Division of Endocrinology and Metabolism, University of California, San Francisco, CA. [3]Professor of Clinical Medicine University of California, San Francisco, CA. [4]Division of Endocrinology, Diabetes & Metabolism, The Ohio State University, Columbus, OH.

DOI: 10.2337/9781580406086.24

intermittently in 20% of hospitalizations. Mean glucose was not significantly different between patients who continued CSII and those who did not. CSII patients, however, had fewer episodes of severe hyperglycemia (>300 mg/dL; $P < 0.02$) and hypoglycemia (<50 mg/dL; $P = 0.03$) than patients who switched from CSII to either intravenous (IV) or subcutaneous (SQ) injections. Compliance with most aspects of CSII guidelines was good, and 100% of CSII patients had an endocrinology consultation. In all of the studies Cook and associates conducted, there was only one instance of an adverse event, which involved a kinked catheter resulting in hyperglycemia.[12,13] Another study of 50 patients at a large medical center demonstrated that even patients who lack vital CSII knowledge on admission can safely continue CSII therapy during hospitalization provided they receive education support.[14] There were also no differences in mean glucose or hypoglycemia among those who continued CSII versus those who did not.

Even though these limited CSII studies in the hospital do not show any particular benefit, they do suggest that staying on CSII is not dangerous as long as there is adequate endocrine support. Larger studies in more diverse settings (particularly settings with less CSII expertise) are needed.

BASIC PUMP MECHANICS

CSII typically uses rapid-acting insulin analogs such as lispro, aspart, or glulisine, but U-500 insulin is being used with CSII with increasing frequency for individuals with insulin resistance. Insulin pumps deliver insulin in a more sophisticated basal-bolus pattern, in fractions of a unit, than is possible with MDI. Additional safety features include a maximum basal rate and maximum bolus. Some insulin pumps may be used in conjunction with continuous glucose monitoring, which may allow users to more easily track and address glucose trends. Insulin delivery is divided into basal and bolus (Table 24.1):

1. **Basal insulin:** CSII simulates endogenous insulin secretion with multiple basal rates delivered over the course of the day. These dose variations allow for less basal insulin to be infused overnight to reduce nocturnal hypoglycemia or more basal insulin to be delivered in the early morning hours to counteract a dawn phenomenon. Multiple patterns can be preprogrammed, for example, to address different needs on work days versus nonwork days. The pump allows individuals to suspend basal insulin delivery if hypoglycemia is present. Basal rates can be temporarily increased or decreased to accommodate a variety of situations, such as exercise or illness.
2. **Bolus insulin:** Bolus doses are optimally delivered using a bolus calculator, which utilizes a preprogramed insulin-to-carbohydrate ratio, sensitivity factor, and glucose target, all of which can be customized by time of day. The patient manually enters carbohydrate intake while glucoses are manually entered or wirelessly transmitted directly from the glucose meter. The bolus calculator will add to or subtract from the food-related bolus if the blood glucose is above or below target based on the sensitivity factor. Boluses can be extended using a dual-wave or a square-wave bolus to provide insulin delivery that is better matched for high-fat meals, or in patients with gastroparesis, both of which tend to have delayed absorption. Active

Table 24.1—Insulin Pump Settings

Insulin pump feature	Example
Basal Continuous infusion of rapid acting insulin Multiple rates Temporary basal (set as % of basal, specific duration) Ability to suspend infusion	00:00 0.85 units/h 06:00 0.5 units/h 12:00 0.7 units/h
Bolus	
Carbohydrate setting Carbohydrate-to-insulin Ratio Set by time of day Immediate or extended delivery	00:00 10 (10 g per unit of insulin)
Sensitivity Supplemental correction dose for high glucose Set by time of day	00:00 60 (1 unit for every 60 mg/dL over the upper target)
Target Level of glucose above which correction dose starts and below which insulin dose is reduced Set by time of day	00:00 90–130 mg/dL
Insulin on board (active insulin time) Duration of time in which reduction in successive correction doses occurs; pump-specific formula such that shorter intervals between correction doses result in greater dose reduction	4:00 hours (any correction dose within 4 h of the previous correction is reduced)

insulin time (or insulin on board) is an important safety feature that prevents bolus stacking by reducing the correction dose of insulin provided as a function of the time from the previous correction dose and within the specified window. Bolus stacking occurs when insulin boluses are given in succession to correct hyperglycemia. The original bolus may be actively lowering the blood glucose for several hours after a dose. If another correction bolus is delivered within the active insulin time, boluses may build up, or stack, causing subsequent hypoglycemia. This phenomenon is especially concerning in patients with renal failure.

APPROPRIATE PATIENTS TO CONTINUE PUMP MANAGEMENT

Appropriate patient selection is essential for safe inpatient CSII management.[10,15] Expert opinion differs on precisely which patients should continue CSII during hospitalization, but experts do agree that certain factors should exclude a patient from continuing inpatient CSII, including altered mental status, critical illness or sepsis, and suicide risk. Patients who continue CSII in the hospital should be able to demonstrate that they can navigate the pump safely, including delivering boluses, changing basic settings, changing infusion sites and set-up, and suspending the pump when appropriate. An assessment of the adequacy of self-care behaviors, including glucose monitoring and regular bolus delivery, may be useful for determining whether a patient should continue CSII in the hospital. Patients who are expected to be NPO for prolonged periods or who will undergo major surgery should not continue pump therapy, but should be transitioned to IV insulin or in some cases MDI. Occasionally, a patient admitted with CSII does not routinely manage his or her own pump, in which case the caregiver must be present at all times during the hospitalization for CSII to safely continue. Patients may need to temporarily remove the pump for certain radiographic testing or short procedures but can resume therapy after the procedure is completed. Transition strategies are discussed later in this chapter.

In one study of 50 patients admitted to the hospital with CSII, nearly 25% were unable to demonstrate vital pump settings, including where to find basal rates or bolus settings, >20% were unable to use the built-in pump calculator program, and 44% could not suspend their pump.[14] Fifty percent of patients could not demonstrate how to set a temporary basal rate. Despite the discrepancy in knowledge, only ~12% of patients did not continue pump therapy during their hospitalization, half of which were discontinued because of patient preference. Instead, patients with insufficient knowledge received CSII education on vital features and the majority were allowed to continue pump therapy throughout their hospitalization. The frequency of follow-up was not reported in this study, but there was no difference in glycemic control while inpatient among those who continued their insulin pump compared with those who did not.

ADVANTAGES AND DISADVANTAGES

There are clear advantages to continuing CSII during a patient's hospitalization. Satisfaction among CSII patients has been reported to be higher when patients are allowed to continue CSII therapy during hospitalization.[10,13,16] In addition, continuing CSII during hospitalization allows for adjustments to pump settings in a controlled environment. The advanced features on CSII provide clear advantages over MDI in several other ways. Unlike MDI therapy, CSII allows for basal insulin to be temporarily increased or decreased in real time for a variety of situations (such as NPO status) using the temporary basal feature. CSII also improves the timing of insulin delivery because patients do not have to rely on nursing staff to administer prandial boluses with meals.

By far, the greatest disadvantage of continuing CSII therapy during hospitalization is unfamiliarity of staff and lack of expert involvement. This lack of understanding creates a situation in which the patient, regardless of the depth of their knowledge regarding CSII, is independently responsible for managing their diabetes in the hospital environment. This inevitably raises safety concerns.[15] In addition, when patients adjust insulin doses without informing the medical staff, potential safety and liability concerns arise. Mental status and overall condition can change quickly in the hospital setting, and thus ongoing surveillance of the patient's capacity to operate the pump is needed. The development of an infrastructure to safely manage pumps in the inpatient setting is multifaceted and involves a multidisciplinary approach, including input from legal services and risk management.

ROLES AND RESPONSIBILITIES

Guidelines describing proper implementation and oversight of CSII have been proposed and are summarized here.[10] Communication among all parties involved is essential for safe and effective inpatient management of CSII. Comanagement involves cooperation among the patient, the diabetes experts, the primary team, and nursing staff.

- **Patient:** The patient must agree to communicate all bolus doses, setting adjustments, site changes, and any problems related to CSII use to nursing.[10] Patients are responsible for the care and maintenance of the pump and for all pump supplies, and they should have an extra set of supplies at the bedside. At a minimum, patients must be able to independently insert and initiate CSII and to bolus independently. The patient may keep their home blood glucose meter at the bedside for monitoring between meals, but all treatment decisions should be based on the hospital-grade meter. These results should be entered manually into the pump for use of the bolus calculator.
- **Primary Provider:** The primary provider or primary team is responsible for initial and ongoing assessment of appropriateness of continued CSII. If CSII is discontinued, then an alternative insulin regimen must be administered. The primary provider or diabetes consult service is responsible for writing insulin pump orders, which include the following: *1*) type of insulin, *2*) basal rates and time periods, *3*) insulin-to-carbohydrates ratios, *4*) sensitivity for correction bolus doses, and *5*) frequency of blood glucose testing.[10] When diabetes expert consultation is not available, the primary team is responsible for monitoring glycemic control and, along with the patient, making any needed adjustments.
- **Nurse:** The nurse is responsible for continual assessment of the patient's mental and physical capability to manage CSII. The nurse is responsible for documentation of glucose levels, carbohydrate counts, and prandial and correction boluses. This requires ongoing patient dialogue. The nurse also must assess and document the location and condition of the infusion site, along with documentation of CSII site changes. Nursing education has been shown to improve overall knowledge and confidence regarding CSII.[17]
- **Diabetes Educator:** Patients may need reinforcement of basic pump principles to ensure safe use in the hospital setting.[15] Patients who present in diabetic ketoacidosis (DKA) could benefit from reinforcement of basic pump DKA prevention strategies once the acute medical crisis is resolved.
- **Diabetes Consult Team:** As discussed before, diabetes and CSII expertise is recommended by expert individuals and teams for the safe comanagement of CSII in the inpatient setting.[3–5] The diabetes consult team assesses patient's level of pump sophistication and glucose control, and makes initial and ongoing adjustments to pump settings. The consult service assesses the patient's overall level of pump sophistication and provides education on vital pump features. If expertise in the management of diabetes and CSII is not available during hospitalization, then the patient's outpatient pump

prescriber should be contacted for dosing recommendations and guidance, if possible.[3]

- **Hospital:** Hospital guidelines, order sets, and policy development are critical if CSII is to be managed safely in the inpatient setting, because most general providers are unfamiliar with how to prescribe insulin pump orders and adjust therapy.[10] We recommend that institutions develop patient contracts or waivers that specify patient responsibilities during hospitalization, set the expectation that settings may be adjusted during the hospital stay, and inform the patient that they may be transitioned off CSII for changes in the individual's medical condition (Figure 24.1).[10] Depending on the hospital, the components of this infrastructure may require approval by an inpatient safety committee or legal or risk management official.

HOSPITAL MANAGEMENT

GENERAL APPROACH FOR THE HOSPITALIZED CSII PATIENT

On admission, it is important to assess whether initial adjustments need to be made to the pump settings for safe glycemic control during hospitalization. Glucose targets for noncritically ill patients are premeal <140 mg/dL and all other

ADULT GUIDELINES FOR USING YOUR SUBCUTANEOUS INSULIN PUMP WHILE IN THE HOSPITAL

LOCATION DATE

While you are in the hospital, it is the hospital staff's responsibility to ensure that your blood sugars are controlled as well as possible. The decision that you will remain on the insulin pump in the hospital will be determined by your medical team in consultation with the endocrine service as well as your medical status. It is against hospital policy and state regulations to keep insulin vials at the bedside and to use insulin from home. You will be asked to change your pump reservoir and infusion set (using your own supplies) and use a new bottle of insulin (will be supplied by the hospital pharmacy).

Your responsibilities:

1. Bring all the supplies needed for use of your pump. Include extra infusion sets, reservoirs and batteries.
2. Change the infusion site every 72 hours while hospitalized. You will need to do this sooner than 72 hours if you experience unexplained hyperglycemia (repeated blood sugar greater than 300mg/dL) or if there are signs of infection at the insertion site.
3. Show the nurse the settings on your pump whenever he/she requests.
4. Disconnect from your pump for mammograms,bone density tests, radiation treatment, CT scan, MRI,and x-rays. The infusion set can remain in place.
5. Do not change pump settings without MD direction.
6. Do not give boluses without RN supervision.

Informed Consent/Waiver of Liability

I hereby request that the University of California at San Francisco Medical Center(UCSF Medical Center) make available to me my own insulin until I am able to switch my pump reservoir to insulin supplied by the hospital pharmacy. I understand that my own medication can not be identified and verified as to type of insulin, previous storage or expiration date. It is the policy of UCSF Medical Center to clearly identify all medications provided by a patient before they may be administered in the hospital. I understand that UCSF Medical Center staff cannot verify the contents in my insulin pump and understand that this may present risks to my health, including but not limited to hyperglycemia, Diabetic Ketoacidosis, hypoglycemia, and infection.

I release UC and its employees from any liability regarding my use of the insulin pump during my hospitalization, including but not limited to damage, loss, theft and malfunction.

I understand that my physicians and other health care providers have the right to terminate my use of the insulin pump should they observe any contraindication to its use or for any reason they believe medically necessary.

My signature below is my acknowledgement that I have read, understood, and agreed to the above.

Figure 24.1—Adult guidelines for using your subcutaneous insulin pump while in the hospital.

glucoses <180 mg/dL.[4,5] Patients with excellent, tight control in the outpatient setting may need setting adjustments to prevent hypoglycemia in the inpatient setting. For some patients using CSII, the target blood glucose setting may need to be increased, particularly if oral intake is compromised, or other factors are present that increase the risk of hypoglycemia, such as renal failure. Patients should be asked about recent frequency and precipitating factors of hyperglycemia and hypoglycemia in the home setting.

An assessment of self-management behaviors is important, including the following:

- **Glucose Monitoring:** As with MDI therapy, frequent glucose monitoring is necessary to prevent, recognize, and treat hypoglycemia and hyperglycemia. With CSII, only rapid-acting insulin is used and potential pump malfunction or infusion site problems may lead to DKA more quickly if a patient is not monitoring adequately.
- **Basal and Bolus Calculations:** Patients who infrequently bolus may rely on higher basal rates to cover carbohydrate intake or frequent snacking, and they may be at risk for hypoglycemia in the hospital setting because food intake may vary. Total daily insulin requirements typically are split evenly between basal and bolus insulin, unless carbohydrate intake is very high or low. Initial adjustment of basal rates, either by reapportioning the total daily dose or by using a temporary basal reduction, may be needed in the hospital, where carb-controlled meals are served and intake may differ from home.
- **Manual Boluses vs. Bolus Calculator:** Manually calculated boluses are known to be much less accurate than those using a bolus calculator.[18–20] Occasionally, patients may override the recommended bolus for valid reasons. If, however, the individual is routinely overriding the bolus calculator, then adjustments in settings are generally warranted.
- **Routine Care:** Other potential pitfalls include inappropriate prolonged suspensions of the insulin pump, failure to change infusion sites at least every 3 days, incorrectly timed boluses, dietary indiscretion, and unrecognized pump or infusion site failure.

Not all institutions have the resources or expertise to analyze data that can be downloaded from the pump. The pump download, however, provides a wealth of information that assists in making adjustments in therapy as well as addressing patient adherence and potential educational needs. This information along with the A1C may be helpful in determining initial dosing adjustments on admission.

Subsequent adjustments should be made cautiously, in increments of up to 10–20% of the total daily dose per day. For temporary adjustments in insulin, such as those required for the management of stress-induced hyperglycemia, NPO status, glucocorticoid use, or acute renal failure, it is usually preferable to avoid adjustments in the preprogrammed basal rate settings, because patients may need to access them when the illness resolves. Instead, providers may choose any number of approaches, including the following:

1. Set an alternate basal pattern. Programming this method may require assistance from the diabetes consult team, but it allows the patient to easily switch back to the preadmission basal pattern as the illness resolves.

2. Use temporary basal rates. This method is quickly customizable and needs to be reset at least daily. This may require assistance from the diabetes consult team.
3. Add an injection of basal insulin that is slowly weaned over time. This may be more preferable for patients or providers than changing settings daily. However, this strategy only addresses hyperglycemia, not hypoglycemia.

Anticipatory dose adjustments should be made for changes in clinical status that may affect glucose levels, such as change in oral intake, renal function, or glucocorticoid dose. Management approaches for selected special situations are presented next, and management approaches for additional scenarios are summarized in Table 24.2.

SURGERIES AND PROCEDURES

For elective procedures and surgeries, decisions about insulin management should occur before admission via contact with the patient's diabetes care provider. Patients may continue CSII during short surgical procedures, at the discretion of the surgeon and anesthesiologist. Blood glucose monitoring should be performed hourly in the procedure area. It is important for the pump site to be easily accessible during the procedure and yet placed to avoid interfering with the procedure or surgical site. CSII should not be worn during magnetic resonance imaging or computed tomography scans.[15] Generally, when patients will be disconnected from CSII for more than 1 h, supplemental insulin to replace the missed basal insulin will be needed. When patients will be disconnected for 1–3 h, supplemental insulin can be calculated as an hourly basal rate multiplied by the time disconnected from the pump, and then delivered either as a separate injection or as a bolus just before the device is disconnected.[21] If patients will be disconnected from CSII for longer than 3 h, IV insulin or transition to MDI therapy is required to prevent iatrogenic DKA. Patients are perhaps at greatest risk of intentional or unintentional omission of basal insulin in the postoperative setting. Patients requiring multiple pump suspensions should transition to MDI.

Oral intake is often restricted for testing or procedures. Patients who have basal-heavy regimens are at greatest risk for hypoglycemia when NPO, whereas patients with morning hyperglycemia may not need any reduction in basal rates at all. The temporary basal setting can be initiated at bedtime and adjusted in real time. For patients with type 1 diabetes who require basal insulin reduction, a conservative reduction of 20% is recommended, whereas patients with type 2 diabetes can tolerate a greater reduction of 20–50%.

DKA

In addition to the usual factors that may precipitate DKA, pump or infusion site failure as well as failure to modify pump therapy in response to hyperglycemia may contribute.[16] Patients who are admitted to the hospital in DKA should be managed with IV insulin, and CSII should be removed until acidosis resolves and mental status normalizes.

Nonadherence to glucose monitoring or pump management as potential causes of DKA can be easily identified by downloading the pump's data. Patients should be trained to respond to hyperglycemia promptly and systematically by bolusing

Table 24.2—Management of Common Scenarios among Hospitalized CSII Patients

	Problem	Potential management strategies
Stress hyperglycemia	Illness-related factors cause temporary hyperglycemia	Use increased temporary basal insulin feature Add alternate basal pattern Add basal insulin injection and wean over time IV insulin Increase carbohydrate-to-insulin ratio Reduce insulin sensitivity
NPO status	Risk for hypoglycemia	Temporary basal insulin setting (80% for type 1 diabetes, 50–80% for type 2 diabetes, U-500 insulin, or basal insulin heavy regimens with >50% of total daily dose is basal)
Glucocorticoids (GCs)	Marked but temporary hyperglycemia	*Short-intermediate-acting GCs once daily:* Increase carbohydrate-to-insulin ratio Reduce insulin sensitivity Temporary basal rate to mimic steroid effect Add injection of NPH *Short-acting GCs multiple times per day or long-acting GCs:* Increase carbohydrate-to-insulin ratio Reduce insulin sensitivity Temporary basal increase Add alternate basal insulin pattern Add injection of basal insulin analogue
Renal failure	Multiple derangements increase risk for hypoglycemia	Raise glucose target Increase active insulin time Anticipatory dose reduction
Gastroparesis	Delayed emptying leads to mismatch in peak glucose and insulin concentration, causing early hyperglycemia and delayed hypoglycemia	Use extended duration bolus (square wave or dual wave); dosing the bolus after the meal may be helpful for those with erratic intake because of GI symptoms
U-500 concentrated regular insulin	U-500 is not FDA approved for use with pumps but is commonly used due to limited reservoir size; U-500 has delayed onset and extended duration of action compared to rapid-acting insulin analogues	Bolus 30 min before meals. Extend active insulin time to 6–8 h Avoid interprandial correction Increase carbohydrate-to-insulin ratio and insulin sensitivity later in the day Marked dose reduction with reduced PO intake

via their pump first and by injection and changing the infusion site if the correction is unsuccessful.[16,22] Frequent monitoring is essential. Site issues, including sites left in too long or a kinked cannula, can precipitate DKA if not detected through frequent monitoring. The patient's infusion sites should be assessed for lipohypertrophy, scarring, and signs of infection. Time between site changes as well as insertion technique should be discussed if the patient is having recurring issues with hyperglycemia and DKA.[22] Actual pump malfunction is rare[1] but should be considered. If malfunction is suspected, the pump company should be contacted to report the problem and to request provision of a new or temporary pump (Table 24.3).

TRANSITIONS OF CARE

When patients need to transition from CSII to MDI therapy, a long-acting basal analog such as glargine or detemir should be administered to cover the patient's basal insulin requirements. The patient's total basal dose can be obtained easily from the pump download or from the pump itself. When determining the corresponding long-acting analog dose, it is important to consider several factors. Patients typically need 20% less insulin when delivered via CSII than via basal insulin analog injection.[22] Therefore, it is reasonable to initially increase the total basal dose by 20% when converting to long-acting insulin injection. For patients with frequent hypoglycemia, decreased PO intake or with basal-heavy insulin regimens (basal insulin dose >50% of the total daily dose) a reduction of 10–20% from the CSII total basal may be reasonable. Long-acting insulin analogs should be given at least 2 h before discontinuation of CSII whenever possible to avoid rebound hyperglycemia. Patients can continue the insulin-to-carbohydrate ratio and sensitivity used in their CSII for bolus injections of rapid-acting analogue.

CSII can be resumed 24 h after the last long-acting basal insulin injection. If the pump is restarted less than 24 h after a basal insulin injection has been administered, a temporary basal should be set reducing the basal to 0–10%, and timed to expire 24 h after the last dose of basal insulin.

When patients transition from IV insulin back to CSII, the overnight IV insulin rates can be observed for changes in the patient's insulin requirements. If IV insulin rates vary greatly from previous pump settings, preadmission settings and glucose control, as well as weight-based calculations, should be considered before changing

Table 24.3—Pump Manufacturers

Company	Website	Customer service number
Animas	www.animas.com	1-877-937-7867
Insulet	www.myomnipod.com	1-800-591-3455
Medtronic	www.medtronicdiabetes.com	1-800-633-8766
Roche	www.accu-chekinsulinpumps.com	1-800-688-4578
Tandem	www.tandemdiabetes.com	1-877-801-6901

the preprogrammed settings. A temporary basal increase or decrease, or an alternate pattern, can be set to test out estimated basal rates before permanent changes are made to settings. IV insulin should be overlapped with initiation of CSII by 1–2 h.

HOSPITAL DISCHARGE

Patients using CSII should be followed by providers who are knowledgeable about CSII technology and management and who are able to provide the necessary resources to sustain safe pump therapy.[3] Specialty care may not be available in some rural settings, making management by a primary care provider a necessity. For all patients, regardless of prescriber, education, training, and follow-up are essential.

REFERENCES

1. U.S. Federal Drug Administration. *General hospital and personal use medical devices panel: insulin infusion pumps panel information*. Washington, DC, March 5, 2010
2. Noschese ML, DiNardo MM, Donihi AC, et al. Patient outcomes after implementation of a protocol for inpatient insulin pump therapy. *Endocr Pract* 2009;15(5):415–424
3. Grunberger G, Abelseth JM, Bailey TS, Bode TS, Handelsman Y, Hellman R, Jovanovic L, Lane WS, Raskin P, Tamborlane WV. AACE insulin pump management task force statement by the American Association of Clinical Endocrinologist consensus panel on insulin pump management. *Endocr Pract* 2014;20(5):463–489
4. Moghissi ES, et al. American Association of Clinical Endocrinologists and American Diabetes Association consensus statement on inpatient glycemic control. *Endocr Pract* 2009;15(4):353–369
5. Umpierrez GE, et al. Management of hyperglycemia in hospitalized patients in non-critical care setting: an Endocrine Society clinical practice guideline. *J Clin Endocrinol Metab* 2012;97(1):16–38
6. Weissberg-Benchell J, Antisdel-Lomaglio J, Seshadri R. Insulin pump therapy: a meta-analysis. *Diabetes Care* 2003;26(4):1079–1087
7. Pickup JC, Sutton AJ. Severe hypoglycemia and glycaemic control in Type 1 diabetes: meta-analysis of multiple daily insulin injections compared with continuous subcutaneous insulin infusion. *Diabetes Med* 2008:25:765–774
8. Yeh HC, Brown TT, Maruthur N, Ranasinghe P, Berger Z, Suh YD, Wilson LM, Haberl EB, Brick J, Bass EB, Golden SH. Comparative effectiveness and safety of methods of insulin delivery and glucose monitoring for diabetes mellitus: a systematic review and meta-analysis. *Ann Intern Med* 2012;157(5):336–347
9. Golden SH, Brown T, Yeh HC, Maruthur N, Ranasinghe P, Berger Z, Suh Y, Wilson LM, Haberl EB, Bass EB. Methods for insulin delivery and glucose monitoring: comparative effectiveness [Internet]. Rockville, MD, Agency for Healthcare Rescarch and Quality 2012

10. Cook CB, Boyle ME, Cisar NS, et al. Use of continuous subcutaneous insulin infusion (insulin pump) therapy in the hospital settings: proposed guidelines and outcome measures. *Diabetes Educ* 2005;31(6):849–857

11. Cook CB, Beer KA, Seifert KM, Boyle ME, Mackey PA, Castro JC. Transitioning insulin pump therapy from the outpatient to the inpatient setting: a review of 6 years' experience with 253 cases. *J Diabetes Sci Technol* 2012;6(5):995–1002

12. Nassar AA, Partlow BJ, Boyle ME, Castro JC, Bourgeois PB, Curtiss BC. Outpatient-to-inpatient transition of insulin pump therapy successes and continuing challenges. *J Diabetes Sci Technol* 2010;4(4):853–872

13. Leonhardi BJ, Boyle ME, Beer K, Seifert KM, Bailey M, Miller-Cage V, Castro JC, Bourgeois PB, Curtiss BC. Use of continuous subcutaneous insulin infusion (insulin pump) therapy in the hospital: a review of one institution's experience. *J Diabetes Sci Technol* 2008;2(6):949–962

14. Kannan S, Satra A, Calogeras E, Lock P, Lansang MC. Insulin pump patient characteristics and glucose control in the hospitalized setting. *J Diabetes Sci Technol* 2014;8(3):473–478

15. Lansang MC, Modic MB, Sauvey R, Lock P, Ross D, Coubs P, Kennedy L. Approach to the adult hospitalized patient on an insulin pump. *J Hospital Med* 2013;8(12):721–727

16. Lee SW, Im R, Magbual R. Current perspectives on the use of continuous subcutaneous insulin infusion in the acute care setting and overview of therapy. *Crit Care Nurse Quart* 2004;27(2):172–184

17. Sweeney TJ, Kenny DJ, Schubert CC. Inpatient insulin pump therapy: assessing the effectiveness of an educational program. *J Nurse Prof Develop* 2013;29(2):84–89

18. Shashaj B, Busetto E, Sulli N. Benefits of a bolus calculator in pre- and postprandial glycaemic control and meal flexibilty of paediatric patients using continuous subcutaneous insulin infusion (CSII). *Diabetic Med* 2008; 25(9):1036–1042

19. Sussman A, Taylor EJ, Patel M, Ward J, Alva S, Lawrence A, Ng R. Performance of a glucose meter with a built-in automated bolus calculator versus manual bolus calculation in insulin-using subjects. *J Diabetes Sci Technol* 2012; 6(2):339–344

20. Maurizi AR, Lauria A, Maggi D, Palermo A, Fioriti E, Manfrini S, Pozzilli P. A novel insulin unit calculator for the management of type 1 diabetes. *Diabetes Technol Therap* 2011;13(4):425–428

21. Medtronic. Guidelines for temporary disconnection. Available from http://www.medtronic-diabetes.co.uk/help-support/lifestyle/guidelines-for-temporary-disconnection.html. Accessed December 2015

22. Walsh J, Roberts R. *Pumping insulin: everything you need to succeed on an insulin pump*, 5th ed. San Diego, CA, Torrey Pines Press, 2012

Chapter 25

Continuous Glucose Monitoring in the Hospital

Patricia Peter, MD,[1] and Silvio E. Inzucchi, MD[2]

Although the optimal glycemic targets in the inpatient setting remain controversial, glucose control for the hospitalized patient is important because both hyperglycemia and hypoglycemia have been associated with longer length of stay, higher risk of complications, and increased mortality.[1] Quality glycemic management in both inpatient and outpatient settings is contingent upon accurate and reproducible measurements of blood glucose levels. Continuous glucose monitoring (CGM) systems have been demonstrated to improve glycemic control outside of the hospital, and interest is emerging in determining whether similar benefits can be realized in the inpatient arena.[2]

The theoretical advantages of inpatient CGM are numerous. The number of data points offered by CGM over the conventional method of blood glucose measurement with bedside capillary glucose meters potentially could help to more precisely direct insulin infusion protocols in intensive care units (ICUs). The ability of CGM to notify nurses and physicians of trends and rates of blood glucose change is a particularly attractive feature, theoretically allowing for early and timely intervention to prevent hypo- or hyperglycemic events. It is also possible for providers to remotely monitor their patients' CGM data, analogous to telemetry alarms alerting staff about patients' arrhythmias. Patients on insulin infusion protocols would suffer less discomfort if they can be monitored with CGM that uses a subcutaneously inserted sensor instead of hourly fingersticks. The potential effects on nursing workload and hospital costs would be an important consideration as well—although their directionality is not intuitively obvious. Given these potential advantages, there is ongoing interest in determining whether CGM will prove to be a viable and perhaps more effective alternative to our current methods of tracking glycemia in the hospital.

LIMITATIONS OF FINGERSTICKS IN THE INPATIENT SETTING

The current gold standard of inpatient glucose measurement relies on central laboratory processing of plasma glucose. Plasma is preferred over whole blood

[1]Section of Endocrinology, Department of Internal Medicine, Yale University School of Medicine, Yale-New Haven Hospital, New Haven, CT. [2]Section of Endocrinology, Yale School of Medicine, New Haven, CT.

DOI: 10.2337/9781580406086.25

because it is less influenced by the hematocrit.[3] Additionally, sample source also affects the measured glucose value, with arterial blood being typically ~10 mg/dL higher than venous blood and ~5 mg/dL higher than capillary blood in the normal physiological range.[3]

Point-of-care (POC) glucose meters, using capillary blood obtained through the lancing of the skin of the fingertips, have been approved for use in the outpatient self-monitoring of blood glucose. They are the most commonly used glucose measuring tools in the inpatient setting, but before the recent approval of the Nova StatStrip Glucose Hospital Meter System (Nova Biomedical, Waltham, MA), none had been sanctioned formally for use in the hospital. Concerns recently have emerged that POC glucose meters are not sufficiently accurate to guide management in the hospitalized population, particularly in the critically ill, in whom there has been a paucity of validation testing. Standards for accuracy are in flux but the U.S. Food and Drug Administration (FDA) currently uses those of the International Organization for Standardization (ISO) 15197:2003 in which 95% of glucose values measured by the meter must fall within 15 mg/dL of the reference method for glucose concentrations <75 mg/dL or within 20% for glucose concentrations >75 mg/dL.[3] Studies have shown that only 40–83% of currently available glucose meters actually meet these standards in the outpatient setting, and many clinicians feel that even if consistently met, these standards are not rigorous enough to guide the often more intensive management of the hospitalized patient population.[4] The FDA recently has responded to these concerns and issued proposed draft guidelines in early 2014. If adopted, these guidelines would require much more stringent requirements for hospital-use glucose meters with 99% of all values falling within +/–10% of the reference method for glucose concentrations ≥75 mg/dL and within +/–7 mg/dL at glucose concentrations <70 mg/dL.[5]

POC capillary glucose meters typically rely on the glucose oxidase or glucose dehydrogenase reactions, both of which have their own potential sources of inaccuracy. The glucose oxidase reaction converts glucose and water into hydrogen peroxide and gluconic acid.[3] When a mediator is used as the last electron acceptor in this redox reaction, oxygen can compete with the mediator and artificially lower glucose values, especially in situations associated with high oxygen tension as with mechanical ventilation.[3] Reducing agents such as ascorbic acid and acetaminophen also interfere with this enzymatic reaction to underestimate true glucose values.[3] Catecholamines, ibuprofen, uric acid, and bilirubin also have been implicated in interference with glucose-oxidase based systems.[3] By contrast, glucose meters that rely on the glucose dehydrogenase system to detect glucose levels are less subject to error because of oxygen tension or interfering medications. Sometimes, however, they can detect other nonglucose sugars, such as mannose, xylose, and the maltose-polymer icodextrin, to overestimate blood glucose, but only if pyrroloquinoline serves as a cofactor in the reaction.[3]

Hospitalized patients often experience physiologic disturbances that introduce additional error into these POC capillary measurements. Studies have raised concerns regarding the accuracy of fingerstick blood glucose measurement in the hospital setting, finding failure to meet ISO standards 13.7–25.2% of the time.[6,7] Many authors find this unacceptable, especially because these glucose meters tended to overestimate true glucose values, which may prompt the administration of a higher insulin dose than actually required. Hypotension and resultant altered tissue perfusion, acidosis, anemia, and hypothermia in these patients may alter the relationship between blood glucose and POC measurements, providing additional sources of error.[8]

In addition to concerns regarding the accuracy of capillary glucose meters in the inpatient setting, these intermittent measurements may not accurately capture the full extent of glucose fluctuations in a critically ill population, making it difficult to intervene in a timely, effective fashion. Also, more practical problems, such as patient discomfort and the considerable nursing workload, are associated with frequent fingerstick testing. Given the limitations of POC testing in the inpatient setting, there is considerable interest in determining whether CGM could emerge as an alternative that could address at least some of these problems.

OVERVIEW OF CGM TECHNOLOGY: SUBCUTANEOUS DEVICES

Currently, two outpatient CGM systems in the U.S. (DexCom G4™ Platinum and Medtronic Enlite™) are approved by the FDA and one is approved for inpatient use in Europe (Sentrino® by Medtronic). All utilize a subcutaneously inserted sensor to measure interstitial glucose concentrations. After equilibrating with the plasma, glucose and oxygen enter the subcutaneous (SQ) tissue and react with the sensor's glucose oxidase to generate hydrogen peroxide in a redox reaction similar to that used in many capillary blood glucose meters. Hydrogen peroxide subsequently becomes oxidized by the sensor's electrode and releases electrons, creating a current whose strength correlates with the glucose concentration. This information is then communicated wirelessly to a nearby display device that graphically displays the current glucose level as well as trending information. Data typically are updated every 5 min. The sensor needs to be changed every 3–7 days, depending on the model. There is usually at least a 2-h "run-in" period immediately after sensor insertion when the device will not report data, and twice-daily calibration by fingerstick results is required. Importantly, the FDA recommends that insulin-dosing decisions be made only *after* confirmation of the CGM glucose value by fingerstick glucose testing.

An important limitation of CGM is that oxidants, such as uric acid, acetaminophen, and salicylic acid, can interfere with the glucose oxidase reaction that underlies many CGM systems, as can occur in capillary glucose meters that depend on this reaction. Additionally, CGM measures interstitial blood glucose whose equilibration with plasma is influenced by a variety of factors, including blood flow, rate of change of intravascular glucose concentration, capillary permeability, volume status, edema, and metabolic rate of nearby cells. This results in a lag time of anywhere from 10 to 30 min.[9] Finally, deposition of a biofilm on the sensor leads to eventual glucose "drift," introducing a potentially harmful bias in glucose measurement.[9]

OVERVIEW OF CGM TECHNOLOGY: INTRAVASCULAR DEVICES

Though most intravascular CGM devices remain largely in the investigative phase and are more invasive than their SQ counterparts, they have the advantage of increased accuracy.[10] Some intravascular devices consist of an intravascular sensor that measures blood glucose without consuming any blood. For example, the GluCath™ (Glumetrics Inc., Irvine, CA) consists of a small optical fiber impregnated with boronic acid derivatives coupled with fluorescence that becomes quenched after interaction with glucose in the blood.[9] The EIRUS™ microdialysis system (Maquet Critical Care, Rastatt, Germany) utilizes a microdialysis fiber incorporated into a central venous catheter to measure glucose concentration via the glucose oxidase method.[11]

Other intravascular devices extract a blood sample that is then run through an external sensor and is either recirculated or discarded. The GlucoScout™ (International Biomedical Ltd., Austin, TX) is actually now FDA approved for sampling arterial or venous blood every 5 min for up to 72 h. Sampled blood flows through a sterile glucose-oxidase electrochemical sensor and is returned to the bloodstream along with a glucose-salt solution that recalibrates the sensor.[9] GlucoClear™ (Edwards LifeSciences, Irvine, CA) is a similarly designed system that is approved for use in Europe. The investigational OptiScanner™ (OptiScan Inc., Hayward, CA) instead uses midinfrared spectroscopy to measure the glucose concentration in a plasma sample extracted from the blood. It remains to be seen what ultimately will prove to be the most accurate and easily implemented glucose-sensing method for these intravascular devices, which are still in the relatively early stages of their development.

Some concerns that have limited the adoption of intravascular devices thus far include the higher infection risk, potentially stronger foreign body response, biofilm deposition affecting sensor accuracy over time, increased thrombotic risk sometimes necessitating the use of anticoagulation, and interference from other solutions that are running through the shared vascular access.[9] Despite these concerns, early studies investigating the use of these intravascular devices in the inpatient setting have thus far shown acceptable accuracy with low complication rates, although these studies were admittedly small and of short duration.[11–15] Potential advantages include increased accuracy and the theoretical ease of coupling such continuous systems with insulin delivery in the future. This would facilitate the creation of a truly closed-loop system (sometimes referred to as the "artificial pancreas") for diabetes management in the inpatient setting.

STUDIES INVESTIGATING THE USE OF CGM IN THE INPATIENT SETTING

Before any new technology could be considered as a replacement (or enhancement) to the current standard of intermittent fingerstick capillary blood glucose monitoring, randomized trials must conclusively demonstrate its advantage, either through better accuracy, decreased workload, or decreased costs. An impact on actual patient outcomes would be desirable but may be more difficult to prove.

There remains no broad clinical consensus for the evaluation of CGM device accuracy. One of the most commonly used analytic tools for this purpose is the Clarke error grid analysis.[16] This graphical method compares the sensor glucose values on the *y*-axis with the reference glucose values on the *x*-axis and stratifies them into five clinical risk zones, A–E, with A and B considered clinically acceptable (Figure 25.1).[16] Other commonly used methods to measure accuracy include

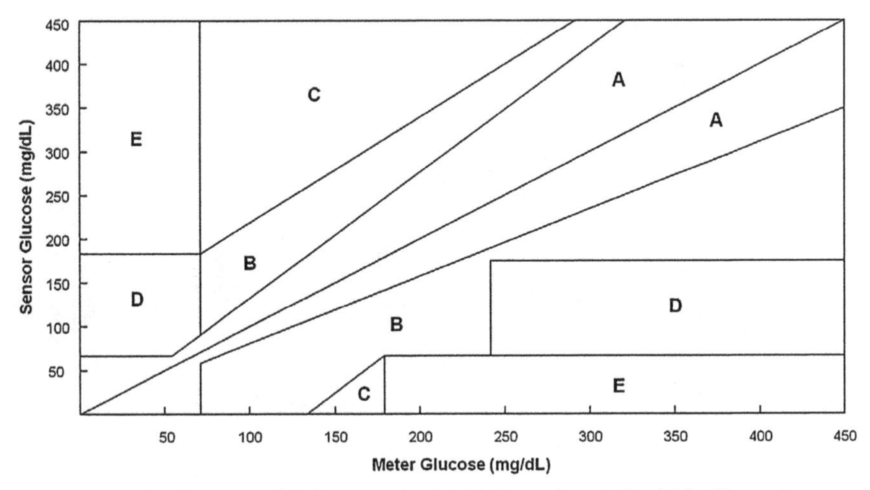

Figure 25.1—Sample Clarke error grid. Values that fall within Zone A are within 20% of the reference value. Zone B deviates from the reference value by greater than 20% but would only lead to benign errors in treatment. Zones C, D, and E would result in clinically significant errors in treatment.[16]

the Bland-Altman plot, the mean absolute relative difference, and the continuous glucose-error grid analysis.[10] Most of the existing clinical studies on CGM have employed one or several of these techniques to report accuracy.

The clinical studies that have investigated CGM in the adult inpatient setting are summarized in Table 25.1. Most have taken place in the ICU and have focused on comparing CGM accuracy to that of reference values, with the majority of studies concluding that the new technology has sufficient accuracy for use in the inpatient setting.[13,17–22] The reference values used in these studies varied widely, but most used either arterial blood glucose analysis or capillary blood glucose values, the latter being an interesting reference standard because, as mentioned previously, POC meters are not formally approved for accuracy in the ICU setting. A retrospective pooled-data analysis of CGM data in 174 ICU patients using arterial blood-gas analysis as the reference echoed these results, finding that 99.1% of all readings fell within the acceptable treatment zone and 92.9% of values met ISO criteria.[23] Several studies have demonstrated that CGM remains reasonably accurate despite the often tenuous hemodynamic status or the pressor requirement of this critically ill population.[13,17,20,21,24] CGM accuracy does not seem to be affected by ketosis, hypothermia, or edema, but most of the investigations reporting on these variables are small and likely underpowered.[8,25]

Other studies, however, have raised serious concerns about the accuracy of CGM in the inpatient setting. For example, Rabiee et al.[26] found that the CGM missed 50% of hypoglycemic episodes as determined by fingerstick, while Boom et al.[27] found that 75% of hypoglycemic events (BG <70 mg/dL) were not detected by CGM when compared with 33% that were not detected by

Table 25.1—Clinical Studies of CGM in the Inpatient Setting

First author and year	Population	Comparison	Clarke A/B (%)	Other outcomes
Goldberg 2004[21]	22 ICU patients	CGMS (Medtronic) vs. CBG	98.7%	-CGM accuracy was not affected by pressors
Corstjens 2006[22]	19 ICU patients	CGMS Gold (Medtronic) vs. arterial POC	100%	
De Block 2006[13]	50 ICU patients	GlucoDay (Menarini) vs. ABG	95–97%	-CGM accuracy was better in AKI, worse in patients on pressors
Price 2008[28]	17 med/surg ICU patients	Guardian RT CGMS (Medtronic) vs. CBG vs. arterial POC	N/A	-Poor agreement among all three methods
Holzinger 2009[17]	50 ICU patients	CGMS Gold (Medtronic) vs. ABG	98.6%	-CGM accuracy was not affected by pressors
Logtenberg 2009[37]	31 patients undergoing cardiac surgery	Paradigm RT CGMS (Medtronic) vs. CBG/ABG	96–99.5%	-Similar glycemic control
Rabiee 2009[26]	19 SICU and burn ICU patients	DexCom STS vs. CBG and plasma glucose	100%	-CGM did not detect 50% of hypoglycemia found by CBG -CGM had 88% false alarm rate for hypoglycemia
Holzinger 2010[30]	RCT of 124 ICU patients	CGMS Gold (Medtronic) vs. ABG	N/A	-Similar glycemic control -86% RRR of severe hypoglycemia in CGM group
Jacobs 2010[29]	29 ICU patients	Guardian RT CGMS (Medtronic) vs. CBG	N/A	-66.6% CGM values met ISO standard for accuracy -Technical difficulties occurred
Dungan 2012[38]	58 non-ICU patients with CHF	CGMS iPro (Medronic) vs. CBG	96.9–99.1%	-CGM was less accurate in CHF inpatients than in outpatients

Kalmovich 2012[35]	32 cardiac surgery patients	CGMS Gold (Medtronic) vs. plasma glucose	N/A	-CGM inaccurately detected hypoglycemic events in one-third of patients
Lee 2012[36]	12 critically ill ER patients	CGMS Gold (Medtronic) vs. CBG	96.8%	-PPV of CGM detecting hypoglycemia was 16.7%
Lorencio 2012[24]	41 med/surg ICU patients	RT CGMS (Medtronic) vs. ABG	N/A	-CGM more accurate in septic shock patients -CGM less accurate in hypoglycemic range than normo- or hyperglycemic ranges
Kopecky 2013[18]	RCT of 24 undergoing elective cardiac surgery	Guardian RT CGMS (Medtronic) vs. ABG	97.5%	-Similar glycemic control -Used eMPC algorithm
Rodriguez-Quintanilla 2013[39]	16 patients with ACS	Guardian RT CGMS (Medtronic) vs. CBG	N/A	-Patients in CGM group took significantly longer to achieve normoglycemia (13 vs. 5.7 h) but all achieved it (vs. 87.5% of controls, not significant)
Schierenbeck 2013[11]	30 cardiac surgery patients	Eirus™ (Maquet) triple lumen catheter with microdialysis vs. ABG	100%	
Siegelaar 2013[25]	60 cardiac surgery patients	Guardian RT CGMS (Medtronic) vs. FreeStyle Navigator (Abbott) vs. ABG	98.4–99.5%	-CGM accuracy decreased with lower peripheral temperature, greater age and higher APACHE scores but was unaffected by microcirculatory variables
Boom 2014[27]	RCT of 178 med/surg ICU patients	FreeStyle Navigator CGMS (Abbott) vs. arterial POC	N/A	-Similar glycemic control -CGM less accurate than POC -CGM costs less and reduces nursing workload
Foubert 2014[12]	10 SICU patients	GlucoClear IVBG system (Edwards) vs. plasma glucose	100%	
Kosiborod 2014[20]	21 CT-ICU patients	Sentrino CGM (Medtronic) vs. ABG and plasma glucose	99.2%	-Alarms missed 25% of hypoglycemic events -53.5–70.2% false alarm rate

continued

Table 25.1—Clinical Studies of CGM in the Inpatient Setting *(continued)*

First author and year	Population	Comparison	Clarke A/B (%)	Other outcomes
Leelarathna 2014[40]	24 ICU patients	FreeStyle Navigator CGMS (Abbott) calibrated with ABG vs. arterial POC	99.2–100%	-CGM accuracy improved with more frequent calibrations
Saur 2014[31]	15 CT-ICU patients	Symphony CGM (Echo, transdermal) vs. ABG	99.6%	-Mean lag time was 10 min
Schuster 2014[19]	24 SICU patients	Guardian RT CGMS (Medtronic) vs. CBG	98.92%	-Accuracy of CGM improved over time
Sechterberger 2014[14]	8 CT-ICU patients	GluCath CGM (GluMetrics) vs. FreeStyle Navigator CGMS (Abbott) vs. ABG	N/A	-Comparable accuracy between the two devices -Intra-arterial device did not interfere with clinical care
Van Hooijdonk 2014[15]	75 ICU patients	OptiScanner (Optiscan) vs. ABG	100%	-One-third of devices had to be disconnected due to malfunction -Identified several commonly used medications that interfered with results

ABG, arterial blood glucose; ACS, acute coronary syndrome; AKI, acute kidney injury; APACHE, acute physiology and chronic health evaluation; CBG, capillary blood glucose; CGMS, continuous glucose monitoring system; CHF, congestive heart failure; CT-ICU, cardiothoracic intensive care unit; eMPC, enhanced model predictive control; ER, emergency room; ICU, intensive care unit: IVBG, intravenous blood glucose; POC, point-of-care; PPV, positive predictive value; RCT, randomized controlled trial; RRR, relative risk reduction; SICU, surgical intensive care unit.

fingerstick. Price et al.[28] found that CGM overestimated blood glucose by 18 mg/dL or more in 25% of actual hypoglycemic events (BG <80 mg/dL). In a rural ICU, only 66.6% of CGM values met ISO standards for accuracy.[29] Also, a study looking at the performance of the Medtronic Sentrino, the first SQ CGM device designed specifically for hospital use, called into question the reliability of CGM alarms, especially in regard to hypoglycemia.[20] The Sentrino CGM system failed to identify 6 out of 24 (25%) hypoglycemic events defined as BG <80 mg/dL as determined by central lab values.[20] Additionally, of the CGM's 47 hypoglycemia alarms, 33 of them were erroneous, resulting in a 70.2% false alarm rate.[20] Similarly, Rabiee et al.[26] found that the CGM detected and alarmed for 167 hypoglycemic events (BG <70 mg/dL), but only 14 of those were found to truly be in the hypoglycemic range based on fingerstick data. Alarm performance was better for hyperglycemia (BG >180 mg/dL), missing <10% of hyperglycemia values but still with a 53.5% false alarm rate.[20]

To date, there have been three randomized trials of CGM in the inpatient setting. Holzinger et al.[30] studied 124 ICU patients comparing glucose control using CGM data points versus arterial blood glucose measurements in their insulin infusion algorithm. The arterial blood glucose values initially were sampled every 1–2 h and then were spaced out to every 4–6 h once the target glucose range was achieved. Although overall glycemic control was similar, the rate of severe hypoglycemia was 1.6% in the CGM compared with 11.5% in the control group, a relative risk reduction of 86%.[30] The authors point out, however, that their glucose control algorithm mandated lowering the insulin infusion rate by half if a steep decline in glucose values was detected (more commonly found in the CGM group), whereas it required a reduction of only 0.5 units/h of the infusion rate for glucose values between 60 and 80 mg/dL, which occurred more often in the control group. This difference in insulin titration strategy potentially contributed to the increased rate of hypoglycemia in controls.[30] Kopecky et al.[18] used a computer-based enhanced model predictive control algorithm to manage hyperglycemia in patients undergoing elective cardiac surgery using CGM versus hourly arterial blood glucoses, and they found no statistically significant differences in glycemic control between the two groups.[18] More recently, Boom et al.[27] studied a population of medical and surgical ICU patients and demonstrated no differences in amount of time in target glucose range, glucose variability, or length of stay in the CGM patients when compared with controls who were monitored by frequent arterial POC measurements. Note, however, that the glucose control algorithms used in these studies were not truly designed for the continuous data feed from CGM. Accordingly, the investigators may not have explored the full potential of this technology in titrating insulin dosing.[18,27] Interestingly, although glucose control was not better in the CGM group, Boom et al.[27] found that nursing time devoted to operationalizing it was significantly decreased from 36 min to 17 min/h and daily blood loss was lower (15.3 mL vs. 60 mL). These investigators also performed a cost analysis and estimated that the total daily cost of CGM was €41 (~$49) versus €53 (~$64) with the conventional care, with the higher cost of the CGM device itself more than compensated for by the cost savings associated with the decreased nursing workload and the avoidance of the material and laboratory costs of POC measurements.[27] In our review of their reported costs, however, the authors assigned a daily cost of the CGM receiver of €1.38 per day, whereas their capillary blood glucose meter was priced at €1.22 per day, both assuming a manufacturer's device lifetime of 2 years. The meter could be used on multiple patients simultaneously, whereas the CGM could be used on only one. Moreover, capillary glucose checks still would be necessary for calibration of the CGM in sensor patients, and these associated costs were not reported. Accordingly, we found the comparative pricing estimates in this report easily arguable.

FUTURE DIRECTION

CGM technology likely will continue to evolve in an effort to improve its accuracy and ease of use. In addition to the SQ and intravascular devices already in existence, companies are developing less-invasive techniques, such as transcutaneous devices that measure transdermal glucose flux and even a temporary tattoo-based glucose sensor that can measure interstitial concentrations.[31,32] As intimated, to better incorporate all of the additional data provided by CGM, new and more advanced control algorithms will have to be developed that can help calculate insulin dose according to a mathematical modeling of the relationship between insulin, glucose, and even perhaps nutritional information, such as tube feeding or total parenteral nutrition composition.[10] In silico models using virtual ICU patients will prove invaluable in testing out these new protocols before their implementation in hospitals.[10]

Ultimately, a large part of the interest surrounding CGM is the vital role it can play in the development of a closed-loop system for more refined and ostensibly safer inpatient glucose management. In addition to CGM, patients would require an insulin infusion, or, conceivably, an SQ insulin pump delivery device, complemented by a computerized algorithm that is able to calculate the appropriate amount of insulin to be delivered based on real-time glucose data. Leelarathna et al.[33] investigated the use of a "closed-loop" glucose control system in 24 ICU patients and found significantly improved efficacy in achieving euglycemia when compared with controls (54.4% of the intervention arm vs. 18.5% in the control group). Ultimately, more studies are needed to determine whether closed-loop systems are viable and, importantly, whether they can lead to not only better biochemical but also improved *clinical* outcomes in the inpatient setting.

CONCLUSION

Until recently, the convenience of POC capillary glucose meters could not be matched by alternative laboratory methods, which were more expensive, required larger amounts of blood, and would not provide the instantaneous data needed to guide management decisions. The increased adoption and improved accuracy of CGM technology in the outpatient setting provides us with a provocative potential alternative, displaying truly continuous glucose values. Although many studies have found that CGM accuracy falls within a clinically acceptable range, there remains no consensus standard by which these systems are being judged.[13,17–23] To date, the improvement in glycemic control proven with CGM use in the outpatient setting has not been consistently replicated in inpatients, and inpatient trials have been small and did not use algorithms designed to accommodate the higher volume of data now provided by CGM.[18,27,30] Some studies have suggested that CGM can decrease nursing workload and increase patient comfort, but much more robust data are needed in this regard.[27,34] The report of cost savings seems overly optimistic, understanding the high current pricing of CGM devices.

Conversely, concerns about inadequate detection of hypoglycemia and a high false alarm rate found in some studies raise doubts about whether current CGM devices are appropriate for use in the hospital.[20,26–28,35,35] Some of this discrepancy in determining whether CGM devices are truly accurate likely is due to the absence of clearly accepted standards for defining accuracy in these systems. The false alarm rate for hypoglycemia or the outright failure to detect hypoglycemic events is particularly troubling especially because part of the appeal of CGM would be the ability of alarms to alert caregivers to hypoglycemia to prompt expeditious corrective measures. These conflicting data formed the basis of the 2011 Endocrine Society's recommendation against the use of real-time CGM in the inpatient setting.[8] Nonetheless, given how technology plays an ever more integral role in the management of patients, from computerized order entry systems that provide decision support to noninvasive monitoring devices that can continuously monitor a patient's cardiopulmonary status, CGM may someday evolve to be an important tool in the glycemic management of hospitalized patients.

REFERENCES

1. Gomez AM, Umpierrez, GE. Continuous glucose monitoring in insulin-treated patients in non-ICU settings. *J Diabetes Sci Technol* 2014;8(5):930–936
2. Juvenile Diabetes Research Foundation Continuous Glucose Monitoring Study, et al. Continuous glucose monitoring and intensive treatment of type 1 diabetes. *N Engl J Med* 2008;359(14):1464–1476
3. Wahl HG. How accurately do we measure blood glucose levels in intensive care unit (ICU) patients? *Best Pract Res Clin Anaesthesiol* 2009;23(4):387–400
4. Grunberger G, et al. Proceedings from the American Association of Clinical Endocrinologists and American College of Endocrinology Consensus Conference on Glucose Monitoring. *Endocr Pract* 2015; 21(5): 522–533
5. Food and Drug Administration. *Blood glucose monitoring test systems for prescription point-of-care use*. Available from http://www.fda.gov/downloads/MedicalDevices/DeviceRegulationandGuidance/GuidanceDocuments/UCM380325.pdf. Accessed 20 December 2015
6. Hoedemaekers CW, et al. Accuracy of bedside glucose measurement from three glucometers in critically ill patients. *Crit Care Med* 2008;36(11):3062–3066
7. Lonjaret L, et al. Relative accuracy of arterial and capillary glucose meter measurements in critically ill patients. *Diabetes Metab* 2012;38(3):230–235
8. Klonoff DC, et al. Continuous glucose monitoring: an Endocrine Society clinical practice guideline. *J Clin Endocrinol Metab* 2011;96(10):2968–2979

9. Joseph JI, et al. Clinical need for continuous glucose monitoring in the hospital. *J Diabetes Sci Technol* 2009;3(6):1309–1318

10. Wernerman J, et al. Continuous glucose control in the ICU: report of a 2013 round table meeting. *Crit Care* 2014;18(3):226

11. Schierenbeck F, et al. Evaluation of a continuous blood glucose monitoring system using a central venous catheter with an integrated microdialysis function. *Diabetes Technol Ther* 2013;15(1):26–31

12. Foubert LA, et al. Accuracy of a feasibility version of an intravenous continuous glucose monitor in volunteers with diabetes and hospitalized patients. *Diabetes Technol Ther* 2014;16(12):858–866

13. De Block C, et al. Intensive insulin therapy in the intensive care unit: assessment by continuous glucose monitoring. *Diabetes Care* 2006;29(8):1750–1756

14. Sechterberger MK, et al. Accuracy of intra-arterial and subcutaneous continuous glucose monitoring in postoperative cardiac surgery patients in the ICU. *J Diabetes Sci Technol* 2015;9(3):663–667

15. van Hooijdonk RT, et al. Accuracy and limitations of continuous glucose monitoring using spectroscopy in critically ill patients. *Ann Intensive Care* 2014;4(1):8

16. Clarke WL, et al. Evaluating clinical accuracy of systems for self-monitoring of blood glucose. *Diabetes Care* 1987;10(5):622–628

17. Holzinger U, et al. Impact of shock requiring norepinephrine on the accuracy and reliability of subcutaneous continuous glucose monitoring. *Intensive Care Med* 2009;35(8):1383–1389

18. Kopecky P, et al. The use of continuous glucose monitoring combined with computer-based eMPC algorithm for tight glucose control in cardiosurgical ICU. *Biomed Res Int* 2013:186439

19. Schuster KM, et al. Continuous glucose monitoring in the surgical intensive care unit: concordance with capillary glucose. *J Trauma Acute Care Surg* 2014;76(3):798–803

20. Kosiborod M, et al. Performance of the Medtronic Sentrino continuous glucose management (CGM) system in the cardiac intensive care unit. *BMJ Open Diabetes Res Care* 2014;2(1):e000037

21. Goldberg PA, et al. Experience with the continuous glucose monitoring system in a medical intensive care unit. *Diabetes Technol Ther* 2004;6(3):339–347

22. Corstjens AM, et al. Accuracy and feasibility of point-of-care and continuous blood glucose analysis in critically ill ICU patients. *Crit Care* 2006;10(5):R135

23. Brunner R, et al. Accuracy and reliability of a subcutaneous continuous glucose-monitoring system in critically ill patients. *Crit Care Med* 2011;39(4):659–664

24. Lorencio C, et al. Real-time continuous glucose monitoring in an intensive care unit: better accuracy in patients with septic shock. *Diabetes Technol Ther* 2012;14(7):568–575

25. Siegelaar SE, et al. Microcirculation and its relation to continuous subcutaneous glucose sensor accuracy in cardiac surgery patients in the intensive care unit. *J Thorac Cardiovasc Surg* 2013;146(5):1283–1289

26. Rabiee A, et al. Numerical and clinical accuracy of a continuous glucose monitoring system during intravenous insulin therapy in the surgical and burn intensive care units. *J Diabetes Sci Technol* 2009;3(4):951–959

27. Boom DT, et al. Insulin treatment guided by subcutaneous continuous glucose monitoring compared to frequent point-of-care measurement in critically ill patients: a randomized controlled trial. *Crit Care* 2014;18(4):453

28. Price GC, Stevenson K, Walsh TS. Evaluation of a continuous glucose monitor in an unselected general intensive care population. *Crit Care Resusc* 2008;10(3):209–216

29. Jacobs B, et al. Continuous glucose monitoring system in a rural intensive care unit: a pilot study evaluating accuracy and acceptance. *J Diabetes Sci Technol* 2010;4(3):636–644

30. Holzinger U, et al. Real-time continuous glucose monitoring in critically ill patients: a prospective randomized trial. *Diabetes Care* 2010;33(3):467–472

31. Saur NM, et al. Accuracy of a novel noninvasive transdermal continuous glucose monitor in critically ill patients. *J Diabetes Sci Technol* 2014;8(5):945–950

32. Bandodkar AJ, et al. Tattoo-based noninvasive glucose monitoring: a proof-of-concept study. *Anal Chem* 2015;87(1):394–398

33. Leelarathna L, et al. Feasibility of fully automated closed-loop glucose control using continuous subcutaneous glucose measurements in critical illness: a randomized controlled trial. *Crit Care* 2013;17(4):R159

34. Aragon D. Evaluation of nursing work effort and perceptions about blood glucose testing in tight glycemic control. *Am J Crit Care* 2006;15(4):370–377

35. Kalmovich B, et al. Continuous glucose monitoring in patients undergoing cardiac surgery. *Diabetes Technol Ther* 2012;14(3):232–238

36. Lee JH, et al. Feasibility of continuous glucose monitoring in critically ill emergency department patients. *J Emerg Med* 2012;43(2):251–257

37. Logtenberg SJ, et al. Pre- and postoperative accuracy and safety of a real-time continuous glucose monitoring system in cardiac surgical patients: a randomized pilot study. *Diabetes Technol Ther* 2009;11(1):31–37

38. Dungan KM, et al. Determinants of the accuracy of continuous glucose monitoring in non-critically ill patients with heart failure or severe hyperglycemia. *J Diabetes Sci Technol* 2012;6(4):884–891

39. Rodriguez-Quintanilla KA, et al. Continuous glucose monitoring in acute coronary syndrome. *Arch Cardiol Mex* 2013;83(4):237–243

40. Leelarathna L, et al. Accuracy of subcutaneous continuous glucose monitoring in critically ill adults: improved sensor performance with enhanced calibrations. *Diabetes Technol Ther* 2014;16(2):97–101

Chapter 26

Noninsulin Therapies

Carlos E. Mendez, MD, FACP,[1] Roma Y. Gianchandani, MD, CDTC,[2] and Guillermo E. Umpierrez, MD, CDE[3]

INTRODUCTION

Hyperglycemia in hospitalized patients is a serious and costly health-care problem associated with increased risk of infections, prolonged hospital stay, disability after hospital discharge, and death.[1] Substantial evidence supports insulin therapy as the most effective approach for treating elevated glucose levels, and it is currently the standard of care for the inpatient management of diabetes and hyperglycemia.[1,2] Randomized controlled studies and meta-analyses, however, have shown that intensive insulin therapy is associated with an increased risk of hypoglycemia, which has been independently associated with adverse cardiovascular outcomes, such as prolonged QT intervals, ischemic electrocardiogram changes/angina, arrhythmias, sudden death, and increased inflammation.[3,4] Hence, alternatives to insulin therapy, such as incretin agents, have been investigated for the management of hyperglycemia and type 2 diabetes (T2D) in the hospital setting. This chapter will review the evidence on the available noninsulin antidiabetic agents and discuss advantages and disadvantages for their use in hospitalized patients.

INPATIENT USE OF ORAL ANTIDIABETICS

The use of oral antidiabetic agents is generally not recommended in hospitalized patients because of the limited data available on their safety and efficacy. Potential adverse effects, including hypoglycemia associated with insulin secretagogues, can increase the risk of complications and mortality in acutely ill patients.[5] In addition, the slow onset of action of some agents preclude their use for achieving rapid glycemic control and timely dose adjustments often required in hospitalized patients.[1,2]

[1]Director, Diabetes Management Program, Stratton Albany VA Medical Center, Assistant Professor of Medicine, Albany Medical College, Albany, NY. [2]Associate Professor, Department of Internal Medicine/Metabolism, Endocrinology and Diabetes, Director, Hospital Hyperglycemia Program, University of Michigan Medical Center, Ann Arbor, MI. [3]Professor of Medicine, Director, Grady Hospital Research Unit, A-CTSI, Emory University, Section Head, Diabetes & Endocrinology, Grady Health System, Atlanta, GA.

DOI: 10.2337/9781580406086.26

Although guidelines and recommendations discourage continuation of home oral diabetes medications in the hospital, their use is common in patients with hyperglycemia across hospitals, presenting a potential source of medication errors.[6] This section discuses the characteristics and considerations for the inpatient use of the most relevant oral antidiabetic medications. Oral dipeptidyl peptidase-4 (DPP-4) inhibitors are discussed in the section on incretin therapies. Table 26.1 summarizes the advantages and disadvantages of the most frequently used antidiabetic agents for the inpatient management of diabetes and hyperglycemia.

METFORMIN

Metformin is the most commonly prescribed medication and is recommended as first-line therapy for the treatment of T2D in the outpatient setting. Although no evidence supports the safety and efficacy for its inpatient use, metformin is commonly used in the hospital setting, and it is estimated that up to 25% of hospitalized patients with T2D are treated with metformin, even in the presence of contraindications.[7]

The antihyperglycemic effects of metformin result from suppression of excessive hepatic glucose production through a reduction in gluconeogenesis. In addition, metformin is thought to increase glucose utilization in skeletal muscle and adipocytes, and it has been suggested to have anti-inflammatory and vasculoprotective effects.

Metformin, when used as monotherapy in the outpatient setting, is effective, resulting in approximately 1 percentage point reduction of HbA_{1c}.[8] Gastrointestinal side effects, specifically abdominal pain, flatulence, and diarrhea, are the most common and are present in ~25% of patients taking metformin.[8] Because metformin does not stimulate endogenous insulin secretion, it does not cause hypoglycemia by itself. Metformin is mainly absorbed from the small intestine, it has an estimated plasma half-life of 1.5 to 4.9 h, and about 90% is excreted through the kidneys.

The association between metformin and lactic acidosis poses the major concern and limitation for its use in the inpatient setting. Metformin was introduced in the late 1950s together with the other major biguanide, phenformin. Phenformin was withdrawn from clinical use in the late 1970s, however, when a significant association with lactic acidosis was recognized. Although early comparative studies showed major differences in the frequencies of lactic acidosis on patients taking phenformin versus metformin (1.76 and 0.13 per million defined daily doses, respectively; $P < 0.001$),[9] increased risk of lactic acidosis with metformin remains an active concern. Since its approval in 1994, metformin has been widely used in the U.S. with a boxed warning about lactic acidosis in the medication package insert.

Recent reports have estimated that the incidence of lactic acidosis in ambulatory patients receiving metformin ranges from 2 to 10 cases per 100,000 patient years; this represents a frequency of lactic acidosis in patients taking metformin similar to that reported in patients with diabetes not receiving the drug. A 2010 Cochrane systematic review also found that the number of cases of lactic acidosis was not increased across 347 clinical trials with 70,490 patient years of metformin use in the ambulatory setting.[10] Even though metformin-associated lactic acidosis

Table 26.1—Advantages and Disadvantages of Antidiabetic Agents

Therapy	Advantages	Disadvantages
Metformin	■ Oral route ■ Extensive experience ■ No hypoglycemia	■ Can cause Lactic Acidosis in patients with impaired kidney function, decompensated CHF, hypoxemia, alcoholism, cirrhosis, contrast exposure, sepsis, and shock ■ Can cause abdominal pain, flatulence, and diarrhea
Insulin Secretagogues Sulfonylureas: Glyburide, Glibenclamide, Glipizide, Gliclazide, and Glimepiride Glinides: Repaglinide and Nateglinide	■ Potent blood glucose lowering effect ■ Oral route	■ High rates of hypoglycemia ■ Significant drug-to-drug interactions ■ May increase risk of cardiovascular events
Thiazolidinediones: Pioglitazone	■ Potent blood glucose lowering effect ■ Oral route ■ No hypoglycemia	■ Can take up to 12 weeks for maximal antihyperglycemic effect ■ Contraindicated in patients with CHF, hemodynamic instability, or evidence of hepatic dysfunction
Sodium–glucose cotransporter 2 (SGLT2) inhibitors Canaglifozin and Dapaglifozin	■ Modest blood glucose lowering effect ■ Oral route ■ No hypoglycemia	■ Increase risk of urinary and genital tract infections ■ Can cause dehydration and hypotension
Glucosidase inhibitors Acarbose	■ Mild blood glucose lowering effect ■ Oral route ■ No hypoglycemia	■ Increased gas production and gastrointestinal symptoms ■ Contraindicated in patients with gastrointestinal disease such as inflammatory bowel disease, partial bowel obstruction, and in severe renal or hepatic disease
GLP-1 RAs Exenatide, Liraglutide, Albiglutide, and Dulaglutide	■ Potent blood glucose lowering effect ■ Low risk for hypoglycemia by itself ■ Improve postprandial glucoses and may decrease glycemic variability ■ Decrease insulin requirements	■ Subcutaneous injections ■ GI side effects (nausea/vomiting) ■ Concern for acute pancreatitis
DPP-4 Inhibitors Sitagliptin, Saxaglitpin, Linagliptin, and Alogliptin	■ Oral route ■ Modest blood glucose lowering effect ■ Low risk for hypoglycemia by itself ■ Improve postprandial glucoses and may decrease glycemic variability ■ Decrease insulin requirements ■ Studied in non-critically ill patients	■ Acute upper respiratory infections as side effect (usually mild) ■ Concern for acute pancreatitis

is rare, mortality estimates are high, ranging from 25 to 50% of cases.[11] Patients with diabetes, in addition, have a higher risk of developing lactic acidosis when compared with patients without diabetes.[10] In acutely ill hospitalized patients, conditions such as renal failure, decompensated heart failure, hypoxemia, alcoholism, cirrhosis, contrast exposure, sepsis, and septic shock significantly increase the risk of lactic acidosis.[12] Therefore, the noted conditions are considered absolute contraindications for the use of metformin therapy in hospitalized patients.[1]

Recommendations to withhold metformin at least 48 h before surgery previously were endorsed based on case reports of patients developing lactic acidosis in the perioperative period.[13] A large retrospective study involving 1,284 patients undergoing cardiac surgery with recent oral ingestion of oral antidiabetics (presumed 8–24 h preoperatively, but discontinued in the hospital) reported that metformin-treated patients had fewer postoperative complications when compared with patients with diabetes who did not receive metformin. The study suggested that recent metformin ingestion was not associated with an increased risk of adverse outcomes in cardiac surgical patients and that metformin treatment could instead have beneficial effects.[14]

In patients with preserved kidney function, metformin may decrease insulin requirements, possibly reducing risk of hypoglycemia from insulin therapy. Therefore, the individualized use of metformin could be considered in stable patients without absolute contraindications hospitalized to nonacute settings, such as nursing homes or rehabilitation units. Because sudden changes in renal function and volume status are common in acutely or critically ill patients, we do not recommend the use of metformin in these patients.

INSULIN SECRETAGOGUES (SULFONYLUREAS AND GLINIDES)

Sulfonylureas are the second most commonly prescribed antidiabetic agents in the outpatient setting. These agents enhance endogenous insulin production by binding to a receptor-like structure on the β-cell surface, resulting in closure of the adenosine triphosphate (ATP)-dependent potassium channels in the β-cell. This leads to the depolarization of the cell membrane, influx of calcium, and subsequent stimulation of insulin secretion.

Sulfonylureas are effective in decreasing glucose levels, often leading to a reduction of HbA_{1c} of 1 to 2 percentage points.[8] Because of the long duration of action, sulfonylureas increase the risk of hypoglycemia, particularly in elderly patients, in patients with impaired renal function, and in those with poor oral intake.[5] Additionally, there is concern that sulfonylurea agents may worsen cardiac and cerebral ischemia by inhibiting ATP-sensitive potassium channels, resulting in cell membrane depolarization and increased intracellular calcium concentration.[15]

Use of sulfonylureas in the inpatient setting is discouraged because of the increased risk of hypoglycemia.[1,2] The prevalence of sulfonylurea-induced inpatient hypoglycemia was reported in 130 out of 692 (19%) of patients treated with sulfonylureas in a single-center retrospective study.[5] Hypoglycemia was most common with the use of glyburide (22%), followed by glimepiride (19%), and glipizide (16%), particularly in patients >65 years and in those with a glomerular filtration rate lower than 30 mL/min.

Significant drug-to-drug interactions have been described with the use of sulfonylureas in hospitalized patients. The use of sulfonylureas in patients treated with fluoroquinolone antibiotics increases the risk of hypoglycemia. Additionally, drugs that inhibit hepatic cytochrome CYP2C9, such as metronidazole, fluconazole, amiodarone, miconazole, trimethoprim-sulphamethoxazole, valproate, and gemfibrozil, also can amplify the effect of sulfonylureas and increase the risk of hypoglycemia.

Repaglinide and nateglinide are the two glinides available in the U.S. They also enhance β-cell insulin production, but differ from sulfonylureas in the absorption and elimination rates, binding sites, and receptor affinity. These differences result in faster onset of action and in shorter duration of action, offering the advantage of better postprandial insulin response. The incidence of hypoglycemia in hospitalized patients treated with repaglinide and nateglinide, however, was reported as 7% in a prospective observational study.[16] Because of the increased risk of hypoglycemia and significant drug-to-drug interactions, the use of sulfonylureas or glinides is not recommended for the inpatient management of hyperglycemia and should be discontinued in most hospitalized patients.

THIAZOLIDINEDIONES

Pioglitazone is the only thiazolidinedione (TZD) available for clinical use in the U.S. It is considered to be an insulin sensitizer, and it exerts its antidiabetic effect through direct activation of the nuclear receptor peroxisome proliferator–activated-receptor γ (PPARγ).[8] TZD agents are effective in improving glycemic control, with an average reduction in HbA_{1c} of 1 to 2 percentage points. Because it can take up to 12 weeks to observe its maximal antihyperglycemic effect, these agents are less attractive when initiating therapy for the inpatient management of hyperglycemia.[2] In addition, TZD therapy is associated with fluid retention, leading to edema and worsening heart failure in predisposed individuals.[8] TZDs are contraindicated in patients with congestive heart failure, hemodynamic instability, or evidence of hepatic dysfunction and should be discontinued in the hospital in patients at risk of these conditions.[2,17]

GLUCOSIDASE INHIBITORS

Acarbose and miglitol are the two α-glucosidase inhibitors available in the U.S. Acarbose has been the most widely studied drug of its class and exerts its antihyperglycemic effect by decreasing the absorption of oligosaccharides in the gut through the competitive inhibition of the enzyme α-glycosidase.[17] Although acarbose can significantly reduce postprandial glucose excursions with low risk of hypoglycemia, the increased delivery of carbohydrates to the colon commonly results in increased gas production and gastrointestinal symptoms, resulting in intolerance to these agents in 25–45% of patients.[8] The use of these agents in the inpatient setting is not recommended because of their mild antihyperglycemic effect, with most studies reporting a reduction in HbA_{1c} of ~0.5% with minimal reduction in fasting plasma glucose.[8] Glucosidase inhibitors are contraindicated in patients with gastrointestinal disease, such as inflammatory bowel disease, partial bowel obstruction, and severe renal or hepatic disease.[15]

SODIUM–GLUCOSE COTRANSPORTER 2 INHIBITORS

Sodium-glucose cotransporter 2 (SGLT2) inhibitors are a newer class of oral antidiabetic medications. They decrease blood glucose levels through the increase of urinary glucose excretion by reducing renal glucose reabsorption in the proximal convoluted tubules.[18] Canaglifozin, dapaglifozin, and empaglifozin are the three drugs approved by the U.S. Federal Drug Administration (FDA) to date for the management of patients with T2D. The SGLT2 inhibitors are effective in reducing HbA_{1c} by ~0.6% to 0.8% with a low risk of hypoglycemia. The use of SGLT2 inhibitors, however, has been associated with increased risk of urinary and genital tract infections compared with placebo therapy (odds ratio, 1.34 to 3.50, respectively). In addition, because of the glycosuric effects, dehydration and hypotension have been reported, and these agents are contraindicated in patients with significantly impaired renal function.[18] Therefore, the potential side effects of SGLT2 inhibitor therapy make the use of these agents less attractive in acutely ill hospitalized patients with hyperglycemia.

INCRETIN THERAPIES AND EMERGING USES

MECHANISM OF ACTION AND SAFETY PROFILE

The term *incretin effect* is used to describe the difference in the amount of insulin produced from the β-cells of the pancreas after an oral glucose load as compared with equivalent intravenous (IV) glucose. Ninety percent of the incretin effect is exerted by glucagon-like peptide-1 (GLP-1) and glucose-dependent insulinotropic polypeptide (GIP), which are secreted by the l and k cells, respectively, of the gastrointestinal tract in response to nutrient ingestion. The major incretin effects are insulinotropic, insulinomimetic, and glucagonostatic, all of which are ambient glucose dependent. Therefore, in response to a nutrient load, incretin hormones increase insulin secretion and sensitivity, while inhibiting glucagon secretion. When normoglycemia is reached, glucagon suppression declines, as does β-cell insulin stimulation; this interplay reduces the risk of hypoglycemia. Other effects of incretin hormones include delayed gastric emptying, increased satiety, reduced β-cell apoptosis (not proven in human studies), and cardioprotection (Figure 26.1). Incretins are rapidly inactivated by DPP-4, resulting in their short half-life. Patients with T2D are known to have low levels of GLP-1, therefore raising its levels is a therapeutic target of diabetes treatment.

Two major classes of drugs engineered to target the incretin axis increase levels of GLP-1 or reduce its degradation. GLP-1 receptor agonists (GLP-1RA) are injectable incretin mimetic peptides, which act on the GLP-1 receptor and also are resistant to degradation by DPP-4.[19] GLP-1RA drugs approved for use in the U.S. to date include exenatide, liraglutide, albiglutide, and dulaglutide. DPP-4 inhibitors, or incretin enhancers, are oral drugs, which competitively and reversibly bind to the active site of DPP-4 enzyme and prevent breakdown of endogenous GLP-1 and GIP. The DPP-4 inhibitors currently available include sitagliptin, saxagliptin, linagliptin, and alogliptin.

In addition to reducing mean glucose levels, incretin-based therapies may decrease glycemic variability.[20] High glycemic variability has been linked with

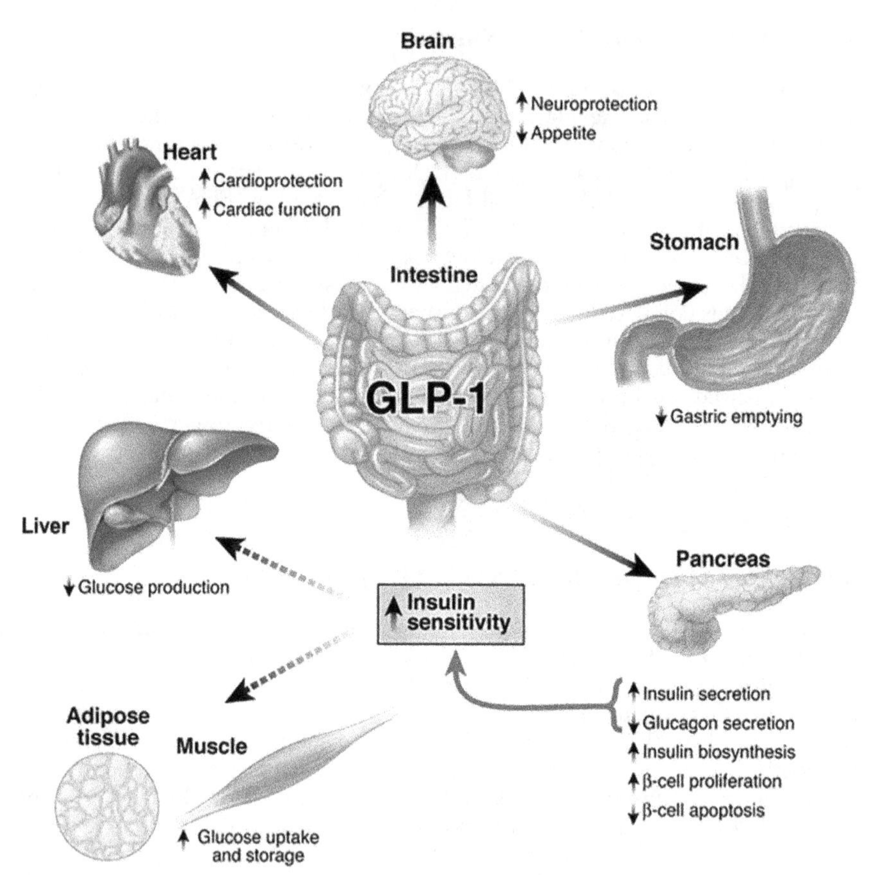

Figure 26.1—Mechanisms of action of incretin hormones.

adverse outcomes in critically ill patients, and with increased length of stay and mortality in noncritically ill hospitalized patients.[21] As incretin-based therapies blunt postprandial glycemic excursions and have a low risk for hypoglycemia, the potential benefits on inpatient glycemic variability and clinical outcomes could be significant, and studies in the hospital setting are needed.

Incretin-based therapies are generally easy to use and titrate; have a quick onset of action, a low risk of hypoglycemia (especially as monotherapy), and a favorable side effect profile; and target the underlying pathophysiology of stress-induced hyperglycemia. This makes them attractive alternatives to insulin in the inpatient setting when insulin therapy may be associated with increase risk for hypoglycemia.

Adverse side effects of the DPP-4 inhibitors are uncommon and are limited to increased risk of upper respiratory tract infections and headaches. However, GLP-1 receptor agonists are frequently associated with nausea, vomiting, and decreased food intake, which could be undesirable in hospitalized patients.

Because of their insulinotropic and glucagon-antagonistic actions, they also carry an increased risk of hypoglycemia when used with insulin. Increased risk for acute pancreatitis, including fatal and nonfatal hemorrhagic or necrotizing pancreatitis, has been reported with incretin therapies.[22] Although postmarketing reports of these occurrences are exceedingly rare, caution should be used in patients with a history of pancreatitis, abdominal pain, or postsurgical ileus. Although clinical trial data has found no associations between adverse cardiovascular events and the use of GLP-1RA or DPP-4 inhibitors, two prospective cardiovascular outcome trials reported that treatment with alogliptin and saxagliptin had no increased risk for ischemic events, although rates of hospitalization for heart failure were increased with saxagliptin therapy.[23]

USE IN SURGICAL AND CRITICALLY ILL PATIENTS

Pilot feasibility studies of predominantly cardiac and postoperative patients have evaluated the effects of GLP-1 and GLP-1RAs on glucose control against a variety of comparator groups for short durations in the intensive care setting. Despite shortcomings of these trials, GLP-1 and GLP-1RAs have consistently shown a favorable impact on glycemic levels with few side effects, which were limited to nausea, vomiting, and hypoglycemia. The studies, which were conducted in different hospital settings, are described in the following sections.

Use of Intravenous GLP-1 in Cardiac Settings

Several studies of GLP-1 in myocardial infarction have evaluated cardiac outcomes. In a study of postmyocardial infarction patients with poor ejection fractions, improvement in left ventricular ejection fraction as well as in glycemic control was achieved with a GLP-1 infusion, which was given after successful angioplasty and revascularization.[24]

In patients undergoing cardiac surgery, use of IV GLP-1 has been evaluated at various perioperative periods. When started 12 h before surgery and continued for 48 h after surgery, GLP-1 improved plasma glucose levels pre- and intraoperatively but not postoperatively. In the postoperative period, insulin was required to maintain target glucose levels, although in lower doses than in controls. Additionally, inotrope use was lower in the GLP-1 group as was the incidence of arrhythmias.[25] When given intraoperatively during a cardiac procedure, GLP-1 significantly reduced glucose levels in patients both with and without diabetes. At cardiopulmonary bypass, mean glucose was found to be 14 mg/dL lower in the GLP-1 group compared with controls. The incidence of hypoglycemia was similar between the two groups.[26] In a separate study, GLP-1 given postoperatively for 12 h after coronary artery bypass graft was found to have glucose control comparable to the insulin group. In this trial, insulin requirements and need for insulin titration were reduced significantly with GLP-1, as was the incidence of arrhythmias.[27]

Use of GLP-1 in Major Surgical Procedures

GLP-1 infusion given in a cross-over trial to postoperative patients with diabetes reduced plasma glucose significantly within 150 min compared with persistent hyperglycemia in the control period ($P < 0.001$).[28] In a recent study, GLP-1 was compared to a saline infusion in surgical and burn ICU in patients receiving

IV insulin. Insulin infusion rates were similar between the groups, but GLP-1 therapy was associated with better glucose control, lower rates of hypoglycemia, and reduced glycemic variability compared with saline infusion.[29]

Use of GLP-1 in Critically Ill Patients on Enteral Feeding

Plasma glucose levels improved in mechanically ventilated patients with stress hyperglycemia who received postpyloric enteral nutrition and a low dose GLP-1 infusion. Use of GLP-1 reduced hyperglycemia with peak glucose of 180 compared with 216 mg/dL in controls.[30] In a similar study of GLP-1 in patients with diabetes, peak glucose levels were lower in the GLP-1 group (205 vs. 228 mg/dL) and more patients reached a glucose target of <180 mg/dL (50% vs. 36%). Because target glucose was not reached in half the patients with GLP-1 alone, either a higher dose of GLP-1 or concomitant insulin infusion may have been necessary in this group.[31]

When GLP-1 was used in hyperglycemic postsurgical patients receiving total parenteral nutrition, glucose levels were lowered to 150 +/– 24 mg/dL within 4 h of infusion. At 8 h, seven out of nine patients had glucose levels <145 mg/dL.[32]

GLP-1RA (exenatide) has been evaluated in the cardiac ICU. A nonrandomized, uncontrolled, pilot study by Abuannadi et al.[20] compared the safety and efficacy of IV exenatide in 40 cardiac ICU patients, 75% of whom had T2D, using an initial 30-min bolus of 0.05 mg/min followed by 0.025 mg/min for 24–48 h versus placebo.[20] Exenatide resulted in similar mean glucose and frequency of hypoglycemic events when compared with a historic control group treated with IV insulin infusions targeting blood glucose 90–119 mg/dL or 100–140 mg/dL. Hypoglycemia was reported in 10% of patients receiving exenatide compared with 21 and 15% in those treated with IV insulin. A total of 20% patients experienced nausea because of exenatide treatment and 15% requested early termination because of severe nausea. A similar study comparing exenatide to two historic control groups had similar results: mean glucose 139 mg/dL on exenatide, 147 mg/dL in recent controls, and 115 mg/dL in pre-2009 controls. Treatment-limited nausea was present in a fifth of patients receiving exenatide.[33]

Subcutaneous (SQ) exenatide has been evaluated in a pediatric burn unit and compared with insulin. Mean glucose levels, glucose variability, and hypoglycemia rates were similar between the groups, and no cases of severe hypoglycemia were seen with exenatide. Exogenous insulin was required in the exenatide group, but at lower doses. Hypoglycemia and nausea were not major issues.[34]

Small studies of IV and SQ incretins have beneficial effects on glucose control in patients with stress hyperglycemia and insulin naive diabetes in the ICU setting, especially in the nonfasting state. Therefore, these drugs are promising alternatives to insulin in the critical care populations. Patients with diabetes, significant postprandial hyperglycemia, and significant insulin resistance may require insulin as adjunct or rescue therapy along with the incretins. In this combination, insulin doses were lower, needed less titration, and produced less glucose variability. The most common side effect was nausea, which was more prominent in the IV exenatide group and probably was dose related in the GLP-1 group, and can limit the use of these medications.

Use in Noncritically Ill Patients

No randomized controlled studies have assessed the use of GLP-1 receptor agonists in the hospital setting. The safety and efficacy of sitagliptin, a DPP-4 inhibitor for the management of inpatient hyperglycemia, recently was evaluated in a randomized pilot study in hospitalized patients with T2D by Umpierrez et al.[35] In this trial, 90 patients treated with diet, oral antidiabetic agents, or a low daily insulin dose (≤0.4 units/kg/day), were randomized to sitagliptin alone or in combination with low-dose glargine insulin or to a basal-bolus insulin regimen plus supplemental doses of insulin lispro. All treatment regimens resulted in prompt and similar improvement in mean daily BG concentrations after the first day of therapy (Figure 26.2). Of importance, most patients with an admission glucose <180 mg/dL treated with sitagliptin plus correction doses of rapid-acting insulin responded as well as those treated in the basal-bolus group. Patients with admission glucose >180 mg/dL treated with sitagliptin alone had higher mean daily blood glucose compared with patients treated with basal-bolus insulin or sitagliptin plus glargine.

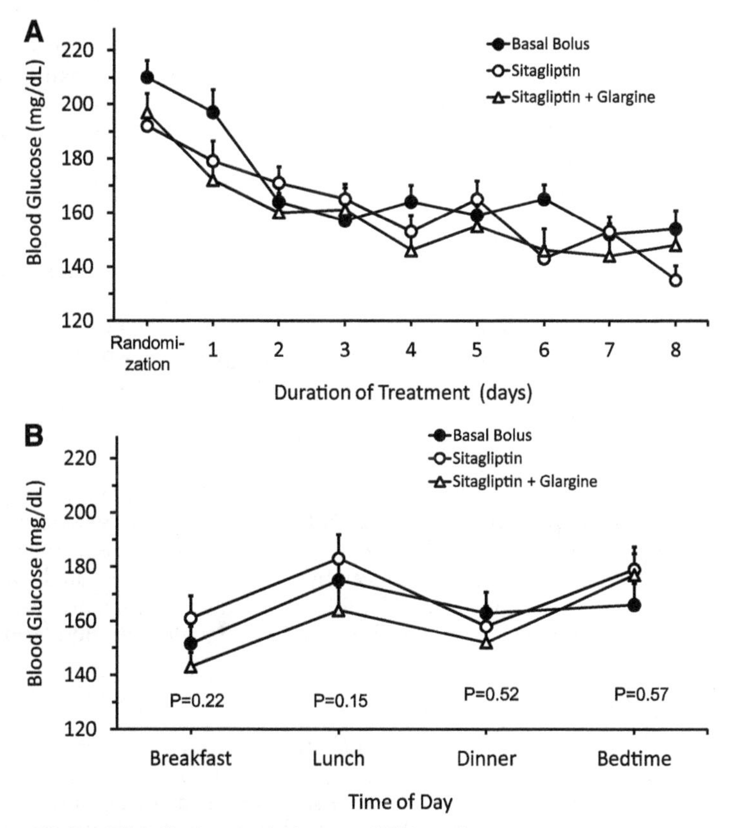

Figure 26.2—Sitagliptin study in non-ICU patients.

In a recent publication, Schwartz and Defronzo outlined a process of care to use incretins for hospitalized patients based on the available evidence and their experience. They endorse the use of DPP-4 inhibitors in noncritically ill patients who are being treated with diet, oral antidiabetic agents, or low doses of insulin. Additionally, these authors recommend use of GLP-1 analogue therapy to control hyperglycemia in the severely ill patients. In their experience, starting GLP-1 analogues before an elective admission or procedure prevents hyperglycemia.[36] During the initial 24 h after initiating GLP-1 analog therapy, a supplemental order for rapid-acting insulin can be included, and after 24 h, this can be changed to a single basal injection of insulin, if necessary. At discharge, patients were transitioned to their home diabetes medications. There are no large prospective studies assessing the safety and efficacy of this approach in the hospital population, and trials validating this approach are needed.

Use in Patients with Steroid-Induced Hyperglycemia

The use of glucocorticoids may lead to or worsen existing hyperglycemia mainly by increasing insulin resistance in the liver and peripheral tissues. In addition, it has been proposed that glucocorticoids impair α-cell function and decrease insulin production by increased Kv channel activity and impaired glucose metabolism inside the β-cell. In an in vitro study, Ranta et al.[37] demonstrated that dexamethasone impairs insulin secretion and induces β-cell apoptosis in INS-1 cells and mouse β-cells through activation of the glucocorticoid receptor.[37] In this same study, the effects of dexamethasone were reversed by the GLP-1 receptor agonist exendin-4 (10 nmol/L), significantly reducing dexamethasone-induced cell death by 82%.

Although no randomized controlled studies have evaluated the safety and efficacy of incretin-based therapies for the inpatient management of steroid-induced hyperglycemia, studies in healthy volunteers and case reports suggest that the benefits of these therapies may be especially important in this patient population. In a randomized controlled study in eight healthy men, treatment with IV exenatide was shown to prevent prednisone-induced hyperglycemia, while significantly decreasing glucagon levels and gastric emptying compared with patients receiving saline infusion.[38] In a recent small case series of hospitalized patients with steroid-induced hyperglycemia, SQ exenatide injections improved glycemic control and decreased hypoglycemic events in one patient.[39]

The use of DPP-4 inhibitors may be attractive in the inpatient management of steroid-induced hyperglycemia, especially because of its positive safety profile and oral route of administration. In a recent study, 11 hospitalized patients with chronic kidney disease and steroid-induced hyperglycemia were treated with alogliptin.[40] The authors reported that alogliptin treatment significantly increased plasma GLP-1 levels, and reduced levels of postprandial glucose and plasma glucagon concentrations.[40]

Use in Long-Term Care Patients

Hypoglycemia in elderly patients with diabetes is known to increase the risk of cardiovascular and cerebrovascular events, progression of dementia, falls, emergency department visits, and hospitalizations. Given the association of intensive insulin therapy with hypoglycemia, the use of DPP-4 inhibitors in patients hospitalized to long-term care settings such as nursing homes or rehabilitation units may be beneficial. On the basis of the positive results observed from the use of sitagliptin in noncritically ill hospitalized patients,[35] an ongoing clinical trial is evaluating the safety and efficacy of linagliptin in combination with metformin compared with basal insulin and metformin in a randomized, open-label, prospective study of elderly, nursing home patients.

Incretin-based therapies also may be used to attempt regimen simplification in patients with diabetes on intensive insulin regimens, in whom tight glycemic control may not be safe or necessary. In an ongoing feasibility study, the use of an algorithm aimed to simplify medication regimens in elderly patients treated with multidose insulin injections is being evaluated. The proposed algorithm uses fasting and stimulated c-peptide to determine eligibility. In patients with positive c-peptide response and no contraindications, linagliptin and metformin are added to their regimen. Subsequently, nutritional insulin doses are reduced and subsequently may be discontinued based on fingerstick blood glucose values and the need for supplemental insulin. Preliminary evaluation of the simplification algorithm in five patients revealed that insulin requirements, hypoglycemic events, frequency of fingerstick blood glucose determinations, and frequency of daily injections significantly decreased ($P < 0.05$).[41] Although results and experience with the use of these medications in stable hospitalized patients seem promising, final analyses of these ongoing trials are necessary before these strategies can be recommended.

CONCLUSION

Inpatient hyperglycemia is common and is associated with an increased risk of complications in patients with and without diabetes. Correction of hyperglycemia with insulin administration has been shown to improve clinical outcomes; however, it is associated with increased risk of hypoglycemia, which is the main limiting factor for achieving glycemic control in the inpatient setting. Preliminary data indicate that incretin therapy has the potential to improve glycemic control with a lower risk of hypoglycemia. Prospective studies are needed to determine the safety and efficacy of these agents in the hospital setting. The other antidiabetic drugs have a limited role in the hospital setting because of the potential for serious adverse side effects: risk of lactic acidosis with metformin, hypoglycemia with sulfonylureas and glinides, edema and heart failure with pioglitazone, and dehydration and risk of urinary and genital infections with the SGLT2 inhibitors.

REFERENCES

1. Moghissi ES, Korytkowski MT, DiNardo M, et al. American Association of Clinical Endocrinologists and American Diabetes Association consensus statement on inpatient glycemic control. *Diabetes Care* 2009;32(6):1119–1131. doi: 10.2337/dc09-9029

2. Umpierrez GE, Hellman R, Korytkowski MT, et al. Management of hyperglycemia in hospitalized patients in non-critical care setting: An Endocrine Society clinical practice guideline. *J Clin Endocrinol Metab* 2012;97(1):16–38. doi: 10.1210/jc.2011-2098; 10.1210/jcem.97.1.zeg16a

3. NICE-SUGAR Study Investigators, Finfer S, Chittock DR, et al. Intensive versus conventional glucose control in critically ill patients. *N Engl J Med.* 2009;360(13):1283–1297. doi: 10.1056/NEJMoa0810625
4. Griesdale DE, de Souza RJ, van Dam RM, et al. Intensive insulin therapy and mortality among critically ill patients: a meta-analysis including NICE-SUGAR study data. *CMAJ* 2009;180(8):821–827. doi: 10.1503/cmaj.090206
5. Deusenberry CM, Coley KC, Korytkowski MT, Donihi AC. Hypoglycemia in hospitalized patients treated with sulfonylureas. *Pharmacotherapy* 2012;32(7):613–617. doi: 10.1002/j.1875-9114.2011.01088.x
6. Scotton DW, Wierman H, Coughlan A, Walters M, Kuhn C. Assessing the appropriate use of metformin in an inpatient setting and the effectiveness of two pharmacy-based measures to improve guideline adherence. *Qual Manag Health Care* 2009;18(1):71–76. doi: 10.1097/01.QMH.0000344595.48510.cb
7. Kosmalski M, Drozdowska A, Sliwinska A, Drzewoski J. Inappropriate metformin prescribing in elderly type 2 diabetes mellitus (T2DM) patients. *Adv Med Sci* 2012;57(1):65–70. doi: 10.2478/v10039-012-0017-7
8. Bolen S, Feldman L, Vassy J, et al. Systematic review: comparative effectiveness and safety of oral medications for type 2 diabetes mellitus. *Ann Intern Med* 2007;147(6):386–399
9. Bergman U, Boman G, Wiholm BE. Epidemiology of adverse drug reactions to phenformin and metformin. *Br Med J.* 1978;2(6135):464–466
10. Salpeter SR, Greyber E, Pasternak GA, Salpeter Posthumous EE. Risk of fatal and nonfatal lactic acidosis with metformin use in T2DM. *Cochrane Database Syst Rev* 2010;(1):CD002967. doi(1):CD002967. doi: 10.1002/14651858.CD002967.pub3
11. Kajbaf F, Lalau JD. Mortality rate in so-called "metformin-associated lactic acidosis": a review of the data since the 1960s. *Pharmacoepidemiol Drug Saf* 2014;23(11):1123–1127. doi: 10.1002/pds.3689
12. Pasquel FJ, Klein R, Adigweme A, et al. Metformin-associated lactic acidosis. *Am J Med Sci* 2015;349(3):263–267. doi: 10.1097/MAJ.0b013e3182a562b7
13. Mercker SK, Maier C, Neumann G, Wulf H. Lactic acidosis as a serious perioperative complication of antidiabetic biguanide medication with metformin. *Anesthesiology* 1997;87(4):1003–1005
14. Duncan AI, Koch CG, Xu M, et al. Recent metformin ingestion does not increase in-hospital morbidity or mortality after cardiac surgery. *Anesth Analg* 2007;104(1):42–50. doi: 104/1/42 [pii]
15. Mendez CE, Umpierrez GE. Pharmacotherapy for hyperglycemia in noncritically ill hospitalized patients. *Diabetes Spect* 2014;27(3):180
16. Varghese P, Gleason V, Sorokin R, Senholzi C, Jabbour S, Gottlieb JE. Hypoglycemia in hospitalized patients treated with antihyperglycemic agents. *J Hosp Med* 2007;2(4):234–240. doi: 10.1002/jhm.212

17. Inzucchi SE, Bergenstal RM, Buse JB, et al. Management of hyperglycemia in T2DM: a patient-centered approach: Position statement of the American Diabetes Association (ADA) and the European Association for the Study of Diabetes (EASD). *Diabetes Care* 2012;35(6):1364–1379. doi: 10.2337/dc12-0413

18. Vasilakou D, Karagiannis T, Athanasiadou E, et al. Sodium-glucose cotransporter 2 inhibitors for T2DM: a systematic review and meta-analysis. *Ann Intern Med* 2013;159(4):262–274. doi: 10.7326/0003-4819-159-4-201308200-00007

19. Lovshin JA, Drucker DJ. Incretin-based therapies for T2DM mellitus. *Nat Rev Endocrinol* 2009;5(5):262–269. doi: 10.1038/nrendo.2009.48

20. Abuannadi M, Kosiborod M, Riggs L, et al. Management of hyperglycemia with the administration of intravenous exenatide to patients in the cardiac intensive care unit. *Endocr Pract* 2013;19(1):81–90. doi: 10.4158/EP12196.OR; 10.4158/EP12196.OR

21. Mendez CE, Mok KT, Ata A, Tanenberg RJ, Calles-Escandon J, Umpierrez GE. Increased glycemic variability is independently associated with length of stay and mortality in noncritically ill hospitalized patients. *Diabetes Care* 2013;36(12):4091–4097. doi: 10.2337/dc12-2430

22. Nauck MA. Incretin-based therapies for T2DM mellitus: properties, functions, and clinical implications. *Am J Med.* 2011;124(1 Suppl.):S3–18. doi: 10.1016/j.amjmed.2010.11.002

23. Schwartz SS, DeFronzo RA, Umpierrez GE. Practical implementation of incretin-based therapy in hospitalized patients with T2DM. *Postgrad Med* 2014:1–7. doi: 10.1080/00325481.2015.996504

24. Nikolaidis LA, Mankad S, Sokos GG, et al. Effects of glucagon-like peptide-1 in patients with acute myocardial infarction and left ventricular dysfunction after successful reperfusion. *Circulation* 2004;109(8):962–965. doi: 10.1161/01.CIR.0000120505.91348.58

25. Sokos GG, Bolukoglu H, German J, et al. Effect of glucagon-like peptide-1 (GLP-1) on glycemic control and left ventricular function in patients undergoing coronary artery bypass grafting. *Am J Cardiol* 2007;100(5):824–829. doi: 10.1016/j.amjcard.2007.05.022

26. Kohl BA, Hammond MS, Cucchiara AJ, Ochroch EA. Intravenous GLP-1 (7-36) amide for prevention of hyperglycemia during cardiac surgery: A randomized, double-blind, placebo-controlled study. *J Cardiothorac Vasc Anesth* 2014;28(3):618–625. doi: 10.1053/j.jvca.2013.06.021; 10.1053/j.jvca.2013.06.021

27. Mussig K, Oncu A, Lindauer P, et al. Effects of intravenous glucagon-like peptide-1 on glucose control and hemodynamics after coronary artery bypass surgery in patients with T2DM. *Am J Cardiol* 2008;102(5):646–647. doi: 10.1016/j.amjcard.2008.06.029

28. Meier JJ, Weyhe D, Michaely M, et al. Intravenous glucagon-like peptide 1 normalizes blood glucose after major surgery in patients with T2DM. *Crit Care Med* 2004;32(3):848–851

29. Mecott GA, Herndon DN, Kulp GA, et al. The use of exenatide in severely burned pediatric patients. *Crit Care* 2010;14(4):R153. doi: 10.1186/cc9222 [doi]

30. Deane AM, Chapman MJ, Fraser RJ, et al. Effects of exogenous glucagon-like peptide-1 on gastric emptying and glucose absorption in the critically ill: Relationship to glycemia. *Crit Care Med* 2010;38(5):1261–1269. doi: 10.1097/CCM.0b013e3181d9d87a

31. Deane AM, Summers MJ, Zaknic AV, et al. Exogenous glucagon-like peptide-1 attenuates the glycaemic response to postpyloric nutrient infusion in critically ill patients with type-2 diabetes. *Crit Care* 2011;15(1):R35. doi: 10.1186/cc9983

32. Nauck MA. A critical analysis of the clinical use of incretin-based therapies: The benefits by far outweigh the potential risks. *Diabetes Care* 2013;36(7): 2126–2132. doi: 10.2337/dc12-2504

33. Abuannadi M, Kosiborod M, Riggs L, House J, Hamburg M, Kennedy K, and Marso M. Management of hyperglycemia with the administration of intravenous exenatide to patients in the cardiac intensive care unit. *Endocrine Practice*: 2013;19:81-90. doi: 10.4158/EP12196.OR

34. Mecott GA, Herndon DN, Kulp GA, et al. The use of exenatide in severely burned pediatric patients. *Crit Care* 2010;14(4):R153. doi: 10.1186/cc9222

35. Umpierrez GE, Gianchandani R, Smiley D, et al. Safety and efficacy of sitagliptin therapy for the inpatient management of general medicine and surgery patients with T2DM: a pilot, randomized, controlled study. *Diabetes Care* 2013;36(11):3430–3435. doi: 10.2337/dc13-0277

36. Schwartz S, DeFronzo RA. The use of non-insulin anti-diabetic agents to improve glycemia without hypoglycemia in the hospital setting: Focus on incretins. *Curr Diab Rep* 2014;14(3):466-013-0466-9. doi: 10.1007/s11892-013-0466-9

37. Ranta F, Avram D, Berchtold S, et al. Dexamethasone induces cell death in insulin-secreting cells, an effect reversed by exendin-4. *Diabetes* 2006;55(5): 1380–1390. doi: 55/5/1380 [pii]

38. van Raalte DH, van Genugten RE, Linssen MM, Ouwens DM, Diamant M. Glucagon-like peptide-1 receptor agonist treatment prevents glucocorticoid-induced glucose intolerance and islet-cell dysfunction in humans. *Diabetes Care* 2011;34(2):412-417. doi: 10.2337/dc10-1677

39. Matsuo K, Nambu T, Matsuda Y, et al. Evaluation of the effects of exenatide administration in patients with T2DM with worsened glycemic control caused by glucocorticoid therapy. *Intern Med* 2013;52(1):89–95. doi: DN/JST.JSTAGE/internalmedicine/52.8622 [pii]

40. Ohashi N, Tsuji N, Naito Y, et al. Alogliptin improves steroid-induced hyperglycemia in treatment-naive Japanese patients with chronic kidney disease by decrease of plasma glucagon levels. *Med Sci Monit* 2014;20:587–593. doi: 10.12659/MSM.889872

41. Mendez et al. unpublished data

Chapter 27

Patient Education

Kellie Rodriguez, MSN, MBA, CDE,[1] Luigi Meneghini, MD, MBA,[2]
Jane Jeffrie Seley, DNP, MSN, MPH, GNP, BC-ADM, CDE, CDTC,[3]
and Michelle F. Magee, MD, MBBCh, BAO, LRCPSI[4]

INTRODUCTION

The increasing prevalence of diabetes and the associated development of acute and chronic complications of the disease result in significant emergency room utilization and hospital admissions. Diabetes is the fourth leading comorbid condition associated with any hospital discharge in the U.S. and is reflected in higher rates of hospitalization across all age-groups.[1] Deficits in diabetes knowledge and effective self-care contribute to diabetes-related hospital admissions.[2,3] Many patients with diabetes do not receive adequate diabetes self-management education (DSME) to support diabetes-related behavioral outcomes. Despite evidence that DSME reduces emergency department visits, hospital admissions, HbA_{1c}, and improves other clinical outcomes,[4–6] <55% of U.S. patients with diabetes receive DSME during the course of their illness and <7% receive it within the first year of diagnosis.[7,8] Although acuity of illness coupled with increased emphasis on shorter hospital lengths of stay may limit the window of opportunity to provide timely and effective diabetes education in the inpatient setting, hospitalization offers an opportunity to provide diabetes patients with the skills and knowledge they need to perform self-care. More attention might be given to diabetes-related issues when patients are admitted for acute glycemic events, but diabetes often is relegated to the status of a near-forgotten comorbidity when other seemingly more acute medical conditions dominate the need for hospitalization. Many inpatient settings, without the availability of designated inpatient diabetes educators, lack the support or infrastructure needed to provide appropriate diabetes care and self-management education before discharge. As a result, the content and consistency of diabetes education services is often variable across hospital settings throughout the country.

[1]Director, Diabetes Education and Community Engagement, Global Diabetes Program, Parkland Health and Hospital System, Faculty Associate, Department of Internal Medicine, Division of Endocrinology, UT Southwestern Medical Center, Dallas, TX. [2]Professor and Executive Director, Global Diabetes Program, Parkland Health and Hospital System, Faculty, Department of Internal Medicine, Division of Endocrinology, UT Southwestern Medical Center, Dallas, TX. [3]Diabetes Nurse Practitioner, Inpatient Diabetes Team, NewYork–Presbyterian Hospital/Weill Cornell Medical Center, New York, NY. [4]Associate Professor of Medicine, Georgetown University School of Medicine, Director, MedStar Diabetes Institute, Washington, DC.

DOI: 10.2337/9781580406086.27

Patient DSME, skill building, and problem solving represent key ingredients for the successful management of diabetes, prevention of acute and chronic complications, and improvement in health status and quality of life. DSME is meant to "support informed decision making, self-care behaviors, problem solving and active collaboration with the health-care team."[9] According to the American Diabetes Association (ADA), patients should receive DSME and diabetes self-management support (DSMS) at diagnosis of the disease and as needed thereafter. The best practice model for diabetes education has shifted from a didactic-type information delivery approach to a more patient-centered, skills-based empowerment experience focused on supporting patients in making better-informed self-management decisions.[10] Successful DSME is associated with better glycemic control; weight management; improved quality of life; healthier coping; decreased utilization of health-care resources, including emergency department (ED) visits and hospital admissions; and lower costs of care. These benefits are enhanced when education interventions are longer in duration and are culturally sensitive and when follow-up education is provided, especially if the message is individualized, and it incorporates behavioral strategies and addresses psychosocial issues.[9]

EVIDENCE FOR THE IMPACT OF INPATIENT EDUCATION ON CLINICAL OUTCOMES AND PROCESSES

Inpatient diabetes education conveys knowledge of diabetes self-care management behaviors and skills to the patient in the short term at the time that it is delivered. To fully assess its impact, intermediate and long-term behavioral and clinical outcomes following discharge should be evaluated. Measures of downstream impact that are clinically meaningful might include an improvement in glycemic control, improved adherence to treatment recommendations and self-management activities, reduction in the need for rehospitalization or acute events requiring emergency intervention, and overall better health and quality of life. A number of studies assessing inpatient diabetes education programs have been published in the literature and provide some guidance on what is possible and what might be effective in this setting. The findings of these trials are summarized in Table 27.1. The trials draw from an adult patient population and provide a number of clinical pearls and strategies that can help providers and educators develop more effective approaches and opportunities to affect patient outcomes via inpatient diabetes education.

DEFINITION OF DIABETES EDUCATION

DSME and DSMS are the ongoing processes of facilitating the knowledge, skills and motivation to undertake effective diabetes self-care, recognizing that patients with diabetes are responsible for ~99% of the success of their diabetes management.[11] DSME is patient-centered, incorporating the values, beliefs, needs, and preferences of the patient into the education experience. The American Association of Diabetes Educators (AADE) developed the AADE7 Self-Care Behaviors™ to provide a framework for outcomes driven diabetes education (Table 27.2). The 2015 ADA Standards of Medical Care in Diabetes outline core recommendations inherent in effective DSME and DSMS (Table 27.3).[1]

Table 27.1—Summary of Key Studies Assessing Inpatient Diabetes Education Programs

Author and reference	Setting	Patient population	Intervention design	Demographics	Outcomes	HbA_{1c} on admission
Koproski et al.[30]	492-bed community teaching hospital	T1D or T2D	Prospective, randomized	*N* = 179, age 60–65, 50% female	Lower length of stay (LOS) for primary diabetes diagnosis and lower 3-month readmission rate	n/a
Davies et al.[32]	UK academic hospital	T1D or T2D referred to the diabetes nurse specialist	Prospective, randomized	*N* = 300 (but data available in much fewer), age 63–64 years, 45–49% female	Lower median LOS and cost; no difference in readmissions, knowledge, or satisfaction with care	n/a
Wexler et al.[29]	Academic medical center	T2D diabetes with HbA_{1c} >7.5%, admitted for nonglycemic reason	Prospective, randomized	*N* = 31, age 55 years, 38–60% female, BMI 33–36 kg/m^2	Better inpatient BG control and lower postdischarge HbA_{1c} in insulin-naïve group	9.7%
Healy et al.[31]	Academic teaching hospital	T1D or T2D and HbA_{1c} >9%	Retrospective review	*N* = 2,265, age ~51 years, ~50% female, 11–16% self-pay	Fewer 30-day and 180-day readmission rates	~11%
Dungan et al.[28]	976-bed academic referral center	T1D or T2D and HbA_{1c} >9%	Prospective, pre-, and postassessment	*N* = 82, age 45 years, 50% female, T2D (74%), BMI 35 kg/m^2, insurance 70%	Predictors of A1C reduction included baseline HbA_{1c}, older age, earlier education and insulin initiation; only 1 readmission for hyperglycemia	11.1%
Magee et al.[33]	900-bed urban teaching hospital	T1D or T2D with admission BG >200 or ≤40 mg/dL	Prospective, pre-, and postassessment	*N* = 125, age 58 years, 66% female, 89% African American, all insured, 84% completed high school or higher	Improvement in medication adherence and diabetes knowledge; fewer readmissions for hyperglycemia	9.4%

Table 27.2—AADE7 Self-Care Behaviors™

- Healthy eating
- Being active
- Monitoring
- Taking medication
- Problem solving
- Reducing risk
- Healthy coping

Source: Haas et al.[11]

Table 27.3—ADA Recommendations for DSME and DSMS

- People with diabetes should receive DSME and DSMS according to the National Standards for DSME and DSMS when their diabetes is diagnosed and as needed thereafter.
- Effective self-management and quality of life are key outcomes of DSME and DSMS and should be measured and monitored as a part of ongoing care.
- DSME and DSMS should address psychosocial issues, as emotional well-being is associated with positive diabetes outcomes.
- Because DSME and DSMS can result in cost-savings and improved outcomes, they should be adequately reimbursed by third-party payers.

Source: Adapted from American Diabetes Association.[9]

DSME is provided by a multidisciplinary workforce, composed of registered nurses, nurse practitioners, physician assistants, dietitians, and pharmacists as the primary instructors of inpatient diabetes education. Multidisciplinary health professionals can obtain certified diabetes educator (CDE) designation following successful completion of a credentialing process developed and maintained by the National Certification Board for Diabetes Educators (NCBDE).[12] CDEs lead DSME services in a variety of health-care settings, including community, outpatient, and hospital settings. In addition, the AADE provides an advanced certification entitled board certified–advanced diabetes management (BC-ADM), designed to validate a health-care professional's specialized knowledge and expertise in the management of people with diabetes.[13] The BC-ADM certification reflects competence in advanced clinical practice and more complex clinical decision making.

The Health-Care Outcomes Continuum (Figure 27.1) illustrates the paradigm shift from cursory survival education to ongoing education that includes knowledge and skill acquisition through to behavior change, improved clinical indicators, and health outcomes.[14] Hospital systems and providers must recognize their roles and responsibilities to patients with diabetes, not as isolated episodes of care, but as a part of a care continuum, connecting patients to required services beyond discharge.

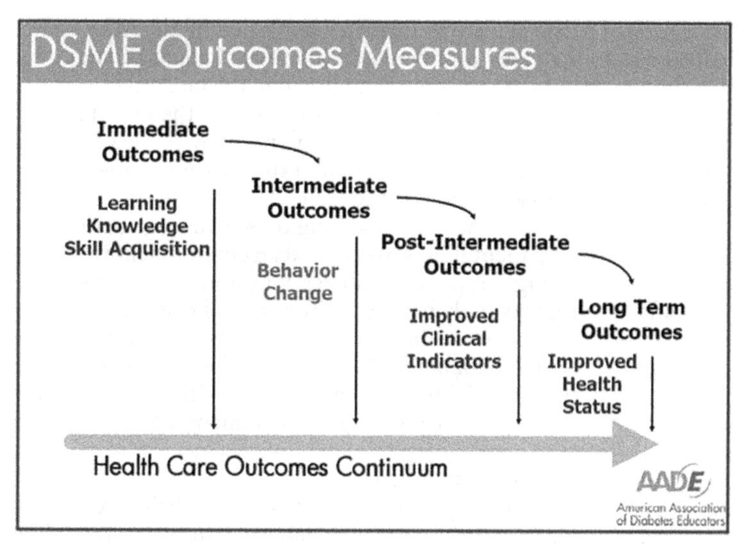

Figure 27.1—DSME outcome measures.

Source: American Association of Diabetes Educators.[14]

CURRENT DEFINITION AND UNDERSTANDING OF DIABETES EDUCATION IN THE HOSPITALIZED PATIENT

The vast majority of studies examining the impact of patient DSME and DSMS on health and other outcomes have occurred in the outpatient environment, with considerably less literature available on the impact of diabetes education in the hospitalized patient. It is anticipated that at any one time, up to 25% of hospitalized patients will have known diabetes and up to an additional 10% will have unrecognized diabetes, demanding provider and health system attention.[15] The inpatient setting represents a unique opportunity to address diabetes care and education by identifying individuals with poorly controlled disease or new-onset hyperglycemia and initiating appropriate therapy, along with DSME and DSMS, before discharge from the hospital. Inpatient diabetes education may be implemented effectively by physicians (e.g., endocrinologists, intensivists, and hospitalists), nurse practitioners, and physician assistants in collaboration with diabetes educators, diabetes resource nurses or champions and bedside nurses, and pharmacists (see Chapter 28).[16]

THEORETICAL FRAMEWORK FOR HOSPITAL-BASED EDUCATION PROGRAMS

There is a paucity of literature that appropriately addresses patient education in the inpatient setting or its potential impact once the patient is discharged. The

2015 Standards of Medical Care in Diabetes published by the ADA dedicate less than half a page to the topic of inpatient diabetes self-management education, with no references cited.[17] A few studies published in the medical literature inform the impact of certain approaches to patient education in the hospital setting and provide a basis for further investigation and exploration with the goal of developing more robust best practices in this vulnerable patient population. These approaches will be discussed later in this chapter.

Hospital-based diabetes education, focusing on self-management, is a difficult undertaking because of patient illness, stress, and an environment that poses challenges to effective learning.[17] Inpatient diabetes educators contribute to the development of effective systems of diabetes care by affecting organizational behavior change toward setting and achieving glycemic targets.[18] In collaboration with other health professionals, diabetes educators in the acute-care setting can enhance care management activities, such as assisting with creating, implementing, and evaluating clinical practice guidelines; recommending changes in diabetes treatment and education approaches; reducing medication errors; and formulating safe and effective discharge regimens.

The acutely ill hospitalized patient presents specific challenges with respect to receptiveness and availability to receive diabetes education, including short lengths of stay, reduced ability to concentrate and retain information, unavailability because of ongoing treatments or diagnostic procedures, and potential language barriers. Whether inpatients can learn while ill and stressed has been questioned, despite evidence that the hospital setting may be effective for providing DSME.[19] One study reported that >80% of medicine service patients felt capable of learning on all days of their hospitalization and 71% of inpatient time was classified as "downtime." Patients expressed a desire to know more about diabetes, self-management, and prevention of disease recurrence or progression.[19] These data suggest that adult inpatients have considerable time and motivation to participate in health education while in the hospital. Other limitations might include lack of time or competency of clinicians to provide appropriate self-management education and instruction regarding use of related technologies[1] (the topic of nursing education is covered in Chapter 28). Self-management education becomes even more critical for patients requiring insulin therapy to control glycemia, especially in the setting of complex basal-bolus insulin regimens.

JOINT COMMISSION REQUIREMENTS FOR ADVANCED DISEASE CERTIFICATION

The Joint Commission's Certificate of Distinction for Inpatient Diabetes Care recognizes hospitals that make exceptional efforts to foster better outcomes across all inpatient settings. In achieving this certification, the Joint Commission (in collaboration with the ADA) has identified that patient education on diabetes self-management is one of the critical elements required in successful inpatient diabetes programs.[20] The Joint Commission developed standards entitled Standards Supporting Self-Management (DSSE) for Inpatient Diabetes Care to offer guidance for inpatient diabetes care (Table 27.4).

Table 27.4—Joint Commission Standards Supporting Self-Management (DSSE) for Inpatient Diabetes Care

DSSE.1: The program involves patients in making decisions about managing their disease or condition
DSSE.2: The program addresses the patient's self-management plan
DSSE.3: The program addresses the patient's education needs

Source: Joint Commission.[20]

The DSSE was developed to promote inclusion of five core focus areas:

- Assessing patients' self-management capabilities
- Providing support for patients in self-management activities
- Involving patients in developing their plan of care
- Educating patients in the theory and skills necessary to manage their disease (Table 27.4)
- Recognizing and supporting self-management efforts

The DSSE supports the need for patients to be actively involved in managing their disease, recognizing that those who learn about their disease, including symptoms and complications, do better in managing long-term health and well-being.

OPTIMIZING DIABETES EDUCATION IN THE HOSPITALIZED PATIENT

In the hospital setting, patient diabetes education should start as soon as feasible following admission, especially in patients who are newly diagnosed, have had severe hypo- or hyperglycemia, or have been started on more intensive diabetes regimens. The key to early education intervention is an effective and streamlined referral pathway to the diabetes education service. Electronic medical record technology is a useful strategy for providing immediate routing to the education service, enabling direct access to the patient record to assist with assessment of clinical need and risk stratification. The AADE suggests that early intervention provides the required time to identify and address barriers, offers opportunity for practice of self-management skills, and facilitates problem solving and coping skills.[18] Educational interventions start with a needs assessment of the patient that includes cognitive ability, language, literacy level, visual acuity, dexterity, cultural context, and identification of barriers to access to diabetes supplies following discharge.[16] Evaluation of numeracy skills in patients is particularly important in diabetes self-management, in which medication management, blood glucose monitoring and interpretation, and dietary recommendations require a great deal of math.[21]

The hospital-based diabetes educator must adapt concepts of diabetes self-management education to the acute care setting. At the very least, the educational intervention should introduce survival skills that will allow the patient to acquire basic knowledge and skills before discharge from the hospital, with the intent of reinforcing and building on those skills in the outpatient setting (Table 27.5).[17,20] If the admission was related to a diabetes crisis such as diabetic ketoacidosis (DKA) or severe hypoglycemia, then information should be provided to help prevent subsequent hospital readmissions.

Patients with established disease who are found to have deficiencies in their understanding of the disease process or in their problem-solving skills also will benefit from self-management education and support. A hospital admission provides an opportunity for medication reconciliation and education, including reevaluating and optimizing the home diabetes medication regimen and promoting healthy self-care behaviors.[22,23] Collaborative efforts among the primary team and the patient should assist in reducing risk and promoting appropriate medication regimen outcomes that the patient is able to follow. As members of the inpatient education team, registered dietitian nutritionists (RDs or RDNs) can address basic to complex nutrition issues. Key responsibilities should include assessment and integration of information to develop a plan of care, including identifying carbohydrates that are counted, appropriate portion sizes, and meal planning. Educating and including caregivers in the provision of care and education during the admission and at the time of discharge will facilitate desired healthy behaviors beyond hospitalization. The hospitalization period presents an opportunity for patients to better understand medication management, the relationship between carbohydrate intake and insulin requirements, and the use of blood glucose monitoring data for pattern recognition as well as to actively participate in treatment decisions. This period also allows clinicians time to verify that the patient is indeed capable of self-managing their diabetes[9] and, if not, what support is needed.

Educational materials and curriculum content should be based on the National Standards for Diabetes Self-Management Education and Support, which provides the framework for quality evidence-based education.[11] As is the case in the outpatient setting, educational content and materials need to be tailored and adapted for individual patient age, diabetes type, cultural factors, health literacy, and numeracy levels. Educational sessions should take place with short, focused sessions.[24] When

Table 27.5—Diabetes Survival Skills for the Hospitalized Patient

- Understanding of diabetes diagnosis
- Self-monitoring of blood glucose (SMBG) and home blood glucose targets
- Purpose, timing, dose, delivery method, and equipment disposal (where appropriate) of glucose-lowering medications—oral and injectable
- Definition, signs and symptoms, treatment, and prevention of hypoglycemia and hyperglycemia
- Sick-day guidelines
- Meal planning, including basics for consistent carbohydrate counting, portion sizes, and role of nutrition in blood glucose management
- Identification and coordination of postdischarge provider and diabetes education
- Guidance for when to call their health-care provider or go to the emergency department

Source: Adapted from American Diabetes Association.[17] Supported by the Joint Commission.[20]

Table 27.6—Durable Medical Equipment, Supplies, and Prescriptions for the Diabetes Patient for Home Use

- Blood glucose meter, test strips, and logbook
- Lancing device and lancets
- Insulin vials or pens
- Insulin syringes or pen needles
- Oral or other injectable diabetes medications
- Alcohol wipes
- Ketone strips (type 1 diabetes)
- Glucagon emergency kit (if required)
- Hypoglycemia treatment (glucose sources)
- Diabetes identification information

Source: Adapted from American Diabetes Association.[17]

developing care plans, the education should emphasize easy-to-understand information at an appropriate reading level. The "teach-back" methodology is a recommended approach to verify participant understanding and to reduce errors, demanding sufficient time to effectively implement.[25] Careful documentation and communication of the education session should be shared and coordinated within the interdisciplinary team and all relevant clinicians and care coordinators. Referrals to community resources for continued DSME and DSMS represent an important element of transitional care.

Upon discharge, it is essential that patients are provided education, access, and instructions for the appropriate durable medical equipment, supplies, and prescriptions required for effective diabetes self-management (Table 27.6). The day of discharge is not always conducive to retention of verbal instructions, especially for insulin and more complex regimens, resulting in an increased risk of medication errors and adverse drug events.[26] Inadequate discharge planning and skills training can lead to confusion about prescribed treatment and medications or follow-up needs, lack of access to recommended treatments because of cost, and anxiety about potential side effects, leading to high personal and financial costs, poor glycemic control, adverse health events, and greater frequency of emergency room use and hospital readmission.[15]

The 2015 National Patient Safety Goals for discharge planning and transitional care recommends care team communication, medication reconciliation, and encouragement of positive patient self-care behaviors.[27] With competing needs, it can be challenging to identify the best way to incorporate diabetes education into the workflow of different hospital units and systems, likely requiring individualization of processes to meet local needs.

IMPACT OF HOSPITAL EDUCATION ON GLYCEMIC CONTROL FOLLOWING DISCHARGE

A few recent trials have shown the impact of an inpatient educational intervention on glycemic control.[28-30] All settings were teaching hospitals and patients enrolled were adults with uncontrolled type 1 diabetes (T1D) or type 2 diabetes (T2D)[28,29] or were adult patients identified on admission as having a primary or secondary diagnosis of diabetes, regardless of prior glycemic control.[30] The educational interventions in these trials focused on basic survival skills, with more advanced concepts reviewed in patients identified as capable of understanding carbohydrate counting and correction insulin scales. In most cases, the educational intervention was part of a multidisciplinary effort involving an endocrinologist and diabetes educator. Improvement in glycemic control as measured by either HbA_{1c} or blood glucose monitoring following discharge was reported in all three studies. The most significant improvement in glycemic control was seen in patients who were either new to insulin or those whose insulin therapy was drastically changed (e.g., the addition of prandial insulin to basal-only regimen). Patients with poorly controlled T1D and those on previously prescribed appropriate insulin regimens did not seem to derive much benefit from the educational intervention. Interestingly, most of the glycemic benefit was evident within 3–6 months from discharge, with a waning effect observed over time. These studies highlight the possible need to address psychosocial and self-care challenges in patients poorly controlled on insulin therapy, as opposed to reinforcing basic survival skills, in the subgroup of insulin-experienced patients. These results highlight the potential advantage of initiating or intensifying insulin therapy in the hospitalized patient as a viable strategy to overcome the barriers of limited time and resources encountered in the primary care setting.

IMPACT ON HOSPITAL LENGTH OF STAY, READMISSION, OR EMERGENCY ROOM VISITS

Another important measure of risk for patients is the frequency of admission or readmission to the hospital or the use of the emergency room department. A retrospective study[31] showed the benefit of CDE-led inpatient diabetes education in reducing 30-day and 6-month readmission rates for patients with diabetes admitted to the hospital with HbA_{1c} >9%. The authors concluded that programs likely to reduce readmission rates need to include education as well as assistance from a nurse navigator (care coordinator), follow-up appointment coordination, medication reconciliation, and close communication with primary care providers to support an effective transition to the outpatient setting. A second prospective, randomized study[32] using a diabetes specialist nursing service reduced the hospital length of stay on average by 3 days, resulting in a reduction in the per patient cost per admission, even after factoring in nursing costs. Readmission rates or time to readmission, however, were not decreased. Other studies showed that incorporating diabetes education alone, or as part of specialist team management, can positively affect hospital readmission and emergency room visits, especially in patients admitted with poor control or a primary diagnosis of severe hyperglycemia.[28,30,33]

Other important benefits of inpatient diabetes education include improvement in knowledge and medication adherence,[33] greater satisfaction with diabetes treatment,[32] and more frequent documentation of patient instruction on various self-management modalities.[30]

An interesting approach to reducing length of stay and hospital readmissions for patients with diabetes made use of a survey to assess patient needs, categorizing them into one of five levels (Table 27.7).[34] The intervention was then specifically geared toward addressing the identified category of needs. The intervention identified a considerable proportion of patients needing social service and

Table 27.7—Categorization of Need for Inpatient Diabetes Education

Level	Result (*N* = 308)	%
1	Comprehensive diabetes education required	11
2	Social and economic supports required	22
3	Focused diabetes education required	26
4	Diabetes education review after discharge	17
5	Unwilling or unable to participate in education	10

Source: Maldonado et al.[37]

financial assistance. The latter ranged from assessing homecare resources and competence of caregivers, to reviewing daily schedules and evaluating resource barriers to diabetes self-management. The group reported that compared with the year prior to implementation, they were able to substantially reduce hospital length of stay and rehospitalizations, resulting in net cost savings of $630,000 by the second year of operation, even after adding in the costs of two nurse educators and a part-time assistant.

Another reported approach to reducing length of stay involved identifying hospitalized patients that needed additional glycemic monitoring, but who otherwise were "fit for discharge."[35] Identified patients were randomized to either usual care or received basic survival skills education before "early discharge," which was followed by weekly or biweekly phone contact with a diabetes nurse specialist until it was deemed that their diabetes was under control. Compared with usual care, the patients supported through this approach had a shorter hospital stay (2.2 vs. 5.9 days) and lower per patient cost of admission (~$1,533 per patient compared with usual care), even after factoring in the cost of the diabetes nurse specialist contacting the patient by phone for an average of 64.8 minutes per patient (10 calls averaging 6.48 minutes in duration).

ADHERENCE TO MEDICATION TREATMENT AND POSTDISCHARGE CLINICAL FOLLOW-UP

Adherence, or how closely a patient follows a mutually agreed upon medication regimen, is a process measure that has been tied to clinical outcomes, including reduction in costs of overall care and hospitalizations.[36] Adherence to insulin is particularly relevant to long-term glycemic control and short-term complications. For example, nonadherence with insulin treatment was responsible for 83% of episodes of diabetic DKA in a large, multiethnic, safety-net hospital, with the cause identified as running out of insulin and substance abuse.[37] In addition, hospitalization may result in an interruption in insulin therapy because of a variety of potential factors, including patient and clinician misunderstanding of appropriate treatment options and challenges with medication reconciliation. Compared with individuals whose insulin treatment is disrupted following hospital discharge, those who continue insulin therapy have been reported to experience fewer readmissions or emergency room visits, better survival rates at 12 months, and lower medical care costs over the 6 months following discharge.[38]

Some of the studies evaluating inpatient education demonstrate some improvement in medication adherence[33] and postdischarge clinic follow-up.[28] Considerable barriers exist to keeping clinic appointments following hospital discharge, even in those patients with the best intentions, including difficulties with transportation or time away from work or usual daily activities, lack of finances, or health insurance.[39] Identifying and addressing barriers as part of the evaluation process in the hospitalized patient should be a component of any education intervention.

OTHER CONSIDERATIONS

Even the best educational interventions might have little impact on the patient who is not ready or receptive to acquiring new knowledge, self-management skills, or problem-solving abilities. For example, patients with chronic, complex diseases such as diabetes may suffer from undiagnosed underlying depression, which could considerably impact the effectiveness of any educational intervention and the ability of the patient to perform self-care.[40] Because depression is two to three times more common in people with diabetes, a quick screening tool such as the Patient Health Questionnaire (PHQ) has the potential to be a valuable addition to any evaluation that is part of an educational intervention.[9]

CONCLUSION

Patient education is an essential component to positively engage patients in healthy habits and effective diabetes self-management activities. Patient activation and engagement have been associated with better health outcomes, lower medical error rates, improved self-care to prescribed treatment, and greater ability of the patient to implement preventive care practices. The inpatient setting offers an opportunity to deliver DSME to patients who may not have access to it in the outpatient setting and who may be uniquely receptive to education during their hospitalization. Optimal diabetes management and education during the short-term hospitalization has the potential to empower the patient to safely and effectively transition to the outpatient setting to improve long-term health outcomes. DSME is best carried out through a multidisciplinary approach that utilizes the full spectrum of expertise of each clinician on the patient's care team. Hospital systems and providers need to recognize their roles and responsibilities to patients with diabetes and to view hospitalizations not as isolated episodes of care but rather as part of a continuum of care that includes survival skills education and connects patients to ongoing outpatient education and support services.

REFERENCES

1. Cook CB, Seifert KM, Hull BP, et al. Inpatient to outpatient transfer of diabetes care: planing for an effective hospital discharge. *Endocr Pract* 2009;15: 263–269

2. Rubin DJ, Donnell-Jackson K, Jhingan R, Golden SH, Paranjape A. Early readmission among patients with diabetes: a qualitative assessment of contributing factors. *J Diabetes Complications* 2014;28:869–873
3. Griffith ML, Boord JB, Eden SK, Matheny ME. Clinical inertia of discharge planning among patients with poorly controlled diabetes mellitus. *J Clin Endocrinol Metab* 2012;97:2019–2026
4. Norris SL, Engelgau MM, Narayan KM. Effectiveness of self-management training in type 2 diabetes: a systematic review of randomized controlled trials. *Diabetes Care* 2001;24:561–587
5. Norris SL, Lau J, Smith SJ, Schmid CH, Engelgau MM. Self-management education for adults with type 2 diabetes: a meta-analysis of the effect on glycemic control. *Diabetes Care* 2002;25:1159–1171
6. Gary TL, Genkinger JM, Guallar E, Peyrot M, Brancati FL. Meta-analysis of randomized educational and behavioral interventions in type 2 diabetes. *Diabetes Educ* 2003;29:488–501
7. Hoerger TJ, Segel JE, Gregg EW, Saaddine JB. Is glycemic control improving in U.S. adults? *Diabetes Care* 2008;31:81–86
8. Li R, Shrestha SS, Lipman R, et al. Diabetes self-management education and training among privately insured persons with newly diagnosed diabetes—United States, 2011–2012. *MMWR* 2014;63:1045–1049
9. American Diabetes Association. Standards of medical care in diabetes—2015: 4. Foundations of care: education, nutrition, physical activity, smoking cessation, psychosocial care, and immunization. *Diabetes Care* 2015;38:S20–S30
10. Marrero DG, Ard J, Delamater AM, et al. Twenty-first century behavioral medicine: a context for empowering clinicians and patients with diabetes: a consensus report. *Diabetes Care* 2013;36:463–470
11. Haas L, Maryniuk M, Beck J, et al. National standards for diabetes self-management education and support. *Diabetes Care* 2013;36(Suppl. 1):S100–S108
12. American Association of Diabetes Educators. The scope of practice, standards of practice, and standards of professional performance for diabetes educators. 2011. Available from http://www.diabeteseducator.org/DiabetesEducation/position/Scope_x_Standards.html. Accessed 13 December 2015
13. American Association of Diabetes Educators. *Candidate handbook for the American Association of Diabetes Educators (AADE) board certified advanced diabetes management (BC-ADM) examination*. 2015:1–20
14. American Association of Diabetes Educators. AADE7™ self-care behaviors, American Association of Diabetes Educators (AADE) position statement. 2014. Available from http://www.diabeteseducator.org/export/sites/aade/_resources/pdf/publications/AADE7_Position_Statement_Final.pdf
15. Umpierrez GE, Reyes D, Smiley D, et al. Hospital discharge algorithm based on admission HbA1c for the management of patients with type 2 diabetes. *Diabetes Care* 2014;37:2934–2939

16. Moghissi ES, Korytkowski MT, DiNardo M, et al. American Association of Clinical Endocrinologists and American Diabetes Association consensus statement on inpatient glycemic control. *Endocr Pract* 2009;15:353–369

17. American Diabetes Association. Standards of medical care in diabetes—2015: 13. Diabetes care in the hospital, nursing home, and skilled nursing facility. *Diabetes Care* 2015;38:S80–S85

18. American Association of Diabetes Educators. AADE position statement: diabetes inpatient management. *Diabetes Educ* 2012;38:142–146

19. Chu ES, Hakkarinen D, Evig C, et al. Underutilized time for health education of hospitalized patients. *J Hosp Med* 2008;3:238–246

20. Joint Commission. Advanced disease-specific care certification requirements for inpatient diabetes care (IDC). January 2014. Available from http://www.jointcommission.org/certification/inpatient_diabetes.aspx

21. Zaugg SD, Dogbey, G et al. Diabetes numeracy and blood glucose control: association with type of diabetes and source of care. *Clin Diabetes* 2014;32(4):152–157

22. Thompson CL DK, Menon MC, Kearns LE, Braithwaite SS. Hyperglycemia in the hospital. *Diabetes Spect* 2005;18:20–27

23. Seley JJ, Wallace M. Meeting the challenge of inpatient diabetes education: an interdisciplinary approach. In *Educating Your Patient with Diabetes*. Weinger K, Carver CA, Eds. New York, NY, Humana Press, 2008, p. 81–96

24. AADE Position Statement: Diabetes inpatient management. *Diabetes Educ* 2012; 38(1):142–146. Available from https://www.diabeteseducator.org/docs/default-source/legacy-docs/_resources/pdf/research/Diabetes_Inpatient_Management_TDE.pdf

25. National Quality Forum. Safe practices for better healthcare–2009 update: a consensus report. 2009. Available from http://www.qualityforum.org/Publications/2009/03/Safe_Practices_for_Better_Healthcare%e2%80%932009_Update.aspx. Accessed 12 December 2015

26. Kripalani S, Jackson AT, Schnipper JL, Coleman EA. Promoting effective transitions of care at hospital discharge: a review of key issues for hospitalists. *J Hosp Med* 2007;2:314–323

27. Joint Commission. 2015 Hospital national patient safety goals. 2015. Available from http://www.jointcommission.org/assets/1/6/2015_NPSG_HAP.pdf. Accessed 12 December 2015

28. Dungan K, Lyons S, Manu K, et al. An individualized inpatient diabetes education and hospital transition program for poorly controlled hospitalized patients with diabetes. *Endocr Pract* 2014;20:1265–1273

29. Wexler DJ, Beauharnais CC, Regan S, Nathan DM, Cagliero E, Larkin ME. Impact of inpatient diabetes management, education, and improved discharge transition on glycemic control 12 months after discharge. *Diabetes Res Clin Pract* 2012;98:249–256

30. Koproski J, Pretto Z, Poretsky L. Effects of an intervention by a diabetes team in hospitalized patients with diabetes. *Diabetes Care* 1997;20:1553–1555

31. Healy SJ, Black D, Harris C, Lorenz A, Dungan KM. Inpatient diabetes education is associated with less frequent hospital readmission among patients with poor glycemic control. *Diabetes Care* 2013;36:2960–2967

32. Davies M, Dixon S, Currie CJ, Davis RE, Peters JR. Evaluation of a hospital diabetes specialist nursing service: a randomized controlled trial. *Diabetic Med* 2001;18:301–307

33. Magee MF, Khan NH, Desale S, Nassar CM. Diabetes to go: knowledge- and competency-based hospital survival skills diabetes education program improves postdischarge medication adherence. *Diabetes Educ* 2014;40:344–350

34. Leichter SB AG, Moore WM. The business of hospital care of diabetic patients: 2. A new model for inpatient support services. *Clin Diabetes* 2003;21: 136–139

35. Wong FK, Mok MP, Chan T, Tsang MW. Nurse follow-up of patients with diabetes: randomized controlled trial. *J Advanced Nurs* 2005;50:391–402

36. Sokol MC, McGuigan KA, Verbrugge RR, Epstein RS. Impact of medication adherence on hospitalization risk and healthcare cost. *Med Care* 2005;43:521–530

37. Maldonado MR, D'Amico S, Rodriguez L, Iyer D, Balasubramanyam A. Improved outcomes in indigent patients with ketosis-prone diabetes: effect of a dedicated diabetes treatment unit. *Endocr Pract* 2003;9:26–32

38. Wu EQ, Zhou S, Yu A, et al. Outcomes associated with insulin therapy disruption after hospital discharge among patients with type 2 diabetes mellitus who had used insulin before and during hospitalization. *Endocr Pract* 2012;18:651–659

39. Wheeler K, Crawford R, McAdams D, Robinson R, Dunbar VG, Cook CB. Inpatient to outpatient transfer of diabetes care: perceptions of barriers to postdischarge follow-up in urban African American patients. *Ethnicity Dis* 2007;17:238–243

40. Akimoto M, Fukunishi I, Kanno K, et al. Psychosocial predictors of relapse among diabetes patients: a 2-year follow-up after inpatient diabetes education. *Psychosomatics* 2004;45:343–349

Chapter 28

Nursing Education

Jane Jeffrie Seley, DNP, MSN, MPH, GNP, BC-ADM, CDE, CDTC, FAAN,[1] Michelle F. Magee, MD, MBBCh, BAO, LRCPSI,[2] and Robert J. Rushakoff, MD[3]

INTRODUCTION

Coordinating diabetes care and self-management education to ensure optimal glycemic control and effective care delivery within workflow processes in the hospital setting can be challenging for nurses. When hospitalized, the majority of diabetes self-management tasks performed by the patient at home are primarily handed off to nursing. No longer in charge of the timing of their own blood glucose monitoring, meals, and insulin delivery or making dosing decisions often leads to patient frustration and conflict, with comments such as "I can take better care of my diabetes at home." Unfortunately, because of a variety of circumstances encountered in the hospital setting, this statement may be true as coordination of the timing of glucose monitoring, medication administration, and meals can be demanding. Whatever may have worked at home may no longer be relevant when a patient becomes acutely ill. In addition, as diabetes self-care becomes more complex and technology driven, educating nurses in the hospital setting to take on the role of implementing the glycemic control regimen and educating their patients about a new and often more intensive regimen is a tremendous challenge. The Joint Commission recommends mandatory nurse education around glycemic management, and teaching diabetes self-care survival skills should be a priority in hospitals.[1–3]

Innovative strategies to ensure that all bedside nurses are consistently taught the basics of inpatient glycemic management are needed. Educating nurses is a costly venture, especially if other nurses must cover for them during training, which is considered "nonproductive time" in many institutions. The use of online learning, shown to be effective for both physicians and nurses for inpatient glycemic management education, is a potentially more flexible and cost-effective strategy to teach and reinforce diabetes management and education to nurses.[4,5]

In addressing the roles of nursing education in the hospital, this chapter will provide an overview of the role of inpatient nurses in diabetes management and

[1]Diabetes Nurse Practitioner, Inpatient Diabetes Team, New York–Presbyterian Hospital/Weill Cornell Medical College. [2]Associate Professor of Medicine, Georgetown University School of Medicine, Director, MedStar Diabetes Institute. [3]Director, Inpatient Diabetes, Professor of Medicine, Division of Endocrinology and Metabolism, University of California, San Francisco, CA.

 DOI: 10.2337/9781580406086.28

self-care education, the role of the diabetes resource or champion nurse, and the role of the diabetes educator. Realistically and depending on the allocation of institutional resources, a combination of these strategies may be needed to provide effective diabetes care and education to inpatients with diabetes and hyperglycemia.

THE HOSPITAL NURSES' ROLE IN DIABETES MANAGEMENT AND SELF-CARE EDUCATION

Nurses have many competing care priorities and struggle with multiple tasks that are often scheduled concurrently. For example, a commonly encountered problem is optimal timing of prandial blood glucose testing, especially prebreakfast, which falls in proximity to shift change from nights to days.[6] When a prebreakfast blood glucose reading is obtained too early and is elevated, the nurse is presented with a decision as to whether or not to immediately administer a correction insulin dose to lower the blood glucose. If that insulin dose is also intended to cover the meal that will not be arriving for an hour or longer, the risk of hypoglycemia associated with insulin administration is a consideration for that patient. Educating nurses that premeal blood glucose checks should be done no more than 1 h before the meal trays are delivered is a key strategy in preventing hypoglycemia.[3,7] Corl et al.[8,9] recommend diabetes education for nurses to increase both their expertise and level of comfort and confidence when caring for patients with diabetes in the hospital setting.

Optimally, bedside nurses should receive education that focuses on core content. Key topics include inpatient glycemic targets, differences in managing patients with type 1 versus type 2 diabetes, basic carbohydrate counting, blood glucose monitoring, insulin administration, coordination of timing of diabetes care, treatment and prevention of hypo- and hyperglycemia, and discharge planning strategies (see Table 28.1).[1–3]

Nurses who have received this education are more capable of assisting the care team in identifying patients who are not achieving glycemic targets and facilitating initiation and adjustments of insulin therapy. Nurses can be on the lookout for inappropriate orders such as not decreasing the basal insulin when steroids are being tapered or a patient with type 1 diabetes who is NPO for a procedure and the basal insulin has been discontinued. Proactive diabetes education before discharge with ample opportunity for the patient to practice skills can lead to lower rates of emergency department visits and readmissions.[10] This is a particularly important cost and quality issue because 30-day readmission rates for patients with diabetes are 1.6 times (20%) higher than for patients without diabetes according to the Elixhauser and Steiner National Healthcare Cost and Utilization Project.[9]

EDUCATING THE PATIENT TO PERFORM DIABETES SELF-CARE

Bedside nurses are in the ideal position to educate patients to perform diabetes self-care behaviors. A teachable moment arises every time a nurse is checking the blood glucose, calculating an insulin dose, or administering insulin. Basic diabetes "survival skills" that should be taught by the bedside nurse include blood glucose self-monitoring; diabetes medication self-administration; hypo- and hyperglycemia recognition, treatment, and prevention; and basic principles of meal planning,

Table 28.1—Key Topics to Consider for Nursing Education

Topic	Minimum Content to Cover
Rationale for improving glycemic control	-how glycemic control prevents short-term complications during acute illness
Difference between Type 1 vs. Type 2 diabetes	-insulin dependent vs. insulin requiring -need for basal insulin for type 1 patients even when NPO
Glycemic Targets	-ICUs vs. general floors -when to notify team to initiate or adjust insulin -outpatient pre and post meals for discharge teaching
Meal Planning	-carbohydrates that are counted -determining portion sizes -carbohydrate servings per meal -spacing meals
Blood Glucose Monitoring & A1c	-how to use home blood glucose (BG) meter -when to check BG based on medication regimen -pre and post meal targets -teaching patients what to do when result is too low or high -need for A1c for pts with *new* hyperglycemia vs. pre-existing diabetes
Diabetes Medications	-mechanism of action of basal, bolus and pre-mixed insulins -teaching patient when, how and how much to take for oral and injectable diabetes medications -coordinating timing of BG monitoring, insulin administration and meal delivery in the hospital and at home -responsible disposal of lancets and syringes/pen needles -patient wearing own insulin pump policy, role of RN
Hypoglycemia	-signs, symptoms, treatment and prevention -importance of re-checking BG every 15–20 minutes until hypoglycemia resolves or dextrose-containing IV is started
Hyperglycemia	-signs and symptoms -treatment -DKA prevention
Discharge Planning	-beginning diabetes education early during hospital stay -teachable moments when performing BG checks, when administering insulin, and around mealtimes -resources for teaching: handouts, practice insulin pens, glucose meters to take home -matching home discharge regimen to each patient's abilities and resources -follow-up appointments for ongoing diabetes education and medication adjustments -when to call the diabetes educator for assistance

including identifying carbohydrates that should be counted and portion sizes.[10,11] Nurses work closely with registered dietitian nutritionists (RDs or RDNs) as colleagues and often depend on them to teach carbohydrate counting; however, the nurse is encouraged to reinforce this teaching to enable the patient to practice the skill and assimilate the knowledge. The patient's meal tray is a great teaching tool to use to identify which foods contain carbohydrates that are counted or appropriate portion sizes. But do nurses feel knowledgeable enough in these topics to teach them to patients? Without additional education in carbohydrate counting, some nurses may not feel competent or comfortable performing these tasks. Munoz et al.[12] provided a comprehensive list of nutrition and other topics to facilitate nurses teaching patients self-management.

DIABETES RESOURCE NURSES

The role of a unit-based resource mentor or specialty nurse has been utilized in a number of nursing specialty areas, such as pressure ulcers, pain management, falls prevention, and diabetes. In the case of diabetes, the nurses' knowledge and confidence in both caring for patients with diabetes and teaching self-management skills to their patients can be enhanced through this model. Modic et al.[13] created a Diabetes Management Mentor Program to empower participants to be glycemic control advocates in an environment in which awareness of glycemic targets was uncertain and resources for diabetes teaching were not well known or utilized. Diabetes management mentors are role models for other unit-based nurses, disseminating new knowledge and resources as they become available.[12] In addition, these mentors are a link between the bedside nurse and diabetes educators—including registered nurses, RDs, doctors of pharmacy, masters of social worker, and other certified diabetes educators (CDEs)—when patients are identified as having complex barriers to learning and require creative adaptations when formulating a sustainable discharge plan.

Diabetes resource nurse or champion programs can range from simple to comprehensive plans. Even in hospitals with a lone inpatient diabetes educator, a simple plan may consist of monthly meetings that cover varying topics and include guest speakers to improve the bedside nurses' working knowledge of glycemic control strategies. Meetings can focus on educating and empowering the unit-based nurse to take on a leadership role in identifying patients with poor glycemic control, notifying the team of the need to make modifications in therapy and maintaining patient education resources on the unit.

The challenge is to convince nursing leadership and hospital administrators to require units to have at least one diabetes *champion* on each unit, or preferably one on each shift. Resource nurses are bedside nurses who also have their normal patient assignments.[14] Administrative support to allow for release time for resource nurses to educate both staff and patients is a key ingredient to the success of the role. One comprehensive diabetes champion program in a multisite health-care system in the Northeast consists of nine 90-min interactive classes that includes instruction in the American Association of Diabetes Educators AADE7 Self-Care Behaviors and use of teaching tools such as blood glucose monitors, insulin saline teaching pens, glucagon emergency kits, monofilaments to measure protective sensation, and carbohydrate counting lists.[15] Upon completion of the course, participants are given a take-home final exam, participate in a graduation ceremony, receive a diabetes champion pin, and receive 15 continuing education credits that can be used toward meeting the requirements to take the CDE exam. Graduates of the program are keenly aware of glycemic control on their unit and are influential in challenging orders and reducing medication errors. In a clinical nurse specialist–run Diabetes Nurse Expert Team (DNET) on the west coast, nurses attended a minimum of one half-day workshop each year and discuss glycemic control issues with peers on their unit.[8] Munoz et al.[12] offered a program that included multiple strategies, including a diabetes nurse *superuser* program, learning-modules that could be completed at any time, and scheduled nursing grand rounds and case presentations. Continuing education credit or advancement on the nursing clinical ladder should be offered to encourage participation. The benefit of resource nurses well placed throughout the hospital in these programs has the potential to improve quality of care, safety, and patient and nurse satisfaction while reducing clinical inertia when glycemic targets are not being met.

THE ROLE OF THE DIABETES EDUCATOR

The availability of an inpatient diabetes educator varies widely from hospital to hospital, ranging from none to several. Similarly, the education background experience and role of the educator may vary and may include glycemic management decisions.[16] As content expert, the diabetes educator often plays a pivotal role in planning and implementing nursing education activities related to inpatient glycemic control and patient self-management education. Table 28.1 lists key topics to consider when educating inpatient nurses to increase their competence in diabetes care and self-management education.

CONCLUSION

Ensuring that hospital-based nurses have a working knowledge of inpatient glycemic management strategies and diabetes self-management education is an important strategy to improve the quality of inpatient diabetes management. Nurses who have received additional diabetes-specific education are better able to assist the care team in identifying patients who are not achieving glycemic targets and to facilitate, initiate, and adjust insulin therapy. Investing in nursing education to improve nurse knowledge and confidence in caring for patients with hyperglycemia or diabetes should be a priority in every acute care setting.

REFERENCES

1. Joint Commission. Advanced disease-specific care certification requirements for Inpatient Diabetes Care (IDC). Available from http://www.jointcommission.org/certification/inpatient_diabetes.aspx. Accessed 20 December 2015
2. Magee MF, Khan NH, Desale S, Nassar CM. Diabetes to go: knowledge- and competency-based hospital survival skills diabetes education program improves postdischarge medication adherence. *Diabetes Educator* 2014;40:344–350

3. Seley JJ, Wallace, M. Meeting the challenge of inpatient diabetes education: an interdisciplinary approach. In *Educating Your Patient with Diabetes*, Weinger K, Ed. New York, NY, Humana Press, 2008, p. 81–96
4. Sullivan MM, O'Brien CR, Gitelman SE, Shapiro SE, Rushakoff, RJ. Impact of an interactive online nursing educational module on insulin errors in hospitalized pediatric patients. *Diabetes Care* 2010;33:1744–1746
5. Tamler R, et al. Durability of the effect of online diabetes training for medical residents on knowledge, confidence, and inpatient glycemia. *J. Diabetes* 2012;4:281–290
6. Cohen LS, Sedhom L, Salifu M, Friedman EA. Inpatient diabetes management: examining morning practice in an acute care setting. *Diabetes Educ* 2007;33:483–92
7. Seley JJ. Diabetes care in the inpatient setting. In *Complete Nurse's Guide to Diabetes Care*, 3rd ed. Childs BP, Cypress M, Spollett G, Eds. Alexandria, VA, American Diabetes Association, 2016 (in press)
8. Corl DE, McCliment S, Thompson RE, Suhr LD, Wisse BE. Efficacy of diabetes nurse expert team program to improve nursing confidence and expertise in caring for hospitalized patients with diabetes mellitus. *J Nurses Prof Dev* 2014;30:134–142
9. Corl DE, Guntrum PL, Graf L, Suhr LD, Thompson RE, Wisse BE. Inpatient diabetes education performed by staff nurses decreases readmission rates. *AADE In Practice* 2015:19–23
10. Healy SJ, Black D, Harris C, Lorenz A, Dungan K. Inpatient diabetes education is associated with less frequent hospital readmission among patients with poor glycemic control. *Diabetes Care* 2013;36:2960–2967
11. Dungan K, Lyons S, Manu K, Kulkarni M, Ebrahim K, Grantier C, Harris C, Black D, and Schuster D. An individualized inpatient diabetes education and hospital transition program for poorly controlled hospitalized patients with diabetes. *Endocr Pract* 2014;20:1265–1273
12. Munoz M, Pronovost P, Dintziz J, Kemmerer T, Wang N, Chang Y, Efird L, Berenholtz SM, Golden SH. Implementing and evaluating a multicomponent inpatient diabetes management program: putting research into practice. *Jt Comm J Qual Patient Saf* 2012;38(5):195–206
13. Modic MB, Canfield C, Kaser N, Sauvey R, Kukla A. Outcomes of a clinical nurse specialist initiative to empower staff nurses. *Clin Nurs Special* 2012:263–271
14. Quinn-O'Neil B, Kilgallen ME, Terlizzi JA. Creating a unit-based resource nurse program. *Am J Nurs* 2011;111:46–51
15. Jornsay DL, Garnett ED. Diabetes champions: culture change through education. *Diabetes Spect* 2014;27:188–192
16. Rodriguez A, Magee M, Ramos P, Seley JJ, Maynard G, Nolan A, Kulasa K, Caudell A, Lamb A, MacIndoe J. Best practices for interdisciplinary care management by hospital glycemic teams: results of a society of hospital medicine survey among 19 US hospitals. *Diabetes Spect* 2014;27:97–205

Chapter 29

Resident Education

Robert J. Rushakoff, MD,[1] Cecilia Low Wang, MD,[2] Jane Jeffrie Seley, DNP, MSN, MPH, GNP, BC-ADM,CDE, CDTC,[3] and Alicia Lynn Warnock, MD, FACP[4]

INTRODUCTION

Management of inpatient hyperglycemia is quite distinct from management of outpatient diabetes in the following ways: (1) blood glucose goals are different, (2) patients are not in their usual clinical state, (3) nutritional intake may be unpredictable, (4) patients may be given intravenous fluids or medications that can alter glucose levels, and (5) many diabetes medications commonly used in the outpatient setting are not recommended for use in the inpatient setting. Thus, patients often require a drastically different regimen for glycemic control in the hospital setting as compared with the outpatient regimen. Even for clinicians who have adequate knowledge of outpatient diabetes management, inpatient management may present significant challenges and require additional knowledge and skills.

In academic teaching institutions, residents are most often responsible for managing the complex spectrum of medical and surgical conditions for which the patient has been admitted, as well as the patient's diabetes or newly discovered hyperglycemia, if present. To date, surveys show medical and surgical residents have substantial deficits in basic diabetes knowledge and inpatient diabetes management skills.[1–4] For example, Latta et al.[2] surveyed 135 medical residents in four teaching hospitals and found that only 65% thought glucose management in noncritically ill patients was important, and 43% were uncomfortable and unfamiliar with ordering prandial and basal insulins. In an educational intervention with medical and surgical residents in an academic medical center in the northeast, Lubitz et al.[5] found that medical residents had a significantly better initial knowledge base than surgical residents as demonstrated by pretest scores ($P < 0.001$); yet post-test results showed only a modest improvement in scores and no longer any difference between the medical and surgical residents. If these knowledge gaps are not addressed, perpetuation of mismanagement may occur after residency as training in residency markedly influences future practice.[6]

[1]Director, Inpatient Diabetes, Professor of Medicine, Division of Endocrinology and Metabolism, University of California, San Francisco, CA. [2]Associate Professor of Medicine, Director, Glucose Management Team, University of Colorado School of Medicine/University of Colorado Hospital, Aurora, CO. [3]Diabetes Nurse Practitioner, Inpatient Diabetes Team NewYork–Presbyterian Hospital/Weill Cornell Medical Center, New York, NY. [4]Director, Walter Reed Diabetes Institute, Endocrinology Service, Department of Medicine, Walter Reed National Military Medical Center, Bethesda, MD.

 DOI: 10.2337/9781580406086.29

EDUCATIONAL EFFORTS

Traditionally, clinical diabetes training for residents may be limited and inconsistent, limited to informal teaching during clinic or inpatient rounds, or perhaps during a noon teaching conference. To address this deficit, groups at some institutions have tried a variety of more formal approaches to training. The results, as summarized in Table 29.1, have been mixed.

In these studies, residents may gain confidence about their knowledge and feel more at ease with inpatient glucose management, but significant improvements in glucose management outcomes generally have not occurred. Meanwhile, clinical inertia continues: the leading factor for this likely rests in the time commitment required to acquire adequate education regarding glucose management amid an already crowded arena of medical knowledge and skills that residents must gain and become proficient in during training. The time required for the interventions noted earlier was often ≥4 h. When the education efforts were primarily voluntary, participation was only 50% despite a $50 incentive. A 3-h course had better participation, but the residents were paid $600. For most hospitals, even a small incentive is not possible. Furthermore, given the current limitations on resident work hours and the ever-increasing number of mandatory administrative and educational online courses, participation in any voluntary education effort will be limited.

LEADING BY EXAMPLE

Baldwin et al.[7] showed that having an endocrinologist round with a member of the medical team improved both insulin order-writing and glucose levels. Similarly, for outpatients, Phillips et al.[8] showed that having an endocrinologist meet with a resident to discuss the management of a specific patient led to greater improvements compared with just giving the resident written suggestions on the day the patient was seen.[8]

RESULTS OF EFFORTS

This section discusses our experiences and describes what has not worked in the past as well as some of the interventions we believe are now making a difference.

THE UNIVERSITY OF CALIFORNIA, SAN FRANCISCO EXPERIENCE

In 2001, the University of California, San Francisco developed and implemented an interactive web-based program to teach medical residents all aspects of outpatient diabetes management. Residents and other providers utilized this as part of a project on chronic disease management. At that time, an online course for inpatient management was developed for both nursing staff and medical housestaff. The course was mandatory, but while nursing staff did participate, housestaff

Table 29.1—Selected Published Studies on Resident Diabetes Education

Clinical setting	Group studied	Intervention	Goal	Findings	Comment
Outpatient					
Lo et al. [10]	Internal medicine residents	4-5 sessions with diabetes team (diabetes educator, endocrinologist, pharmacist)	Increased diabetes knowledge and improved patient outcomes	Minimal change in knowledge and no change in outcomes.	
Cook et al. [11]	Internal medicine residents	Web-based modules compared with printed materials	Increased knowledge	Test scores improved from 66 to 75% for both formats.	
Sperl-Hillen et al. [12]	10 primary care residency programs	18 virtual cases (outpatient)	Satisfaction with training and self-assessed knowledge	Pre- and postsurveys completed by only 65% of 142 participants; 90% of completers gave good marks for the cases as being helpful; 50% found it difficult to find time to participate.	Only 50% of volunteer residents (completed all cases; incentive: $50 gift cards); 20% did not complete any cases.
Phillips et al. [8]	Internal medicine residents	Randomized to four groups: *1)* No intervention *2)* Patient-specific advice was prepared and placed on the chart prior to the visit *3)* Meet with endocrinologist every 2 weeks for feedback *4)* Both 2 and 3	Improved HbA_{1c}, blood pressure, and lipids.	Best outcomes were with combination of chart reminders plus feedback. Feedback was independently associated with improvements.	

Cook et al.[13]	Family medicine, internal medicine, and surgery residents	7 online modules	Acceptance of training method	Modules took about 30 min each. Residents felt learning objectives met.	No data yet on clinical impact.
DeSalvo et al.[14]	Pediatric residents	4 sessions over 8 weeks: first session online with basic information; others each 1 h live and combination question/answer sessions and case discussions	Decreased inpatient diabetes-related errors and increased adherence to diabetes pathway	Decreased errors from 19.4% to 6.6%. The types of errors were 43% insulin orders 49% communication 15% IV fluids.	>90% of residents participated in sessions.
Desimone et at.[15]	Internal medicine residents	Formal lectures on institution-specific insulin management at the beginning of 4-week rotation; intervention group also received detailed written/PDA information	Knowledge improvement at end of 4-week rotation; glucose control improvement (% of capillary blood glucose values within goal range in a 2-day period after 4-week rotation)	Knowledge test scores improved in both groups from 69–76% to 84%. No improvement in capillary blood glucose values within goal range.	Short study with small sample size (n = 22).
Tamler et al.[16–18] / inpatient	Internal medicine residents	Two 90-min case conferences vs. 10 online case discussions (total 3 h)	Increased knowledge, increased confidence, glucose control	Initially, median blood glucose decreased from 152 to 139 mg/dL. Hypoglycemia (glucose <70 mg/dL) increased. In long-term follow-up, patient admissions with glucoses at target increased from 19 to 22%.	Participants received $600.

participation was limited. Updates of these courses have been made, but use remained voluntary and usage remained spotty. Following a complete infrastructure update for diabetes management in 2005, mandatory case-based training for both medical and surgical residents began with support from the residency leaders. Cases were tailored to the respective residency programs. In each case, small groups led by endocrinologists or diabetes nurses and pharmacists went through a series of cases. The residents demonstrate how to write initial insulin orders and how to adjust doses. Web-based versions of this training are available, but they rarely are utilized because of time constraints. The case-based sessions are 90 min long. Our data showed that glucoses did significantly improve after the initiation of the training (with the percentage of glucoses within target increasing by 30%), but subsequent audits continued to show significant clinical inertia. In 2013, we initiated our virtual inpatient glucose management service. For patients who do not have appropriate insulin orders written and two or more glucose levels are >225 mg/dL in the previous day, a glucose management note is placed in the chart, giving specific recommendation for adjustment of insulin and the reasons for this change. This real-time learning, adding to their previous case-based training, has led to the residents in all specialties learning by doing. To the present, the number of patients listed on this daily report because of elevated glucose levels had decreased by >60% (from about 30/day to 12/day).

THE UNIVERSITY OF COLORADO HOSPITAL AND SCHOOL OF MEDICINE EXPERIENCE

Over the past 10–15 years, the University of Colorado Hospital has instituted a number of glycemic management protocols for hypoglycemia, basal-bolus insulin therapy, and intravenous insulin infusions in a variety of clinical settings, as well as for patients receiving tube feeding or parenteral nutrition. Housestaff traditionally have received training regarding inpatient glycemic management through "on-the-fly" teaching at the bedside and clinical conferences, such as morning report or noon conference. Hospital-wide education efforts have included housestaff, but formal training through these efforts has not been targeted toward them. Inpatient diabetes management was added to the formal resident curriculum in 2006, and because of time constraints, both diabetic emergencies and inpatient hyperglycemia management were covered in a single 1-h lecture, and beginning in 2009, these lectures were scheduled to be given only every other year. Starting in 2011, a 3-h time slot was allotted to the management of inpatient diabetes, glycemic emergencies, and outpatient diabetes. Unfortunately, this change has not provided the time, setting, or frequency needed to improve clinical knowledge or skills in inpatient hyperglycemia management in an enduring fashion.

Taking into account resident time constraints, a new curriculum for management of inpatient hyperglycemia for internal medicine was developed for delivery during noon conference sessions for residents on inpatient rotations. Two 1-h sessions were developed: basic and advanced. The basic session is focused toward interns and fourth-year medical student externs and includes basic diabetes knowledge and elements of professional society guidelines[1,2] and the advanced session is focused toward second- and third-year residents and includes more complex management situations, such as steroid-induced and tube-feeding or parenteral nutrition-associated hyperglycemia. The sessions consisted of specific learning objectives, pre- and post-tests, and short didactics interspersed with small-group discussion of cases. Pre- and post-tests were administered at the beginning and end of each 60-min session, with self-assessment of clinical skills and level of comfort incorporated into the post-test. This curriculum was piloted in February 2015, and 38 learners participated (20 in the basic session, 18 in the advanced session). Medical knowledge after the education session improved in 64% of the domains assessed, and 41.3% of residents in the basic session versus 75% of residents in the advanced session felt that their clinical knowledge and ability to manage inpatient hyperglycemia improved after the session. Ninety-four percent of learners felt that this format "worked for them." Going forward, these modules will be packaged to include learning objectives, cases, detailed answer keys, teaching points, and key published references that can be delivered by chief medical residents and attending physicians.

WALTER REED NATIONAL MILITARY MEDICAL CENTER EXPERIENCE

The recent 2011 merger of two major military medical centers (National Naval Medical Center and Walter Reed Army Medical Center) into a single medical campus served as a unique opportunity to redesign and implement new innovative strategies to improve diabetes-related care at the newly integrated Walter Reed National Military Medical Center. Hospital-wide improvements have included updated instructions for inpatient management of hyperglycemia; implementation of standardized insulin order sets; reconfiguration of the electronic medical record interface (user-friendly visualization of medications, blood glucose, and carbohydrate intake); development of transitions of care algorithms; direct booking for patient education classes; and improvements to bedside patient diabetes education with electronic flow sheets. From the outset, medical residents, interns, and nurses, who form the backbone of day-to-day patient care and hospital processes, were recruited and engaged in hospital systems change and the ongoing education efforts, which have continually reinforced the implemented changes. Specific elements of program sustainment include the following:

- Internal Medicine Education
  - Diabetes Ambassadors: so-named resident members of the multidisciplinary hospital-level committee (this satisfies graduate medical education [GME] requirements for hospital-level involvement/patient safety projects)
    - Each ambassador serves as a liaison between the internal medicine program and other (primarily surgical) residency programs
    - Several residency process improvement projects have involved diabetes-related care processes
  - Informal, voluntary weekly education sessions lead by endocrinology staff and fellows
    - Case-based interactive teaching using past or current inpatients (i.e., curb-side consultation)

NEW YORK–PRESBYTERIAN/WEILL CORNELL MEDICAL COLLEGE EXPERIENCE

A popular education strategy at the Weill Cornell campus of New York–Presbyterian Hospital has been diabetes nurse practitioner-led small-group 1-h inservice with medicine interns that included the review and distribution of a diabetes pocket card. Clinical tools such as dosing algorithms to initiate and titrate insulin, perioperative diabetes medication adjustment guidelines, a transition guide from inpatient to outpatient, and instruction for writing diabetes prescriptions for discharge were included. Hyperglycemia rates were significantly reduced from baseline (37.12%) compared with postintervention (34.79%, $P = 0.004$).[9]

Table 29.2—Suggestions for Effective Resident Education

General
1. Mandatory education beginning during internship
2. An education plan that balances educational needs and time constraints
3. Basic content on management and glycemic goals, medications, insulin types, and pharmacodynamics

Specific
1. Specialty-specific case-based training
2. Cases covering common day-to-day situations, not "interesting" or esoteric cases
    a. Patient admitted who had been on basal insulin at home, now NPO
    b. Patient admitted who had been on oral agents or diet alone; now eating or NPO
    c. How and when to initiate basal and bolus insulin
    d. Transition from IV insulin to SQ insulin
    e. How to make daily adjustments in IV and SQ insulin
    f. Patients on glucocorticoids
    g. Patients on enteral feeding or parenteral nutrition
    h. Perioperative/NPO procedure adjustments for insulin
    i. Guidelines for patients wearing an insulin pump at home
3. Cases generally should be institution-specific
    a. Examples should use the insulins on formulary
    b. Cases should use the format of insulin order sets used
    c. When residents rotate through multiple hospitals with different order sets and insulin formularies, attempts should be made to include cases utilizing those formats.

Feedback
1. Ongoing reports back to residents about glucose management (generally service-specific)
2. Daily prompts to assist with management.
    a. Autogenerated alerts for high glucose levels to signal providers that an intervention is required (with caution to avoid "alert fatigue")
    b. Oversight monitoring by glucose management team or service to assist in educating and supporting the resident regarding potential causes of hypo- and hyperglycemia, and the specific changes that should be made

ONGOING CHALLENGES

Although improving resident knowledge of inpatient diabetes is important, additional interventions that utilize innovative approaches are needed to advance this effort. As discussed, a multipronged approach is required, which may include the following:

1. Institution and specialty-specific case-based training
2. Electronic prompts within the EMR for appropriate intervention (while respecting the potential for "alert fatigue")
3. Real-time patient-specific guidance and support using cases the residents have learned about in prior educational interventions to apply that knowledge to the patient they currently are managing.

Additional details regarding specific interventions are listed in Table 29.2.

CONCLUSION

Insulin is the medication that is most frequently involved in medication errors, the average length of stay is short, and clinical inertia is common in the inpatient setting. With the restrictions in residency time, the case needs to be made to residency leaders to prioritize mandatory inpatient diabetes management training. There may need to be a combination of live and online learning, with available assistance at the time that orders are written, to have the greatest impact on resident awareness, knowledge, and skills in this area. This education must not be limited to medical residents, but also should include surgical, obstetrical, and any resident that may be involved in managing a patient with hyperglycemia in the inpatient setting.

REFERENCES

1. Rubin DJ, Moshang J, Jabbour SA. Diabetes knowledge: are resident physicians and nurses adequately prepared to manage diabetes? *Endocr Pract Off J Am Coll Endocrinol Am Assoc Clin Endocrinol* 2007;13:17–21
2. Latta S, et al. Management of inpatient hyperglycemia: assessing knowledge and barriers to better care among residents. *Am J Ther* 2011;18:355–365
3. Ahmed A, Jabbar A, Zuberi L, Islam M, Shamim K. Diabetes-related knowledge among residents and nurses: a multicenter study in Karachi, Pakistan. *BMC Endocr Disord* 2012;12:18
4. Gosmanova A, Gosmanov N. Assessing diabetes-related knowledge among internal medicine residents using multiple-choice questionnaire. *Am J Med Sci* 2009;338:348–352
5. Lubitz CC, Seley JJ, Rivera C, Sinha N, Brillon DJ. The perils of inpatient hyperglycemia management: how we turned apathy into action. *Diabetes Spectr* 2007;20:18–21

6. Maheux B, Beaudoin C, Jacques A, Lambert J, Lévesque A. Effects of residency training in family medicine v. internship training on professional attitudes and practice patterns. *CMAJ Can Med Assoc J J Assoc Medicale Can* 1992;146:901–907

7. Baldwin D, Villanueva G, McNutt R, Bhatnagar S. Eliminating inpatient sliding-scale insulin: a reeducation project with medical house staff. *Diabetes Care* 2005;28:1008–1011

8. Phillips LS, et al. An endocrinologist-supported intervention aimed at providers improves diabetes management in a primary care site: improving primary care of African Americans with diabetes (IPCAAD) 7. *Diabetes Care* 2005;28:2352–2360

9. Seley JJ, Brillon DJ, Chiu Y, Sinha-Gregory N, Gerber LM. Using an educational intervention to improve inpatient glycemic control one intern at a time. American Diabetes Association 73rd Annual Scientific Sessions, Chicago, Il. Abstract P699 published in abstract book (2013). *Am Diabetes Assoc 73rd Annu Sci Sess Chic Il Abstr P699 Publ Abstr Book 2013*

10. Lo MC, Freeman M, Lansang MC. Effect of a multidisciplinary-assisted resident diabetes clinic on resident knowledge and patient outcomes. *J Grad Med Educ* 2013;5:145–149

11. Cook DA, Dupras DM, Thompson WG, Pankratz VS. Web-based learning in residents' continuity clinics: a randomized, controlled trial. *Acad Med J Assoc Am Med Coll* 2005;80:90–97

12. Sperl-Hillen J, et al. Using simulation technology to teach diabetes care management skills to resident physicians. *J Diabetes Sci Technol* 2013;7:1243–1254

13. Cook CB, et al. Development of computer-based training to enhance resident physician management of inpatient diabetes. *J Diabetes Sci Technol* 2009;3:1377–1387

14. DeSalvo DJ, Greenberg LW, Henderson CL, Cogen FR. A learner-centered diabetes management curriculum. *Diabetes Care* 2012;35:2188–2193

15. Desimone M, et al. Effect of an educational inpatient diabetes management program on medical resident knowledge and measures of glycemic control: a randomized controlled trial. *Endocr Pract* 2012;18:238–249

16. Tamler R, et al. Effect of case-based training for medical residents on confidence, knowledge, and management of inpatient glycemia. *Postgrad Med* 2011;123:99–106

17. Tamler R, et al. Effect of case-based training for medical residents on inpatient glycemia. *Diabetes Care* 2011;34:1738–1740

18. Tamler R, et al. Durability of the effect of online diabetes training for medical residents on knowledge, confidence, and inpatient glycemia. *J Diabetes* 2012;4:281–290

Chapter 30

Transition of Care: Discharge from the Hospital

Daniel J. Rubin,[1] Luigi F. Meneghini, MD, MBA,[2] Jane Jeffrie Seley DNP, MSN, MPH, GNP, BC-ADM, CDE, CDTC,[3] Enrico Cagliero, MD,[4] Linda M. Gaudiani, MD, FACP, FACE,[5] and Janice L. Gilden, MS, MD, FCP, FACE[6]

The transition of care upon discharging a patient from the hospital presents both an opportunity to optimize diabetes care and a challenge to prevent adverse outcomes. Gaps in transitional care are common. Nearly half of patients may experience a medical error after discharge.[1] A poor care transition can undermine patient satisfaction and put a patient at risk for preventable morbidity and hospital readmission.[2–5]

Historically, less attention has been focused on the transition out of the hospital than the transition into the hospital.[6] When primary care physicians cared for their own patients during hospitalization, transition issues were addressed more easily in the context of provider continuity. The rise of dedicated hospitalists and the limits in work hours of medical house staff have decreased continuity of providers between inpatient and outpatient settings.[3,7] In addition, many patients are discharged to subacute facilities in the interim between acute and outpatient care, introducing another layer of provider discontinuity. This discontinuity increases the likelihood of communication failures, making effective communication about hospital discharge ever more important. Further challenges in accomplishing comprehensive discharge planning and timely postdischarge follow-up are presented by the pressure to discharge patients rapidly. Coupled with the increasing complexity of hospitalized patients, recognition has been growing that a poor transition of care represents a patient safety issue.[2,3] The transition from inpatient to outpatient has become a national priority. Several medical societies representing internal medicine, hospital medicine, emergency medicine, and care management have published policy papers to facilitate better discharge processes.[6,8]

[1]Assistant Professor of Medicine, Temple University School of Medicine, Section of Endocrinology, Diabetes, and Metabolism, Philadelphia, PA. [2]Professor and Executive Director of the Global Diabetes Program, Parkland Health and Hospital System, Department of Internal Medicine, Division of Endocrinology, University of Texas Southwestern Medical Center, Dallas, TX. [3]Diabetes Nurse Practitioner, Inpatient Diabetes Team, NewYork–Presbyterian Hospital/Weill Cornell Medical Center, New York, NY. [4]Associate Professor of Medicine, Harvard Medical School, Associate Physician, Massachusetts General Hospital, Boston, MA. [5]Medical Director, Braden Diabetes Center, Marin Endocrine Care and Research, Associate Clinical Professor Medicine, University of California–San Francisco, San Francisco, CA. [6]Diabetes/Endocrinology Division, Department of Medicine, Rosalind Franklin University of Medicine and Science/Chicago Medical School, Captain James A. Lovell Federal Health Care Center, Presence Saints Mary and Elizabeth Medical Center, Chicago, IL.

DOI: 10.2337/9781580406086.30

Similarly, recognition also has been growing that the inpatient to outpatient transition of patients with diabetes deserves more attention and research.[7,9] Recently professional health-care organizations, including the American Diabetes Association, have published guidelines on optimizing the transition out of the hospital setting.[9–11] Key aspects of these guidelines are discussed in the following section.

THE SCOPE OF AN EFFECTIVE HOSPITAL-TO-HOME TRANSITION

The hospital-to-home transition of care includes not only the discharge but also the postdischarge period. Herein, we focus on the transition from hospital to home rather than discharges to nonacute facilities, because these facilities provide support not generally available to patients discharged home. An effective hospital discharge is one in which the patient or caregivers have received appropriate individualized education during the hospitalization and have been provided with an agreed-on clear, understandable, and accurate postdischarge plan. This plan must be documented and accessible to the patient's outpatient providers, most importantly the primary care provider.[7] An effective transition of care mitigates the risk of preventable medical errors, readmissions, and emergency care.

Readmission risk factors among patients with diabetes include lower socioeconomic status, racial or ethnic minority, comorbidity burden, public insurance, emergent or urgent admission, and a history of recent prior hospitalization.[5,12] Hospitalized patients with diabetes are at higher risk of readmission than those without diabetes as reflected by 30-day readmission rates of 14.4–22.7%,[12,13] compared with 8.5–13.5% for those without diabetes.[14,15] Potential interventions to reduce readmission risk are inpatient diabetes self-management education (DSME), specialty care, diabetes-specific discharge instructions, coordination of care, and postdischarge support.[12,16–18]

Successful coordination of the inpatient to outpatient transition requires a team approach involving physicians, nurse practitioners, physician assistants, nurses, dietitians, care managers, clinical pharmacists, social workers, certified diabetes educators (CDEs), and, in some cases, language- and ethnic-appropriate home educators or promoters.[9,19] The inpatient diabetes educator, who may be a CDE and often is a registered nurse, registered dietitian nutritionist, nurse practitioner, physician assistant, or clinical pharmacist, is a key member of the team. Responsibilities of the inpatient diabetes educator relevant to the transition of care include *1*) assessing the patient's current diabetes knowledge and self-management skills in relation to the reason(s) for hospitalization, *2*) initiating DSME for those newly diagnosed with diabetes, *3*) providing information on basic self-management skills with the goal of safety, *4*) coordinating inpatient and postdischarge diabetes care with other health professionals, *5*) providing information on community resources and outpatient diabetes education programs, and *6*) serving as a resource for nursing staff and other health care providers.[19] The methods for achieving these goals should be tailored to patient preferences and needs.

CHALLENGES TO AN EFFECTIVE TRANSITION OF CARE

Numerous challenges must be overcome to achieve an effective transition of diabetes care after hospitalization.[7] First, the average length of hospital stay for patients with diabetes has decreased dramatically, from 9.0 days in 1988 to 4.8 days in 2009.[20] This has shifted more of the acute care component to the outpatient setting, adding greater complexity and burden of care on patients and caregivers when returning home than in years past. In addition, the shorter length of stay means that less time is available during hospitalization to address the discharge transition. Second, bedside nurses have competing priorities that may not allow sufficient time to educate patients. Third, hospitalized patients may be unable or unwilling to participate in education and transitional planning because of impairment of mental status, acute illness, pain, anxiety, tests or procedures that require them to be away from the hospital room, or knowledge deficits. Fourth, family, caregivers, or outpatient providers may be difficult to contact and meet. Fifth, the medical management of diabetes is complex and expensive. Prescriptions required for all the medications and supplies, such as a blood glucose meter, lancets, test strips, a glucagon emergency kit, insulin syringes, or insulin pen needles, might be overlooked.[21] Furthermore, patients may not have health insurance that covers the prescribed medications and supplies, and thus financial barriers must be addressed. Patients lacking financial resources also may have difficulty attending follow-up appointments because of cost and limited transportation means.[22] Lastly, elderly patients, especially those lacking family support, may need greater social services.

Part of the complexity of diabetes management in the transition to home is that most patients have an inpatient regimen that is quite different from their home regimen, and these need to be reconciled to ensure optimal glycemic control.[18] Any adjustment of therapy often is best made soon after discharge, perhaps within days. Yet another barrier to an effective transition of care is clinical inertia, the reluctance to change disease management despite not meeting therapy goals. Many patients with uncontrolled diabetes do not have their outpatient regimens intensified before discharge. For example, a retrospective cohort study of 2,025 admissions of male veterans receiving medical therapy for diabetes with an admission HbA_{1c} >8% found that only 22.4% of discharges had a change in diabetes medication during hospitalization.[23] Nearly one-third of the cohort had no change in diabetes therapy upon discharge, no documentation of HbA_{1c} within 60 days of discharge *and* no follow-up appointment within 30 days of discharge.

ELEMENTS OF AN EFFECTIVE TRANSITION OF CARE

To overcome these barriers to an effective transition of diabetes care, multiple strategies are required (Table 30.1).[9–11]

DIABETES DISCHARGE PLANNING

Because the inpatient-to-outpatient transition of care for patients with diabetes is complex, planning should begin at the time of admission. A key component of

Table 30.1—Strategies to Successfully Transition Patients with Diabetes from Hospital to Home

- Start diabetes discharge planning at admission; include the patient and family or caregivers whenever possible
- Obtain an HbA_{1c} at admission if none is available within the prior 1–2 months
- Confirm preadmission diabetes regimen and reconcile with postdischarge diabetes regimen
- Consider the type and severity of diabetes (HbA_{1c}) and the capabilities and motivation of the patient when establishing a postdischarge diabetes regimen
- Assess the need for and provide inpatient diabetes education on survival skills
- Consider a referral for ongoing outpatient DSME[34]
- Provide a written postdischarge plan for diabetes management to the patient
- Provide a written discharge summary and transition plan for outpatient providers
- Fill and review prescriptions for new or changed medications before discharge
- Assess barriers to transition plan and self-care behaviors
- Before discharge, schedule a follow-up appointment with the outpatient diabetes provider within 1 month (sooner if insulin adjustments are anticipated)
- Provide postdischarge support in the form of phone calls or and in-home nurse visit

discharge planning is a current HbA_{1c}. An HbA_{1c} should be obtained upon admission if one is not available within the prior 2 to 3 months.[10,11] The admission HbA_{1c} provides critical information to guide diabetes therapy during hospitalization and upon discharge.[11,19] In general, patients with an HbA_{1c} at goal (usually <7% or <8% for patients who are older or have serious comorbidities) may be discharged on their prior outpatient diabetes regimen unless relevant clinical circumstances changed during hospitalization (e.g., contraindication to previous diabetes medications, renal impairment, or need for glucocorticoids). Patients with an elevated HbA_{1c} probably would benefit from therapy revision or require intensification of the outpatient regimen. As in the outpatient setting, providers should be aware of the situations in which HbA_{1c} may not accurately reflect glycemic control, such as anemias, end-stage renal disease, or if receiving a blood transfusion.[11]

Several recent studies provide support for this recommendation. A retrospective cohort of 732 patients with poorly controlled diabetes newly initiated on insulin during hospitalization, found that continuation of insulin after discharge was associated with a lower risk of all-cause and diabetes-related readmission at 12 months postdischarge compared with discontinuing insulin.[24] In a retrospective cohort study of 1,949 patients with type 2 diabetes, intensification of diabetes therapy was associated with a 67% lower risk of readmission or an emergency department visit within 30 days in the subgroup of medicine inpatients with a baseline HbA_{1c} ≥8%.[25] In addition, postdischarge HbA_{1c} decreased by 1.8% in this subgroup compared to 0.6% in patients who did not have their diabetes therapy intensified. Lastly, in a prospective multicenter open-label one-arm trial in 224 patients with type 2 diabetes discharged from general medical or surgical services, admission HbA_{1c}-based adjustment of diabetes therapy plus postdischarge monitoring and titration over 12 weeks reduced the mean HbA_{1c} from 8.7% to 7.3% ($P < 0.001$).[26] In this study, patients with an HbA_{1c} <7% were discharged on their preadmission diabetes regimen. Patients with an HbA_{1c} between 7% and 9% were discharged on their preadmission regimen plus insulin glargine at 50% of their last hospital dose. Those with an HbA_{1c} >9% were discharged on their preadmission regimen plus insulin glargine at 80% the glargine hospital daily dose, or on basal-bolus insulin at 80% the inpatient dose.

Another component of discharge planning that should begin at admission is medication reconciliation. Accurate accounting of the outpatient regimen is critical for diabetes medication safety during hospitalization and a safe and effective transition home, especially for patients on insulin. Lack of attention to medication reconciliation at discharge may lead to inadvertent discontinuation of antihyperglycemic therapy, which is associated with adverse outcomes.[24,27]

Other aspects of care coordination that should be considered well before discharge are outpatient services, such as the need for DSME or a home nursing visit. Assessment of barriers to self-care, including financial resources and access to health insurance, food, and transportation, may improve outcomes.[5,22,28] Ideally, the patient and family or caregivers should be involved at every step of the transition to optimize performance of self-care.[6,28] A standardized clinical pathway with a checklist to document progress with transition planning may help ensure that all aspects of a comprehensive care plan are individualized and met for each patient.[7] For the elderly, effort should be made to simplify medication regimens upon discharge to meet individualized glycemic goals.

INPATIENT DIABETES EDUCATION

Inpatient DSME is discussed in detail elsewhere (see Chapter 27). Inpatient education is addressed in this section as it relates to the hospital discharge transition. Every patient's need for diabetes education during hospitalization should be assessed as early as possible to maximize the time available to address barriers to a smooth transition home.[9] This assessment should address prior management of diabetes, especially if it may have led to the current admission and the level of glycemic control, as well as the patient's motivation, cognition, literacy, numeracy, visual acuity, dexterity, cultural context, and financial resources as they relate to diabetes self-management behaviors. Those new to diabetes, insulin therapy, or self-monitoring of blood glucose need particular attention.[7]

An important reason for early assessment of the need for inpatient diabetes education is the day of discharge may not be the optimal time for learning, especially if the patient needs time to practice new skills. Patients and families may be distracted by the anticipation of discharge, and providers may feel rushed by competing priorities.[28] A study of 100 inpatients given medication education by pharmacists suggested that educating on the day of discharge may not be as conducive to recall of verbal instructions as educating the patient 1 to 3 days before discharge.[29] Advance education also allows for time to review new knowledge and skills, and it provides the patient with an opportunity for questions to be addressed.

Data support the assertion that inpatient diabetes education is an important component of an effective transition from the hospital to home. Inpatient diabetes education among poorly controlled patients has been associated with a lower risk of readmission and improved glycemic control.[16,30,31] Two small pilot trials of inpatient diabetes education and transition planning for patients with poor glycemic control reduced HbA_{1c} by >2% over 6 to 12 months of follow-up.[30,31] Transition planning may be an important adjunct to inpatient diabetes education because patients who receive the education without additional support may have difficulty obtaining their medications and supplies after discharge.[21] Unfortunately, not every hospital implements such an essential service for patients with diabetes because data are lacking on the potential cost savings of a robust inpatient diabetes education and transition program (e.g., reduction in preventable readmissions or emergency room visits).

OPTIMIZING DIABETES THERAPY UPON DISCHARGE

When determining the diabetes management regimen upon discharge, clinicians should consider the type and severity of diabetes, the effect of illness on glycemia, and the capabilities and interests of the patient.[10] As discussed, a recent HbA_{1c} is useful to guide adjustments in diabetes therapy. Barriers to insulin use, such as cognition, literacy, numeracy, visual acuity, dexterity, cultural context, and financial resources, should be addressed.[32] Ideally, inpatient diabetes education covers the basics of the anticipated outpatient regimen, and feedback obtained by the educator informs the selection of the discharge regimen. Involving patients and their caregivers in this process will help promote self-care. A trial of the anticipated outpatient regimen 1 to 2 days before discharge might enable an assessment of effectiveness and safety albeit with the caveat that food intake and activity levels are frequently quite different between the hospital and home settings.[11]

DISCHARGE INSTRUCTIONS AND COMMUNICATION WITH OUTPATIENT PROVIDERS

Upon discharge, patients should receive both written and verbal instructions regarding their diabetes self-management regimen. These instructions need to be clearly communicated to the person who will administer these medications and have understanding verified.[10,11] Medical errors and adverse drug events have been linked to poor communication of discharge instructions.[2,3] Verbally communicated instructions alone are inadequate. Using illustrations, printed materials, and a teach-back method may improve comprehension of discharge instructions.[3]

Formalized, diabetes-specific discharge instructions for patients with diabetes may be more effective than generic instructions.[17] The following components of glycemic management should be included in the discharge record given to the patient: *1*) the principal diagnosis; *2*) a problem list; *3*) a reconciled diabetes medication list that indicates changes from the preadmission list as well as the name (generic and brand), dosage, dosing schedule of each medication, and circumstances in which each medication should not be taken, if applicable; *4*) recommendations for the timing and frequency of home blood glucose monitoring; *5*) information about the recognition and treatment of hypo- and hyperglycemia; *6*) a blood glucose log annotated with pre- and postmeal targets and when to call

Table 30.2—Glycemic Management Principles for Inclusion in the Patient Discharge Record

- Principal diagnosis and type of diabetes
- Problem list
- Reconciled diabetes medication list
- Blood glucose monitoring recommendations
- Recognition and treatment of hypo- and hyperglycemia
- Blood glucose log with pre- and postmeal targets and when to call provider
- List of pending laboratory results upon discharge
- Contact information of health-care provider responsible for ongoing diabetes care
- Follow-up appointment date and time

a health-care provider; *7*) a list of pending laboratory results and appointments upon discharge; and *8*) the name and contact information of the health-care provider responsible for ongoing diabetes care (Table 30.2). Contact information for the discharging clinician should be provided as a backup.

All of the items listed except for the hypo- and hyperglycemia education and the glucose log should be included in written documentation to the primary care physician and other outpatient providers. In addition, a summary of the inpatient diabetes management and follow-up needs should be included.

PRESCRIPTIONS

Prescriptions for new or changed medications should be filled and reviewed with the patient and caregiver before discharge.[8,10] In addition to the medications themselves, prescriptions may be needed for insulin syringes or pen needles, a blood glucose meter, glucose test strips, lancets and lancing devices, urine ketone strips, a medical alert identification, and a glucagon emergency kit (for those with a history of significant hypoglycemia). Filling prescriptions before discharge ensures that patients will have access to the medications and supplies that they need. To avoid omitting a prescription, a standardized diabetes discharge order set or checklist may be helpful.[17,21]

FOLLOW-UP APPOINTMENTS

All patients should have appropriate follow-up appointments, including with the outpatient diabetes provider within 1 month, scheduled by the time of discharge.[8–10] Scheduling follow-up appointments before discharge makes attendance more likely.[33] Involving the patient and caregivers in scheduling may improve attendance rates, but this has not been formally tested independent of other interventions. The time, date, and location of follow-up appointments should be included in written discharge instructions, along with each provider's name and contact information.

POSTDISCHARGE TRANSITION STRATEGIES

A number of strategies may contribute to a more effective inpatient to outpatient transition. One is a phone call 2 to 3 days after discharge from either a nurse or pharmacist to confirm the medical plan and assess the patient's condition.[7,28] Follow-up by phone at regular intervals postdischarge to adjust diabetes therapy has been shown to promote glycemic control,[26] but it is unlikely that such a model is sustainable within the current payment structures. A transitional care clinic that provides outpatient follow-up within 5 days of discharge may prevent readmissions of indigent patients admitted for diabetes-related problems who do not have primary care providers.[18] Such a clinic would be particularly beneficial for patients who had significant changes to their prehospitalization regimen. Last, an in-home nursing visit to assess safety should be considered for discharged patients who are new to insulin therapy or to an intensive insulin regimen.

CONCLUSION

An effective transition of diabetes care from hospital to home requires a multidisciplinary approach that implements multiple strategies along the continuum of care, including discharge planning starting at the time of admission, DSME, optimizing therapy at discharge and ensuring access to therapy, communicating verbal and written instructions with teach back, and postdischarge short-term and long-term follow-up. Although financial support for this comprehensive approach is a challenge in the current cost-reduction era, data are starting to accumulate showing its value in terms of patient safety, prevention of hospital readmission, and improved diabetes control.

REFERENCES

1. Schnipper JL, Kirwin JL, Cotugno MC, et al. Role of pharmacist counseling in preventing adverse drug events after hospitalization. *Arch Intern Med* 2006;166:565–571
2. Forster AJ, Murff HJ, Peterson JF, et al. The incidence and severity of adverse events affecting patients after discharge from the hospital. *Ann Intn Med* 2003;138:161–167
3. Kripalani S, Jackson AT, Schnipper JL, et al. Promoting effective transitions of care at hospital discharge: a review of key issues for hospitalists. *J Hosp Med* 2007;2:314–323
4. Lipska KJ, Wang Y, Kosiborod M, et al. Discontinuation of antihyperglycemic therapy and clinical outcomes after acute myocardial infarction in older patients with diabetes. *Circ Cardiovasc Qual Outcomes* 2010;3:236–242
5. Rubin DJ, Donnell-Jackson K, Jhingan R, et al. Early readmission among patients with diabetes: a qualitative assessment of contributing factors. *J Diabetes Complications* 2014;28:869–873

6. Snow V, Beck D, Budnitz T, et al. Transitions of care consensus policy statement: American College of Physicians, Society of General Internal Medicine, Society of Hospital Medicine, American Geriatrics Society, American College of Emergency Physicians, and Society for Academic Emergency Medicine. *J Hosp Med* 2009;4:364–370

7. Cook CB, Seifert KM, Hull BP, et al. Inpatient to outpatient transfer of diabetes care: planing for an effective hospital discharge. *Endocr Pract* 2009;15:263–239

8. National Transitions of Care Coalition. *Care Transition Bundle: Seven Essential Intervention Categories*. Washington, DC, National Transitions of Care Coalition, 2011

9. Moghissi ES, Korytkowski MT, Dinardo M, et al. American Association of Clinical Endocrinologists and American Diabetes Association consensus statement on inpatient glycemic control. *Diabetes Care* 2009;9009–9029

10. American Diabetes Association. Diabetes care in the hospital, nursing home, and skilled nursing facility. Section 13. In *Standards of Medical Care in Diabetes—2015*. *Diabetes Care* 2015;38:S80–S85

11. Umpierrez GE, Hellman R, Korytkowski MT, et al. Management of hyperglycemia in hospitalized patients in non-critical care setting: an Endocrine Society clinical practice guideline. *J Clin Endocrinol Metab* 2012;97:16–38

12. Rubin DJ. Hospital readmission of patients with diabetes. *Current Diabetes Reports* 2015;15:1–9

13. Bennett KJ, Probst JC, Vyavaharkar M, et al. Lower rehospitalization rates among rural Medicare beneficiaries with diabetes. *J Rural Health* 2012;28:227–234

14. Pennsylvania Health Care Cost Containment Council. *Hospital Readmissions in Pennsylvania 2010*. 2012, p. 1–24, http://www.phc4.org/reports/readmissions/10/. Accessed 4 January 2015

15. Friedman B, Jiang HJ, Elixhauser A. Costly hospital readmissions and complex chronic illness. *Inquiry* 2008;45:408–421

16. Healy SJ, Black D, Harris C, et al. Inpatient diabetes education is associated with less frequent hospital readmission among patients with poor glycemic control. *Diabetes Care* 2013;36:2960–2967

17. Lauster CD, Gibson JM, DiNella JV, et al. Implementation of standardized instructions for insulin at hospital discharge. *J Hosp Med* 2009;4:E41–E42

18. Seggelke SA, Hawkins RM, Gibbs J, et al. Transitional care clinic for uninsured and Medicaid-covered patients with diabetes mellitus discharged from the hospital: a pilot quality improvement study. *Hosp Pract* 2014;42:46–51

19. Dombrowski NC, Karounos DG. Pathophysiology and management strategies for hyperglycemia for patients with acute illness during and following a hospital stay. *Metabolism* 2013;62:326–336

20. Centers for Disease Control and Prevention. *Average Length of Stay (LOS) in Days of Hospital Discharges with Diabetes as Any-Listed Diagnosis, United States, 1988–2009*. Washington, DC, U.S. Department of Health and Human Services, 2014

21. Kimmel B, Sullivan MM, Rushakoff RJ. Survey on transition from inpatient to outpatient for patients on insulin: what really goes on at home? *Endocr Pract* 2010;16:785–791

22. Wheeler K, Crawford R, McAdams D, et al. Inpatient to outpatient transfer of diabetes care: perceptions of barriers to postdischarge follow-up in urban African American patients. *Ethn Dis* 2007;17:238–243

23. Griffith ML, Boord JB, Eden SK, et al. Clinical inertia of discharge planning among patients with poorly controlled diabetes mellitus. *J Clin Endocrinol Metab* 2012;97:2019–2026

24. Wu EQ, Zhou S, Yu A, et al. Outcomes associated with post-discharge insulin continuity in US patients with type 2 diabetes mellitus initiating insulin in the hospital. *Hosp Pract* 2012;40:40–48

25. Wei NJ, Wexler DJ, Nathan DM, et al. Intensification of diabetes medication and risk for 30-day readmission. *Diabet Med* 2013;30:e56–62

26. Umpierrez GE, Reyes D, Smiley D, et al. Hospital discharge algorithm based on admission HbA1c for the management of patients with type 2 diabetes. *Diabetes Care* 2014;37:2934–2939

27. Wu EQ, Zhou S, Yu A, et al. Outcomes associated with insulin therapy disruption after hospital discharge among patients with type 2 diabetes mellitus who had used insulin before and during hospitalization. *Endocr Pract* 2012;18:651–659

28. Cain CH, Neuwirth E, Bellows J, et al. Patient experiences of transitioning from hospital to home: an ethnographic quality improvement project. *J Hosp Med* 2012;7:382–387

29. Calabrese Donihi A, Yang E, Mark S, et al. Scheduling of pharmacist-provided medication education for hospitalized patients. *Hosp Pharm* 2008;43:121–126

30. Dungan K, Lyons S, Manu K, et al. An individualized inpatient diabetes education and hospital transition program for poorly controlled hospitalized patients with diabetes. *Endocr Pract* 2014;1–24

31. Wexler DJ, Beauharnais CC, Regan S, et al. Impact of inpatient diabetes management, education, and improved discharge transition on glycemic control 12 months after discharge. *Diabetes Res Clin Pract* 2012;98:249–256

32. Lavernia F. Treating hyperglycemia and diabetes with insulin therapy: transition from inpatient to outpatient care. *Medscape J Med* 2008;10:216; quiz 216

33. Wheeler K, Crawford R, McAdams D, et al. Inpatient to outpatient transfer of care in urban patients with diabetes: patterns and determinants of immediate postdischarge follow-up. *Arch Intern Med* 2004;164:447–453

34. Powers MA, Bardsley J, Cypress M, et al. Diabetes self-management education and support in type 2 diabetes: a joint position statement of the American Diabetes Association, the American Association of Diabetes Educators, and the Academy of Nutrition and Dietetics. *J Acad Nutr Dietetics* 2015;115:1323–1334

Index

Page numbers followed by an *f* indicate figure; page numbers followed by *t* indicate tables

D

F

G

H

J

L

M

N

O

P

Q

R

U

V

W

CPSIA information can be obtained
at www.ICGtesting.com
Printed in the USA
FFHW012310010519
52211623-57581FF

9 781580 406086